MRI Atlas of the Corpus Callosum

Including Diffusion MRI and Proton MR Spectroscopy

Published by

WARREN H. GREEN, INC.
8356 Olive Boulevard
St. Louis, Missouri 63132, U.S.A.

2002 by WARREN H. GREEN, INC.

ISBN No. 0-87527-529-X

Sener, R. Nuri

Printed in the United States of America

MRI ATLAS OF THE CORPUS CALLOSUM

Including Diffusion MRI and Proton MR Spectroscopy

R. Nuri Sener, M.D.
Professor of Radiology
Department of Radiology
Ege University Hospital
Bornova, Izmir, Turkey

formerly
Research Fellow at the University of Texas
Health Science Center
Department of Radiology, Neuroradiology Section
San Antonio, Texas, U.S.A.

WARREN H. GREEN, INC.
St. Louis, Missouri, U.S.A.

Dedication

To Özge Özgürler
  Bahar Sener and
  Dr. Faik Sener

ABOUT THE AUTHOR

R. Nuri Sener, M.D. holds the position of Professor of Radiology at Ege University, School of Medicine, Izmar, Turkey. He worked as a Neuroradiology Research Fellow in 1990-1991 (one year) and 1996-1997 (three months) at the Neuroradiology Section of the University of Texas, Health Science Center in San Antonio, Texas, U.S.A. Dr. Sener served as a visiting professor in the following radiology departments: 1. Ulleval Hospital, Oslo, Norway. 2. Royal Alexandra Hospital, Sydney, Australia. 3. University Hospital, Sao Paulo, Brazil. 4. Tygerberg Hospital, Cape Town, South Africa. 5. University Hospital, Kumamoto, Japan, and 6. P. Stradina Hospital, Riga, Latvia. Dr. Sener's primary field of research is Pediatric Neuroradiology.

FOREWORD

This atlas represents a contribution to an area that has been often overlooked
and considered insignificant by medical imaging specialists and clinicians alike.
Ever since the publication of human studies several decades earlier in which
the corpus callosum was surgically sectioned, principally for the purpose of
seizure propagation limitation, the corpus callosum has been considered largely
functionally inert. This opinion resulted from the observation that the patients who had their respective callosums sectioned manifested relatively few
overt clinical findings on casual inspection. This sentiment was given further
impetus by the observation that patients who had hypogenesis, or even com-
plete agenesis, of the callosum showed very little in the way of gross neuro-
logic findings clinically.

However, this impression misses the point: subtle adaptive changes in cerebral function that allow for relatively normal basic function of the relatively
independent cerebral hemispheres in such cases do not exclude the presence
of underlying profound occult alterations in interhemispheric function. This
alteration may be subclinical, and is often only obvious when the patient is
subjected to critical tests that are sensitive to the types of interhemispheric
functional parameters that have otherwise been adapted to in these patients.

With progressive evolution of clinical and medical imaging based tests of central nervous system function and dysfunction, this complacent attitude surrounding the role of the corpus callosum in brain activity can no longer be
accepted. An in-depth knowledge of the normal and pathologic anatomy
must precede the functional analysis of this important structure. We can de-
pend on researchers like Dr. Sener to forge the way forward in this newly
emerging field.

This textbook is one major step along this pathway, and represents an interesting waypoint that must be mastered in order to move ahead into the future.

J. Randy Jinkins, MD,
FACR, FEC
Philadelphia, PA
USA

Contents

III - Lesions Indirectly Involving the Corpus Callosum 183

NORMAL CORPUS CALLOSUM

Normal corpus callosum

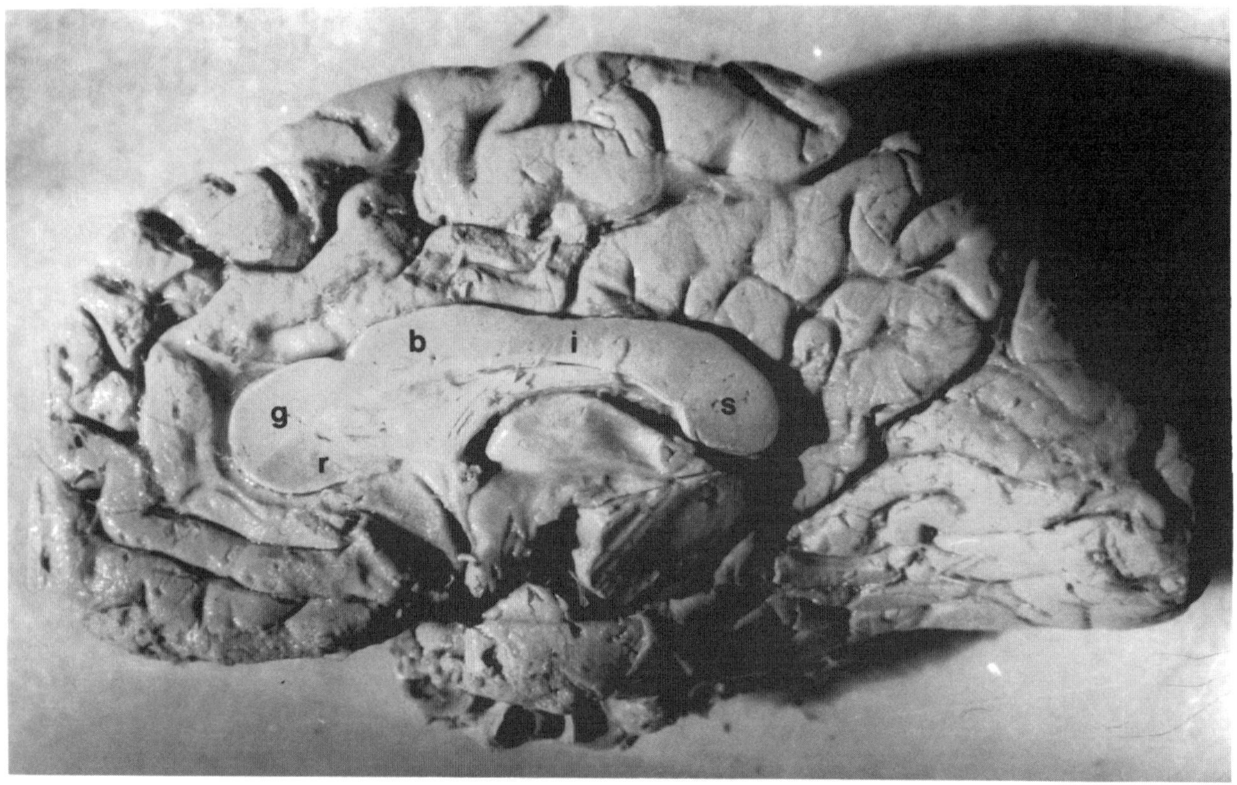

Figure 1.

Figure 1. **Normal corpus callosum**. Anatomic specimen from an adult cadaver shows the normal corpus callosum in sagittal plane. r=rostrum, g=genu, b=body, i=isthmus, s=splenium. According to the currently favoured theories the corpus callosum normally develops in an anterior to posterior direction. The genu forms first followed by posterior growth to form the body and splenium. This process is completed *by approximately 20 weeks gestational age*. The exception to this orderly anteroposterior development is the rostrum which forms latest of all. The corpus callosum assumes a nearly adult configuration approximately by the age 9 to 12 months. It continues to grow during childhood and reaches to adult size approximately by the age of 7 to 10 years.

References:
1. *Hayakawa K, Konishi Y, Matsuda T, et al. Development and aging of brain midline structures: assessment with MR imaging. Radiology 1989; 172: 171*

Figure 2. **Normal corpus callosum.** Adult cadaver. Axial plane g=genu, s=spenium.

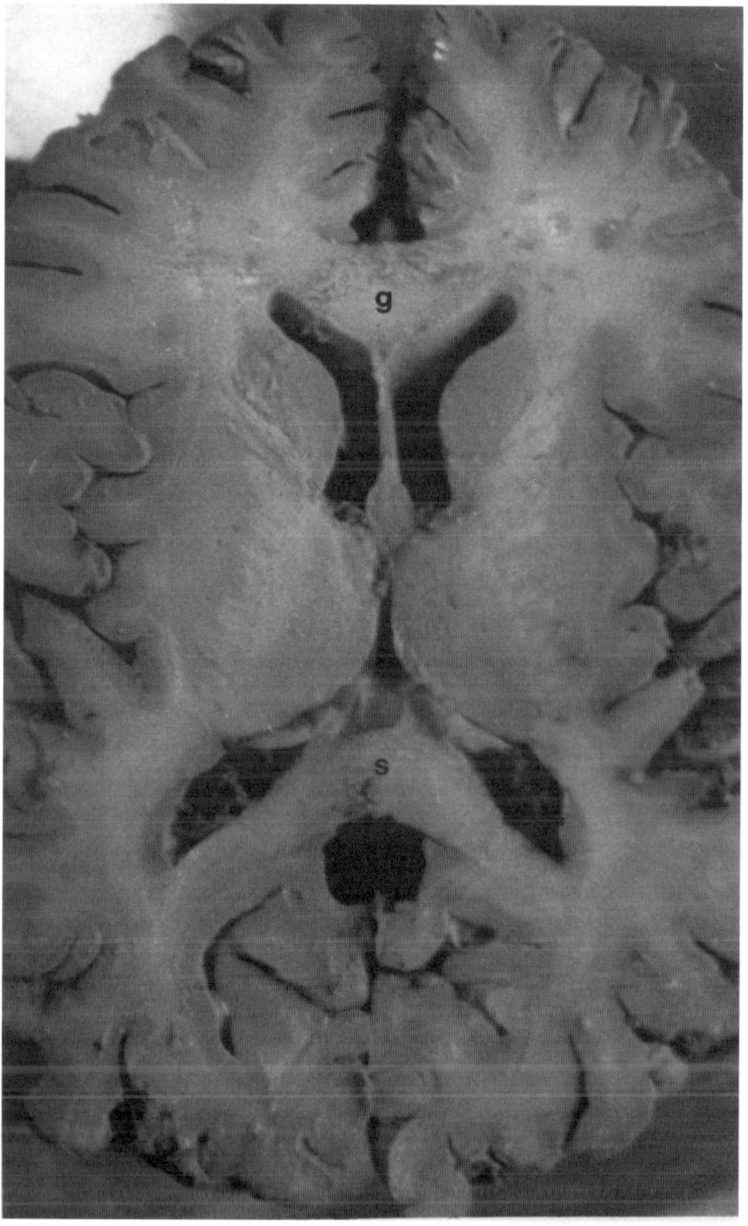

Figure 2.

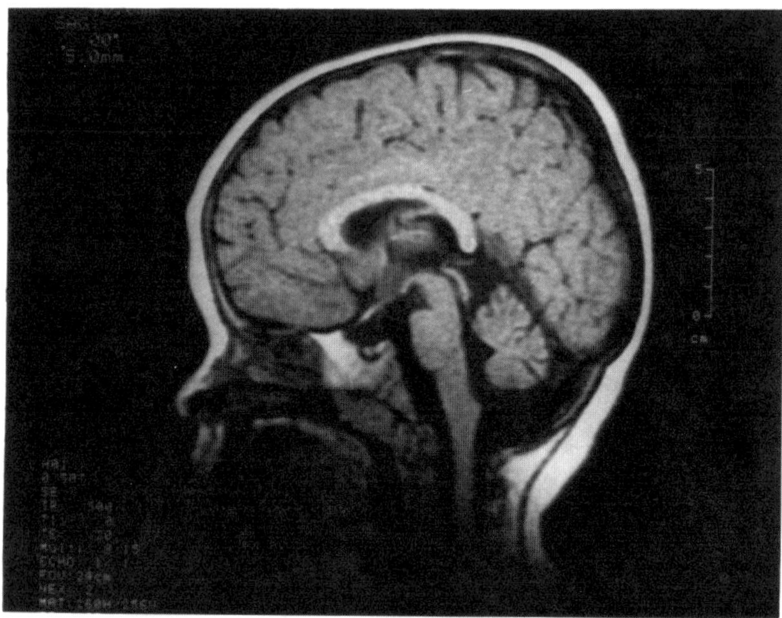

Figure 3.

Figure 3. **Normal corpus callosum.** 8-month-old boy. Sagittal T1-weighted (T1W) MR image shows the normal corpus callosum at this age (8-months). At birth the thickness of the corpus callosum is approximately one third to one fourth of this size. It gradually thickens by growing age. On T1W MR images the myelination of the corpus callosum first becomes apparent in the splenium at approximately 4-5 months, followed by the genu, and the remaining parts at approximately 5-7 months and the remaining parts. The signal pattern of the normally myelinated corpus callosum is identical to that of the white matter throughout the MR imaging sequences (hyperintense on T1W, and hypointense on T2W).

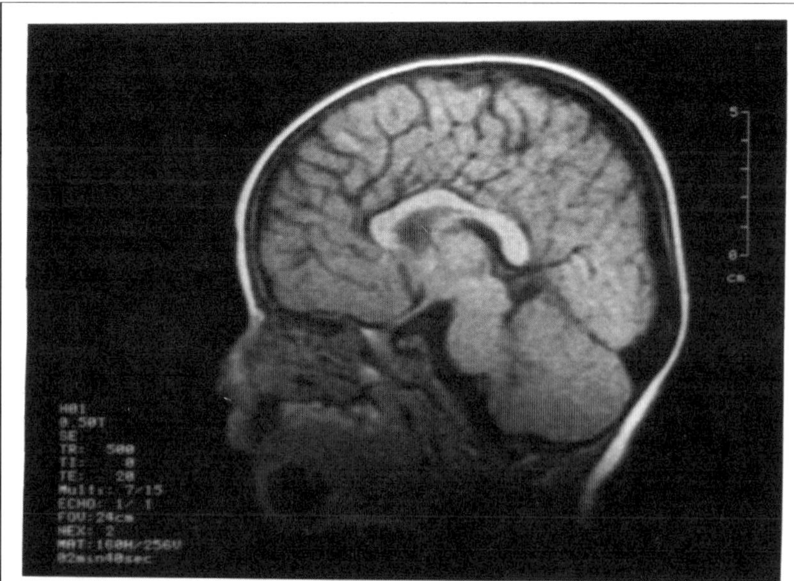

Figure 4. **Normal corpus callosum.** 12-month-old girl. Sagittal TIW MR image. The corpus callosum assumes an adult configuration at approximately this age; however, it continues to grow exponentially up to the age 10.

Figure 4.

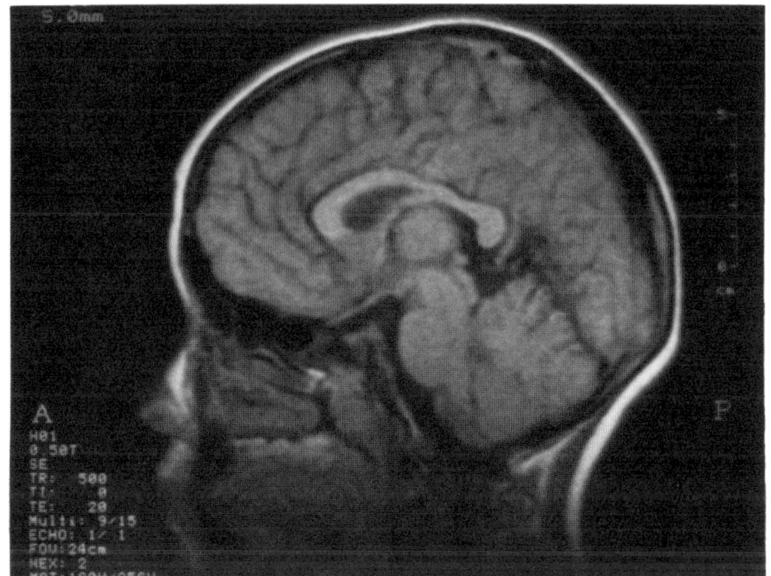

Figure 5. **Normal corpus callosum.** 7-year-old boy. Sagittal T1W MR image shows an adult-size corpus callosum. The corpus callosum reaches to adult size approximately by the age 7 to 10. After this, it shows minimal growth approximately up to the age 40. Then it shows a small decrease at ages 40-60.

Figure 5.

Figure 6. **Normal corpus callosum in an adult** (36-year-old man). Sagittal T1W MR image. r=rostrum, g=genu, b=body, i=isthmus, s=splenium. beyond the scope of this atlas.

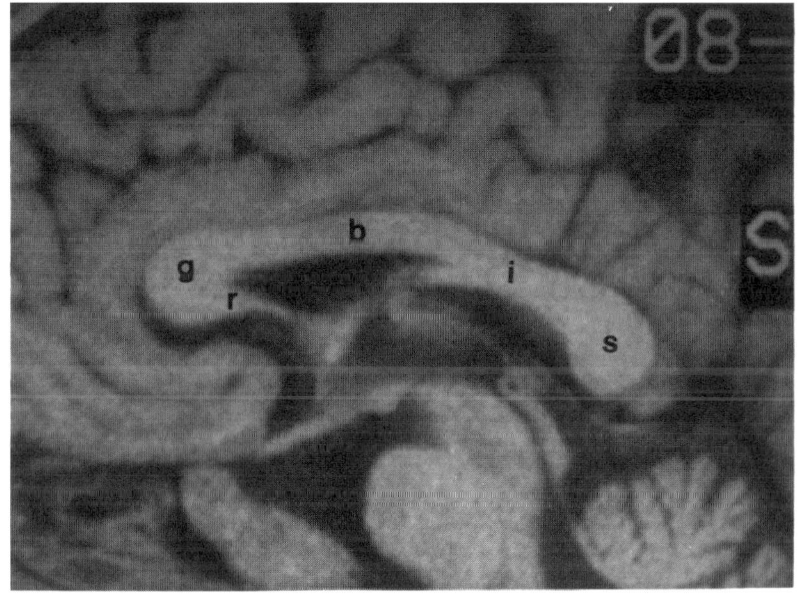

Figure 6.

References
1. *Hayakawa K, Konishi Y, Matsuda T, et al. Development and aging of brain midline structures: assessment with MR imaging. Radiology 1989; 172:171.*
2. *Barkovich AJ: Pediatric neuroimaging. New York, Raven Press, 1995;181*

Normal corpus callosum

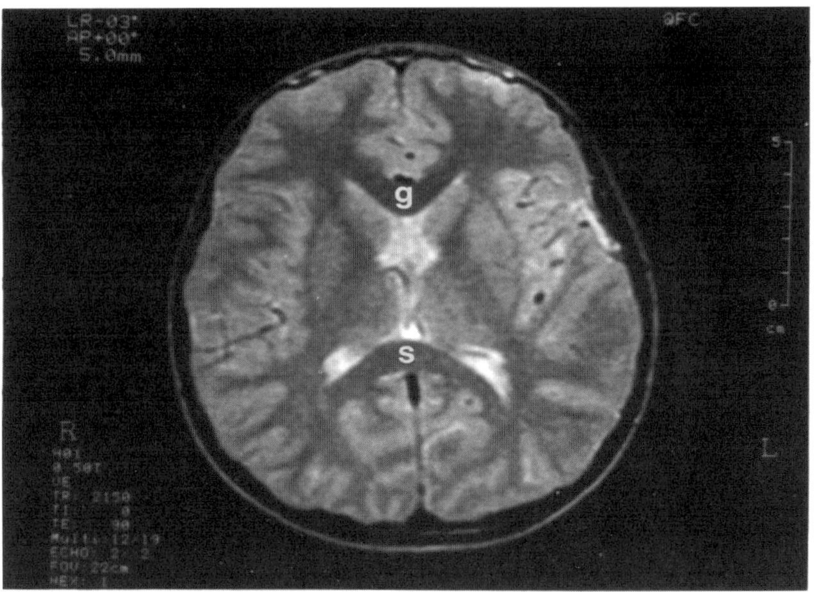

Figure 7.

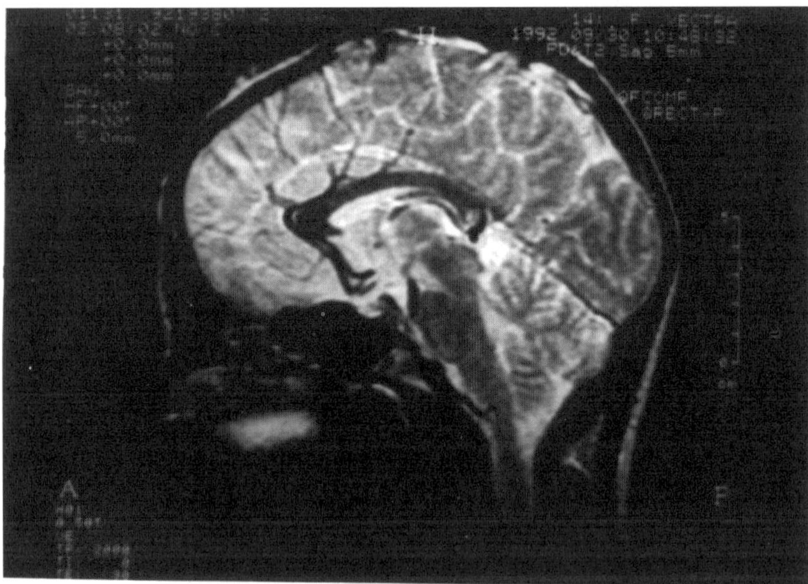

Figure 8.

Figure 7. **Normal corpus callosum on an axial T2-weighted (T2W) MR image.** 8-year-old boy. g=genu, s=spenium. The signal pattern of the corpus callosum is identical to that of the white matter (hypointense on T2W).

Figure 8. **Normal corpus callosum on a sagittal T2W MR image.** 14-year-old girl. It has a signal pattern (hypointense) identical to that of the white matter.

Figure 9 a,b. **Normal corpus callosum.** 16-year-old boy. Sagittal (a), and coronal (b) FLAIR (fluid attenuated inversion recovery) images. The innermost layer of the corpus callosum appears as a thin bright line, approximately 2 mm in thickness. This is best appreciated on sagittal FLAIR images. In conditions associated with hydrocephalus this bright line becomes thicker.

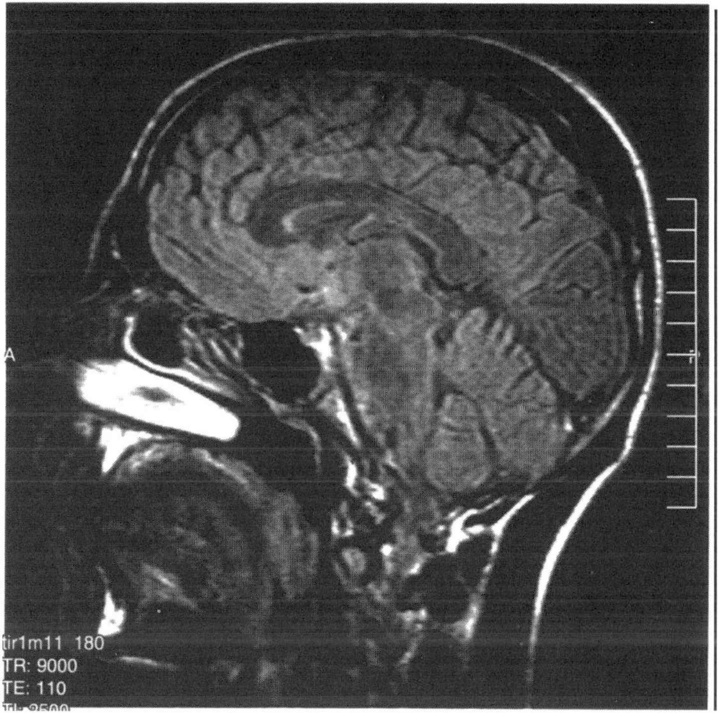

Figure 9a.

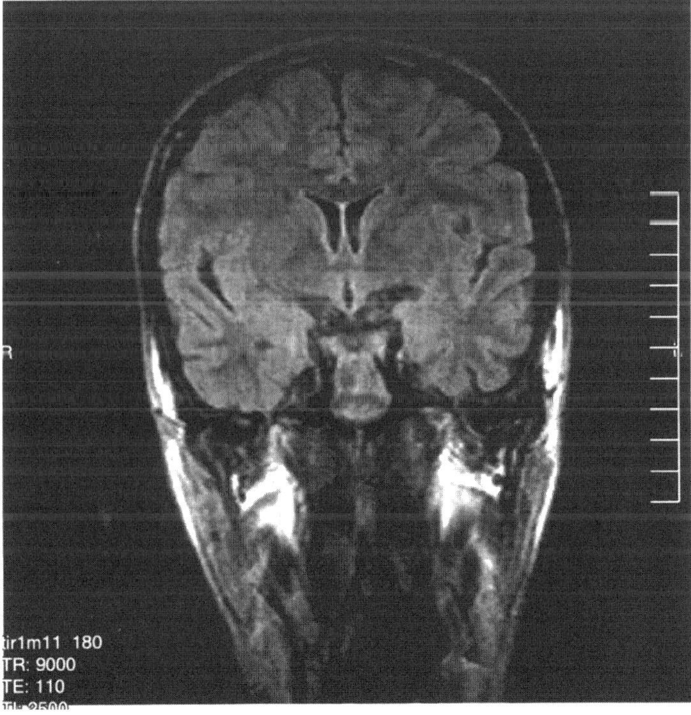

Figure 9b.

Figure 10 a-c. **Normal corpus callosum.** 16-year-old boy. Apparent diffusion coefficient (ADC) maps are shown from an echo-planar diffusion imaging sequence. *(In this sequence obtained on a 1.5 Tesla MR unit diffusion sensitivity values: i.e. b value at b=0, b=500 sec/mm², and b=1000 sec/mm² are applied in section-select, phase-encoding, and readout gradients, or are applied by averaging these referred to as 'Trace' diffusion, and automated ADC maps are generated. These two are also called as isotropic diffusion imaging).*

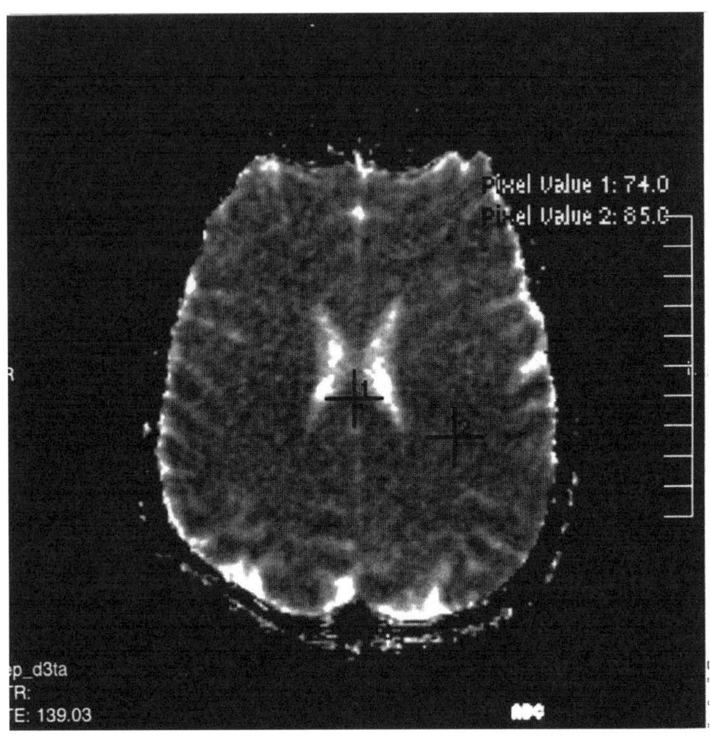

Figure 10a.

Figure 10b.

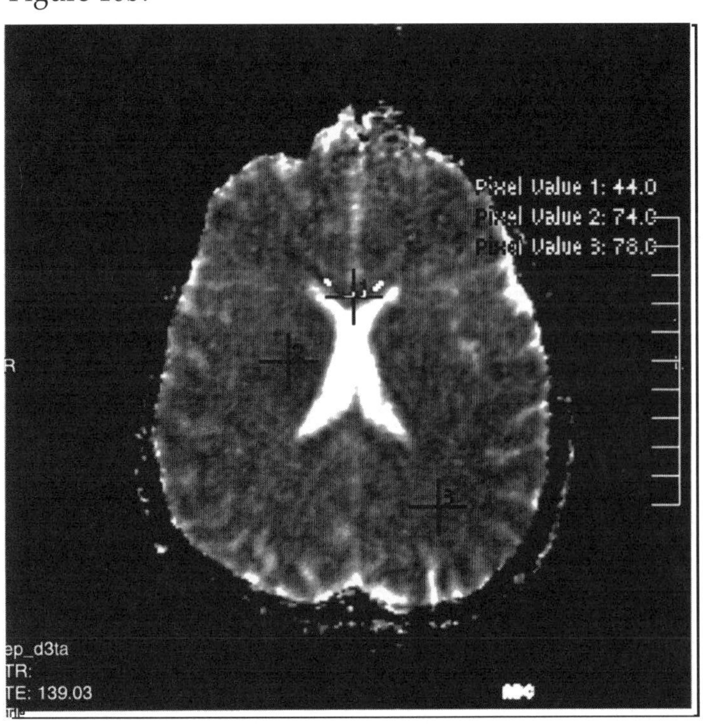

ADC values can be measured directly by pixel lens and/or ROI evaluations from ADC maps, or by using Stejskal-Tanner equation: $ADC = -(1/b) \ln (S/So)$: So is signal intensity with the gradient factors b=0; S is the signal intensity with the gradient factors b=1000 sec/mm²; 1n is natural logarithm, and b in 1/b is 1000. On ADC maps, the ADC values of some parts of the corpus callosum may be similar to the normal white matter: **0.84±0.11** X10⁻³ mm²/sec, ranging between 0.60 and 1.05 X10⁻³ mm²/sec.

This: 0.74 $\times 10^{-3}$ mm^2/sec, and a normal parenchymal value are shown: 0.85 $\times 10^{-3}$ mm^2/sec (a). However, in some parts of the normal corpus callosum anisotrophy effects cause low values. This is shown: 0.44 $\times 10^{-3}$ mm^2/sec, compared to two normal parenchymal ADC values: 0.74 and 0.78 $\times 10^{-3}$ mm^2/sec (b). One low: 0.45 $\times 10^{-3}$ mm^2/sec, and two normal: 0.76 and 0.86 $\times 10^{-3}$ mm^2/sec ADC values are shown from the corpus callosum, compared to normal parenchymal values: 0.87 and 0.83 $\times 10^{-3}$ mm^2/sec (c).

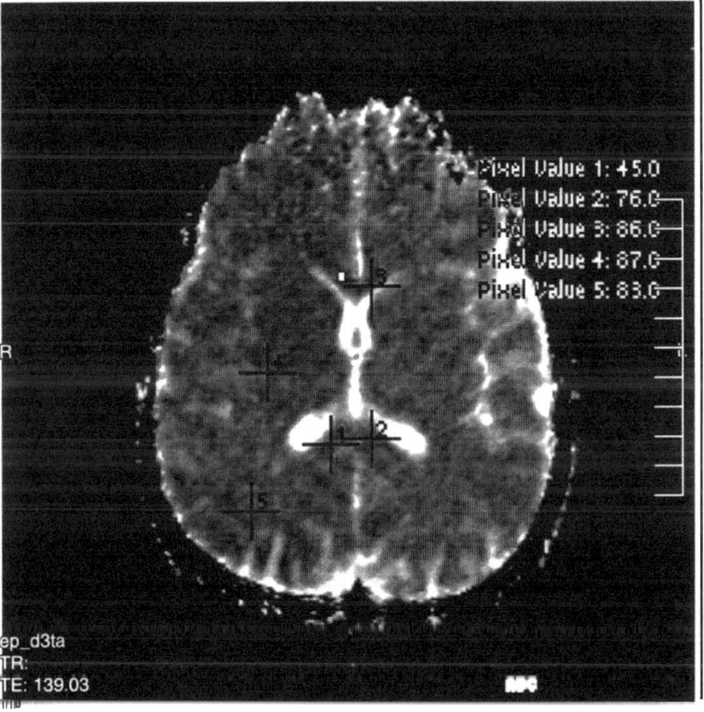

Figure 10c.

References
1. Morriss MC, Zimmerman RA, Bilaniuk, LT, et al. Changes in brain water diffusion during childhood. Neuroradiology 1999; 41:929
2. Sener RN. Diffusion MRI: apparent diffusion coefficient (ADC) values in the normal brain, and a classification of brain disorders based on ADC values. Comput Med Imaging Graph 2001;25:299

Normal corpus callosum

Figure 11 a,b. **Normal corpus callosum.** 21-year-old woman. PSIF images (reverse FISP, fast imaging in steady state precession), which is a gradient-echo sequence (also called anisotropic diffusion sequence) show the normal corpus callosum with low signal, similar to anterior part of the pons.

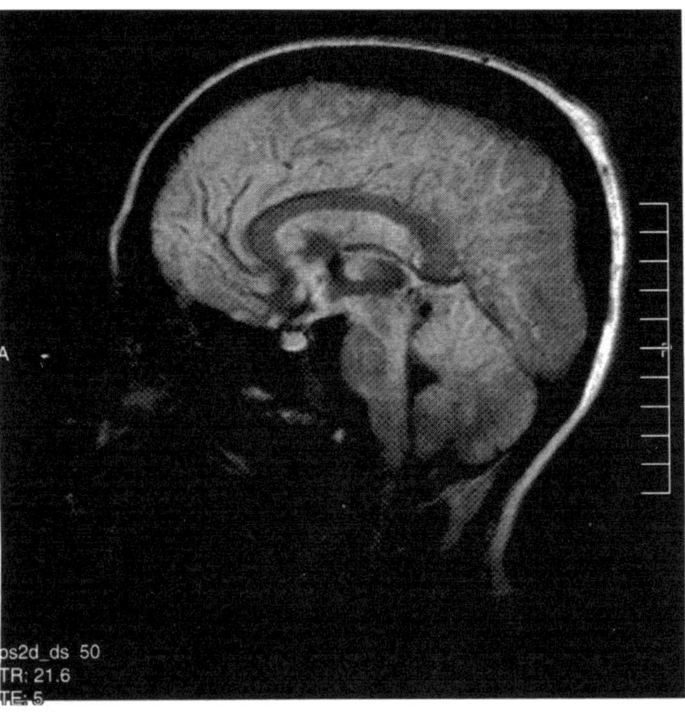

Figure 11a.

Figure 11b.

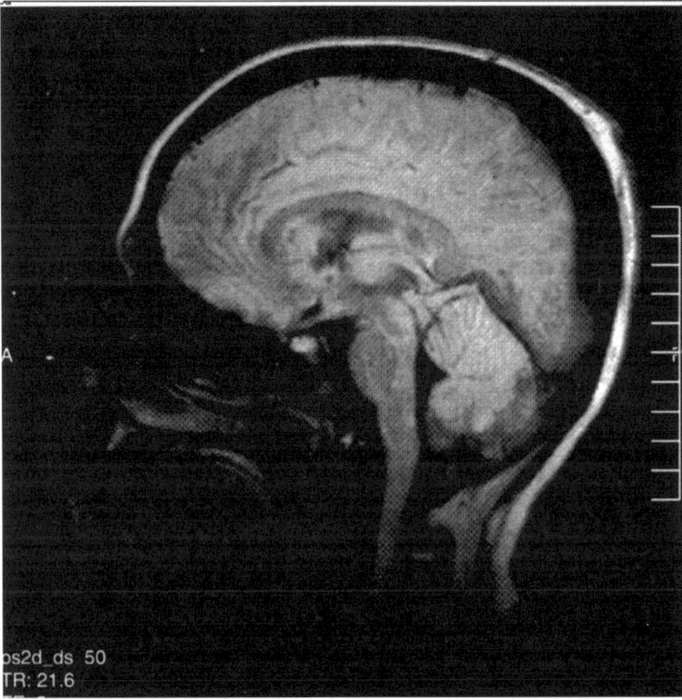

LESIONS DIRECTLY INVOLVING THE CORPUS CALLOSUM

CALLOSAL ABSENCE

Figure 12. **Callosal absence (agenesis) in Dandy-Walker syndrome.** 8-month-old girl. *SE T1W MR image.* There is a large posterior fossa cyst due to cystic dilatation of the fourth ventricle (asterisk), the superior vermis is small and displaced upward. The inferior vermis is absent. The cerebellar hemispheres were hypoplastic (Dandy-Walker syndrome). The condition is associated with total callosal absence (arrow).

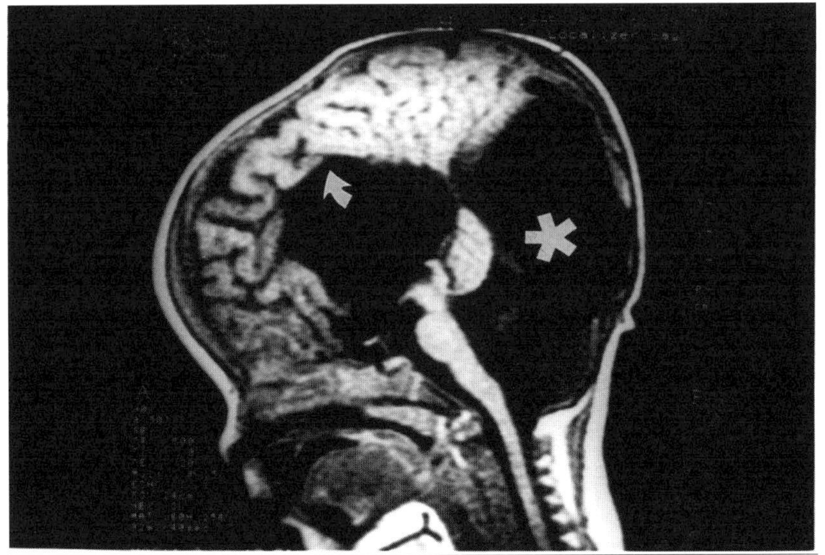

Figure 12.

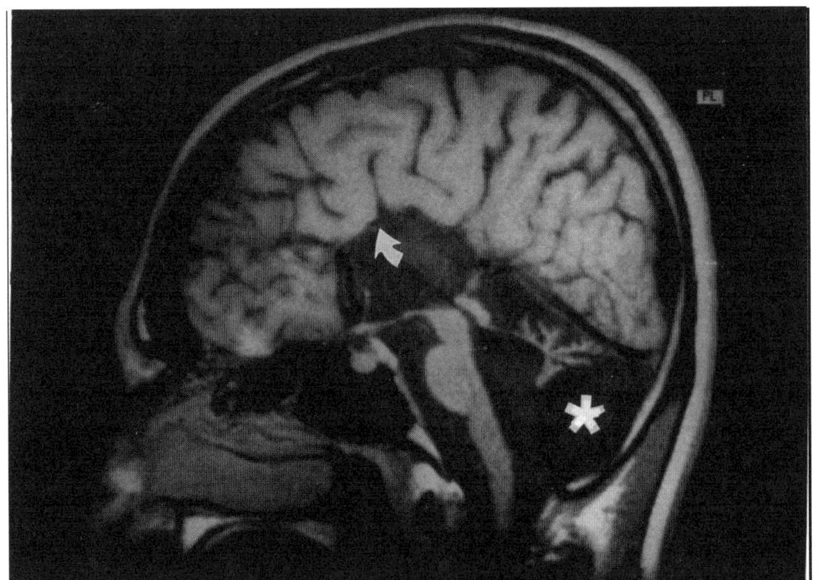

Figure 13.

Figure 13. **Callosal absence in Dandy-Walker variant.** 2-year-old boy. *SE T1W MR image.* The fourth ventricle is dilated, the superior vermis is dysplastic, and the inferior vermis is absent. The posterior fossa is normal in size (asterisk) (Dandy-Walker variant). Note total callosal absence (arrow). Total callosal absence is less common in Dandy-Walker variant compared with those cases with Dandy-Walker syndrome.

References
1. *Osborn AG. Diagnostic neuroradiology. St. Louis, Mosby, 1994;59*
2. *Barkovich AJ: Pediatric neuroimaging. New York, Raven Press, 1995;249*
3. *Wolpert SM, Barnes PD. MRI in pediatric neuroradiology. St. Louis, Mosby, 1992;102*
4. *Barkovich AJ, Kjos BO, Norman D, et al. Revised classification of posterior fossa cysts and cystlike malformations based on the results of multiplanar MR imaging. AJNR 1989; 10:977*
5. *Altman NR, Naidich TP, Braffman BH. Posterior fossa malformations. AJNR 1992; 13:691*
6. *Barkovich AJ, Norman D. Anomalies of the corpus callosum: correlation with further anomalies of the brain. AJNR 1988; 9:493*
7. *Wilson ME, Lindsay DJ, Levi Cs, et al. US case of the day. Dandy-Walker variant with agenesis of the corpus callosum. Radiographics 1994; 14:678*

Figure 14 a-c. **Callosal absence associated with multiple schwannomas.** 17-year-old boy with neurofibromatosis. *a, b, and c, SE T1W MR images after administration of intravenous contrast-medium.* There is a total callosal absence (arrow) (a). Coronal images show the interhemispheric fissure extending to the third ventricle due to callosal absence, and bundles of Probst indenting the medial walls of the lateral ventricles (b, c). The temporal horns and the third ventricle are dilated due to the compression effect of the associated neurogenic tumors located in the cerebellopontine angle, bilateral acustic neurinomas (arrows) (b), and in the vicinity of the foramen magnum, a hypoglossal neuroma, (circles) (b, c).

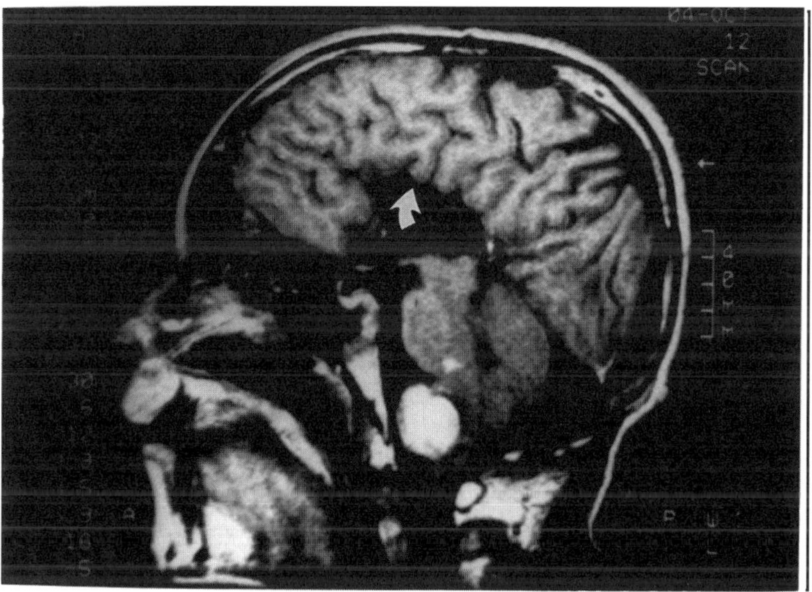

Figure 14a.

Reference
1. Toedt C, Holzinger H, Salbeck R, et al. A combination of generalized neurofibromatosis (Recklinghausen disease) and agenesis of the corpus callosum. Digitale Bilddiagn 1989; 9:105

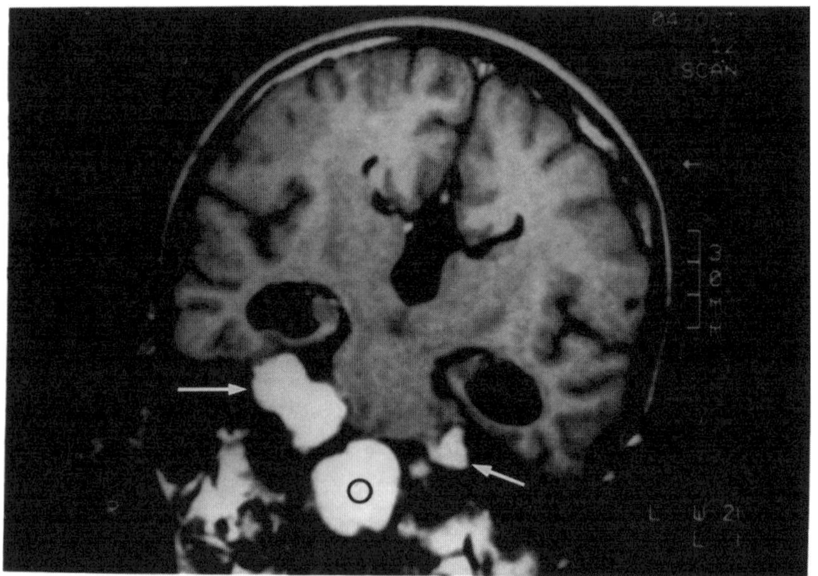

Figure 14b.

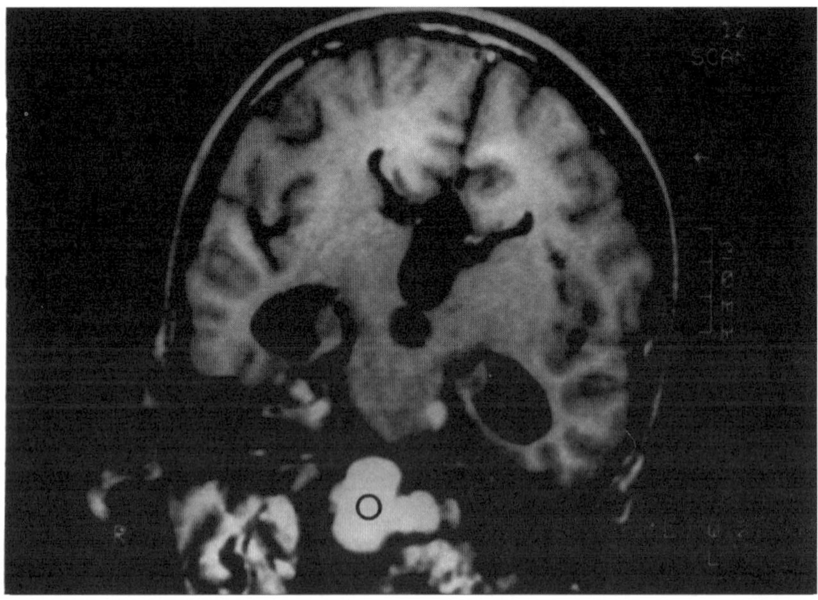

Figure 14c.

Figure 15 a,b. **Callosal absence associated with an interhemispheric cyst and schizencephaly.** 8.5-year-old girl with Aicardi's syndrome. *a) SE T1W, and b) SE T2W MR images.* The corpus callosum is absent. There is an interhemispheric cyst (ct), blending with the third ventricle (a). Note a schizencephalic cleft, lined with heterotopic gray matter, in the right hemisphere (arrow) (b).

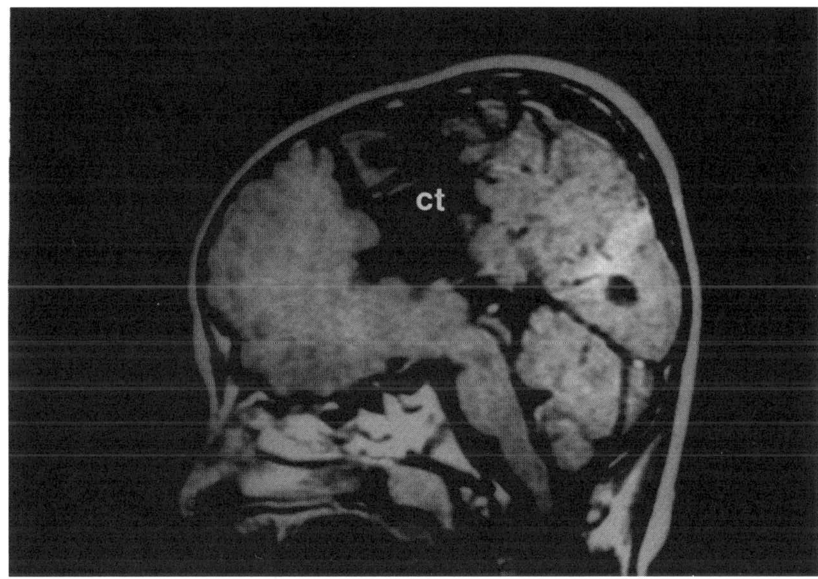

Figure 15a.

References

1. Yamagata T, Mormoi M, Miyamoto S, et al. Multi-institutional survey of the Aicardi syndrome in Japan. Brain Dev 1990; 12:760

2. Hall Craggs MA, Harbord MG, Finn JP, et al. Aicardi syndrome: MR assessment of brain structure an myelination. AJNR 1990; 11:532

3. Mori K. Giant interhemispheric cysts associated with agenesis of the corpus callosum. J. Neurosurg 1992; 76:224

4. Schwartz AM, Ghatak NR. Interhemispheric cysts in association with agenesis of the corpus callosum. Clin Neuropathol 1990; 9:177

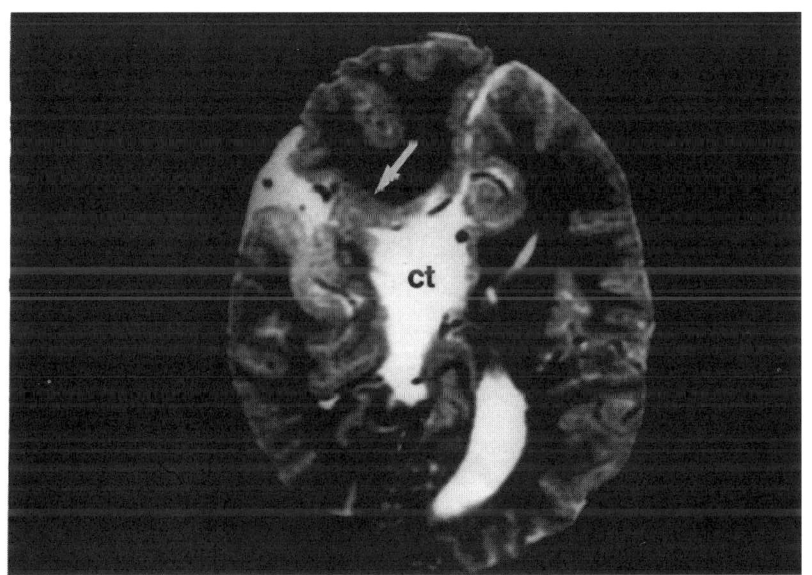

Figure 15b.

Figure 16 a,b. **Callosal absence in septo-optic dysplasia.** 18-month-old girl. *a) SE T1W MR image, and b) direct coronal CT scan.* The corpus callosum is absent (curved arrow) (a), and as a result the falx extends well into the third ventricle (arrow) (b). The optic nerve is thin (straight arrow) (a). Additional views confirmed thinning of the optic nerves, and an ophthalmologic examination revealed optic atrophy and poor vision (septo-optic dysplasia). Total callosal absence is very rare in septo-optic dysplasia (from reference 5).

References
1. *Barkovich AJ, Fram EK, Norman D. Septo-optic dysplasia: MR imaging. Radiology 1989; 171:189*
2. *Filz CR. Holoprosencephaly and related entities. Neuroradiology 1983; 25:225*
3. *Fukutomi T, Masakado M, Takayanagi R, et al. A case of hypopituitarism associated with empty sella and agenesis of corpus callosum, a variant form of septo-optic-pituitary dysplasia. Fukuoka Igaku Zasshi 1990; 81: 396*
4. *Lahat E, Strauss S, Tadmor R, et al. Infantil spasms in patient with septo-optic dysplasia, partial agenesis of the corpus callosum and an interhemi-spheric cyst. Clin Neurol Neurosurg 1992; 94:165*
5. *Sener RN. Septo-optic dysplasia associated with total absence of the corpus callosum: MR and CT features. Eur Radiol 1993; 3:551*

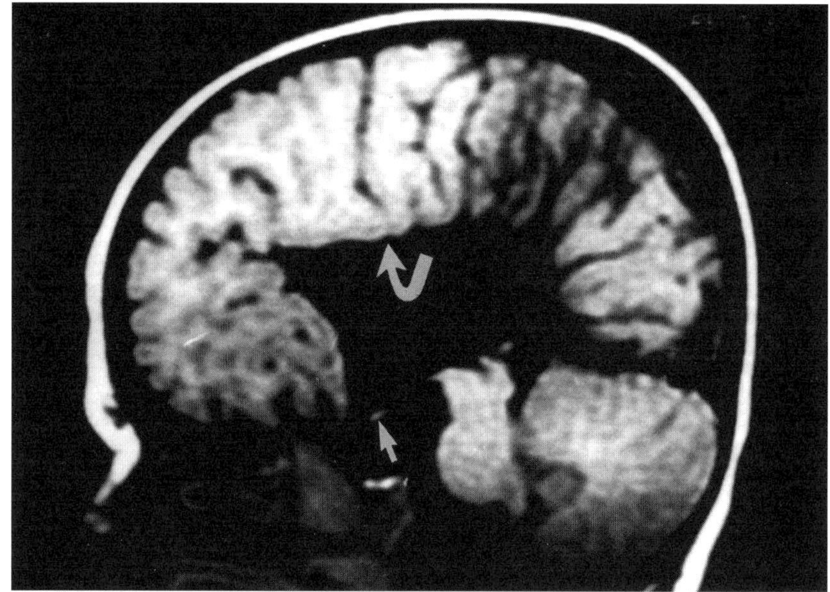

Figure 16a.

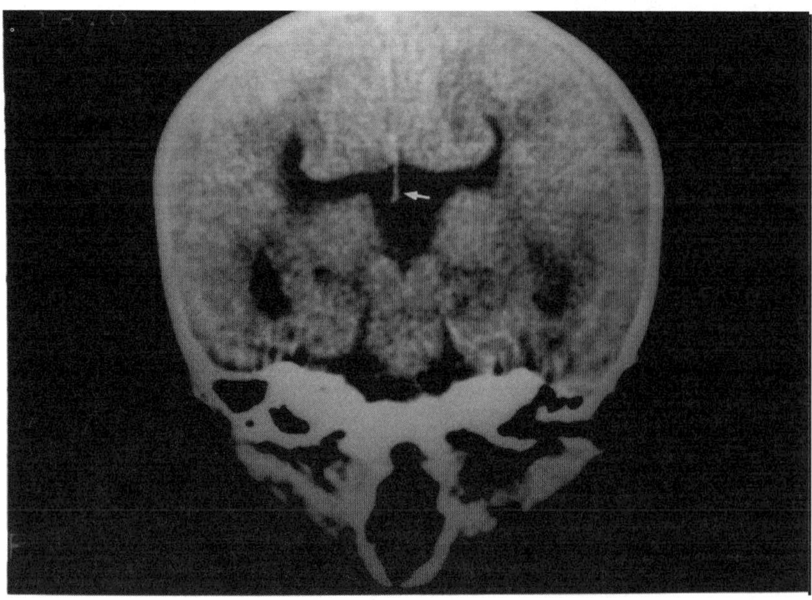

Figure 16b.

Figure 17 a, b. **Callosal absence in septo-optic dysplasia.** 6-month-old boy. *a) SE T1W, and b) inversion recovery (IR) MR image after administration of contrast medium.* Total callosal absence is noted (arrow) (a). The coronal image shows a very thin optic chiasm (arrows) (b), at least three times thinner than that of a normal age-matched individual. Our experience with these two patients (including that in Fig. 13) suggests existence of a different form of septo-optic dysplasia, which may be labeled as calloso-septo-optic or calloso-optic dysplasia.

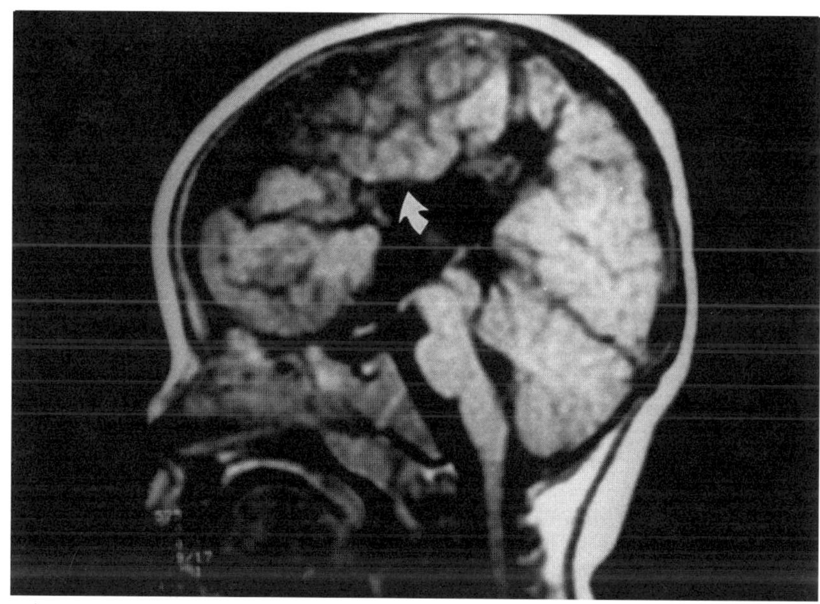

Figure 17a.

References

1. *Barkovich AJ, Fram EK, Norman D. Septo-optic dysplasia: MR imaging. Radiology 1989; 171:189*

2. *Fitz CR. Holoprosencephaly and related entities. Neuroradiology 1983; 25:225*

3. *Fukutomi T, Masakado M, Takayanagi R, et al. A case of hypopituitarism associated with empty sella and agenesis of corpus callosum, a variant form of septo optic pituitary dysplasia. Fukuoka Igaku Zasshi 1990; 81:396*

4. *Lahat E, Strauss S, Tadmor R, et al. Infantil spasms in patient with septo-optic dysplasia, partial agenesis of the corpus callosum and an interhemispheric cyst. Clin Neurol Neurosurg 1992; 94:165*

5. *Sener RN. Septo-optic dysplasia associated with total absence of the corpus callosum: MR and CT features. Eur Radiol 1993; 3:551*

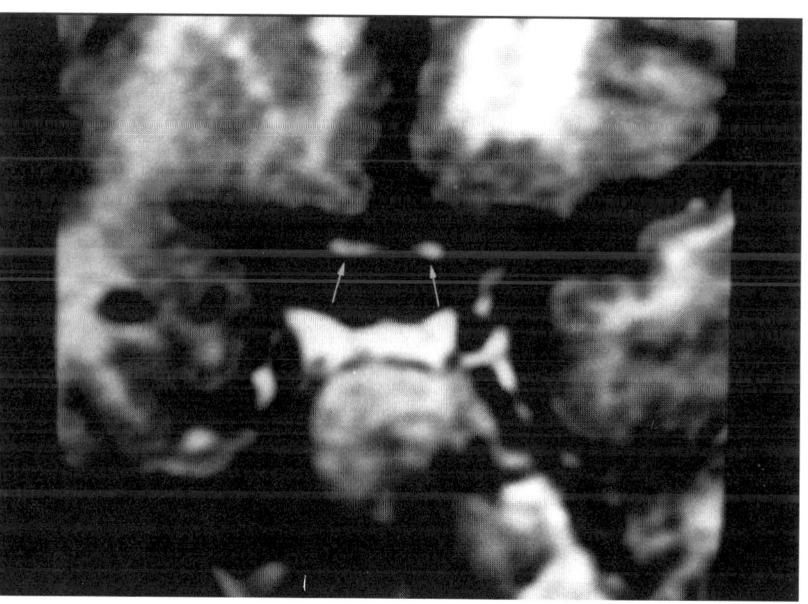

Figure 17b.

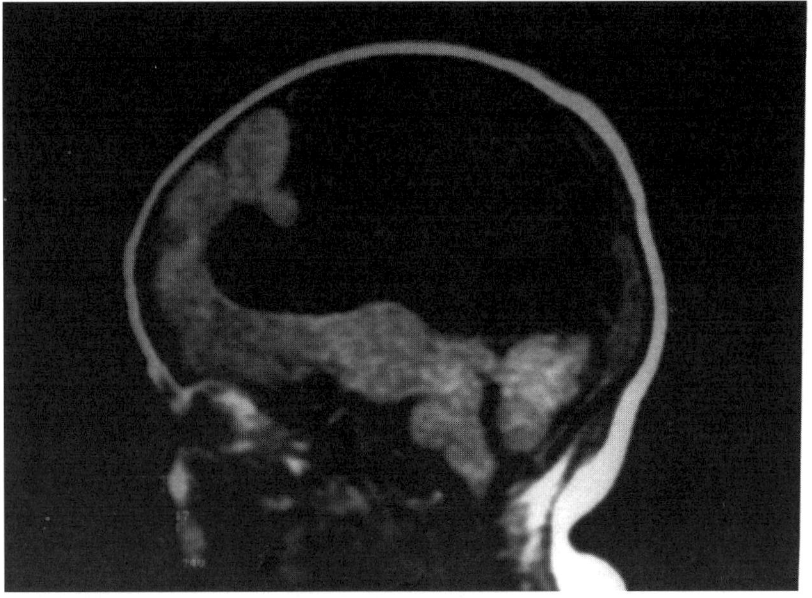

Figure 18a.

Figure 18. a-c. **Callosal absence in alobar holoprosencephaly**. 1-month-old girl. *a) SE T1W, b)SE T2W, and c) IR T1W MR images.* The corpus callosum is usually absent in alobar and semilobar types of holoprosencephaly, as demonstrated in this case. Note interhemispheric fusion (straight arrows) (a, b), and thalamic fusion (curved arrow) (c), characteristic for holoprosencephaly.

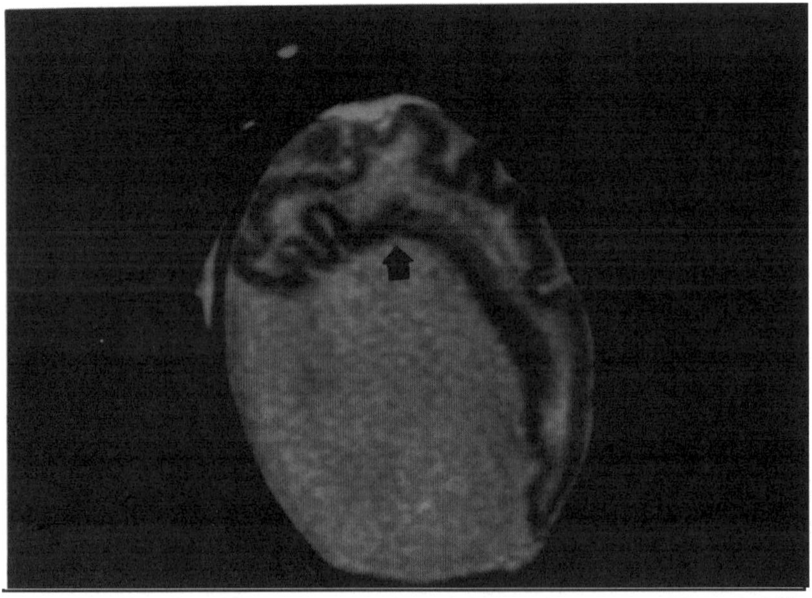

Figure 18b.

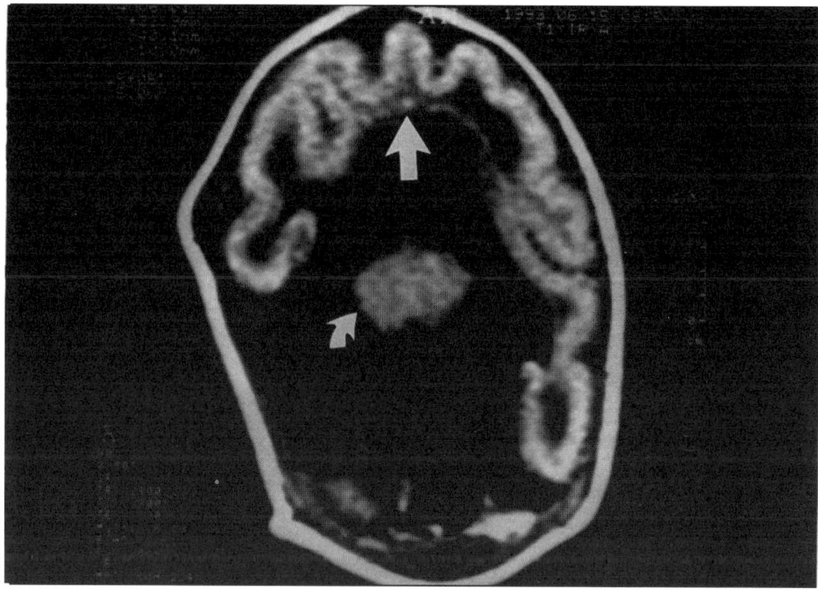

Figure 18c.

References
1. *Fitz CR. Holoprosencephaly and related entities. Neuroradiology 1983; 25:225*
2. *Barkovich AJ, Norman D. Anomalies of the corpus callosum: correlation with further anomalies of the brain. AJNR 1988; 9:493*

Figure 19a.

Figure 19a-i. **Alobar holoprosencephaly (Intrauterine MRI).** 20-week-old fetus. Ultrasound reveals a fetus with cyclopia (a). Intrauterine MRI with the TRUFI (True-FISP=fast imaging with steady state precession) sequence reveals a single ventricle, and fusion of the frontal lobes as well as the thalami, characteristic for holoprosencephaly. Cyclopia is shown (arrow) (b,c). Photograph after delivery reveals cyclopia (d). Azygous anterior cerebral artery is common in holo-prosencephalies, and an example is shown by MR angiography (arrow) (e). In an age-matched fetus (22 weeks) normal brain is demonstrated by using the HASTE (half-fourier single-shot turbo spin echo) sequence in transverse (f,g), coronal (h), and sagittal imaging planes (i). In both imaging sequences TRUFI and HASTE, acquisition time is 11 seconds.

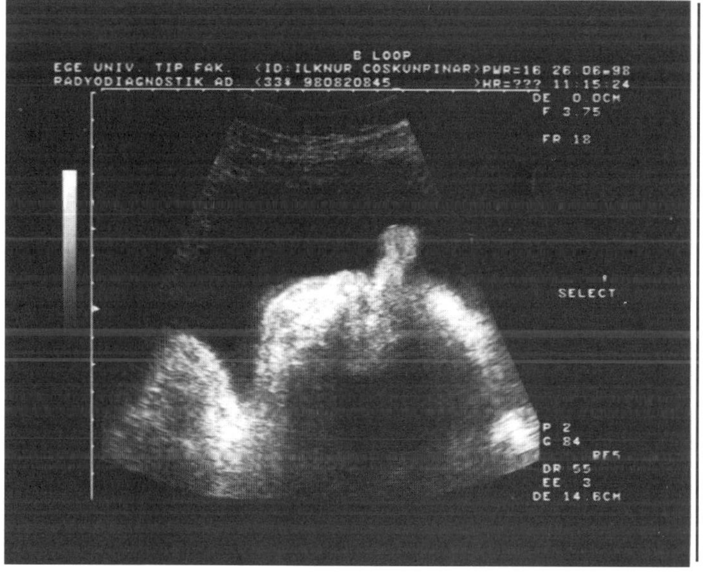

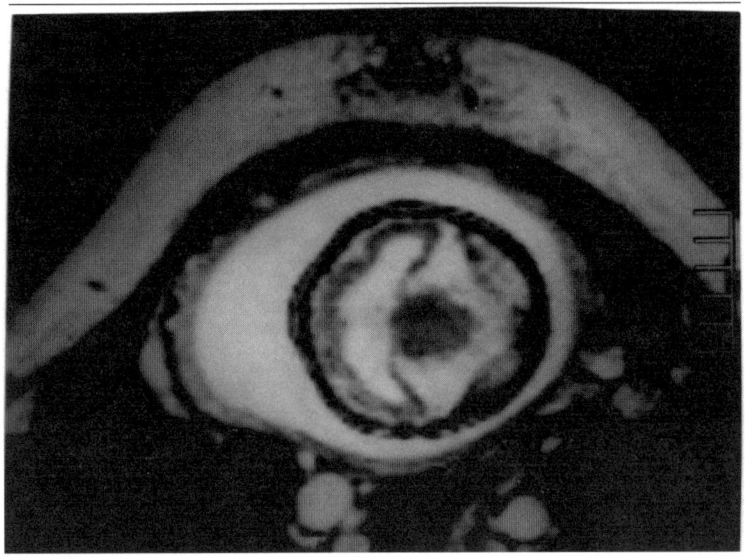

Figure 19b.

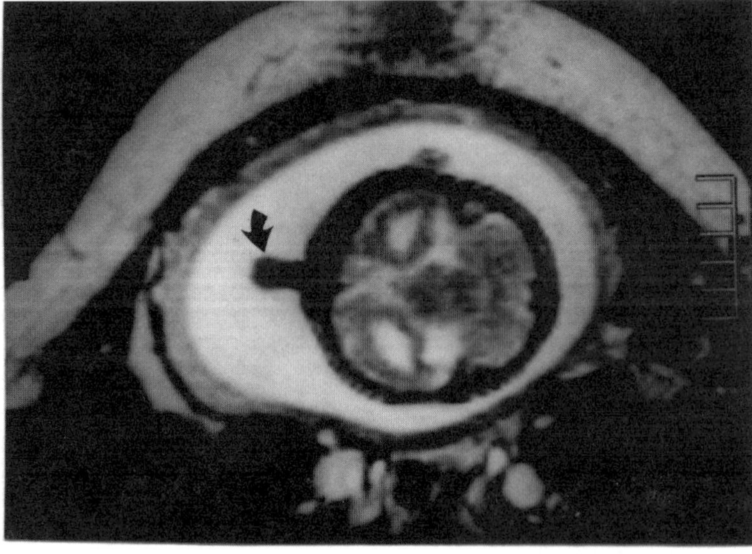

Figure 19c.

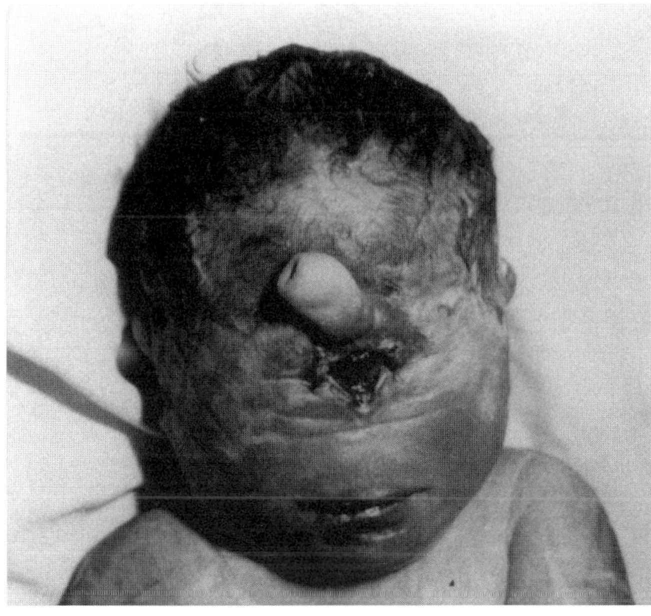

Figure 19d.

Figure 19e.

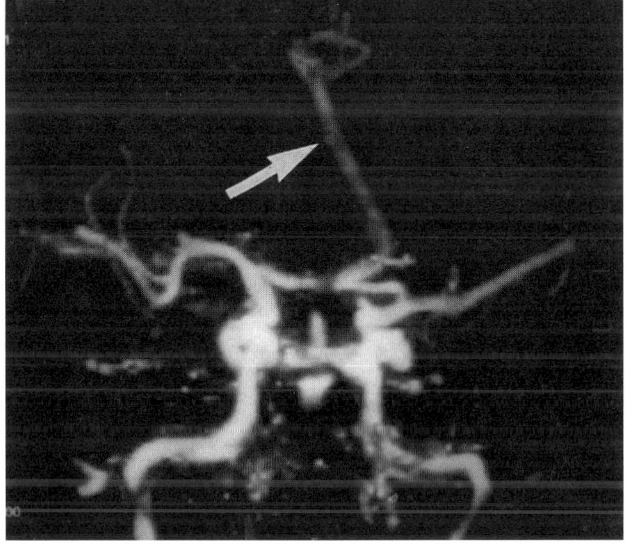

Figure 19f.

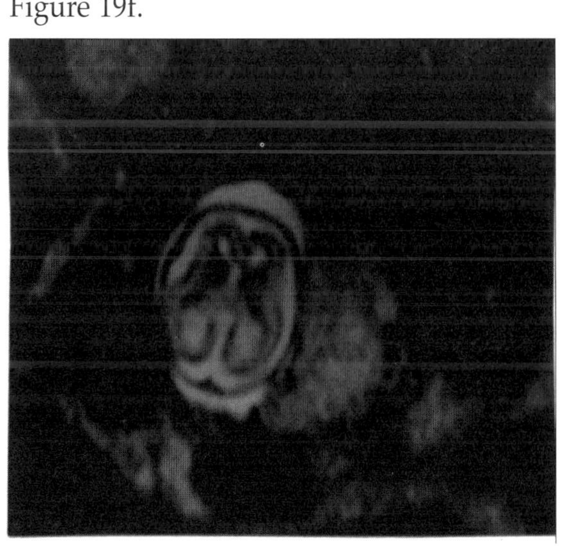

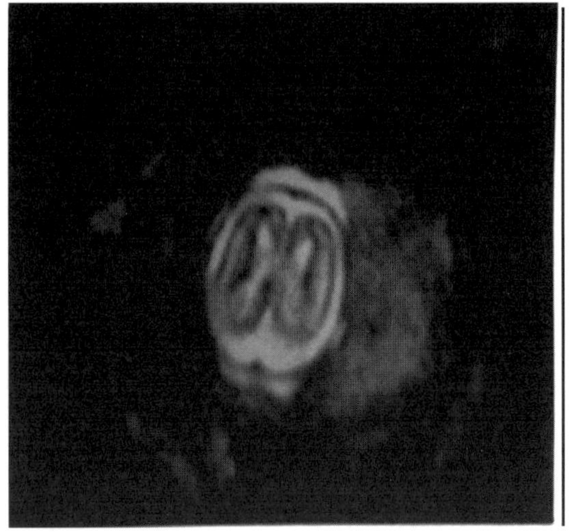

Figure 19g.

Figure 19h.

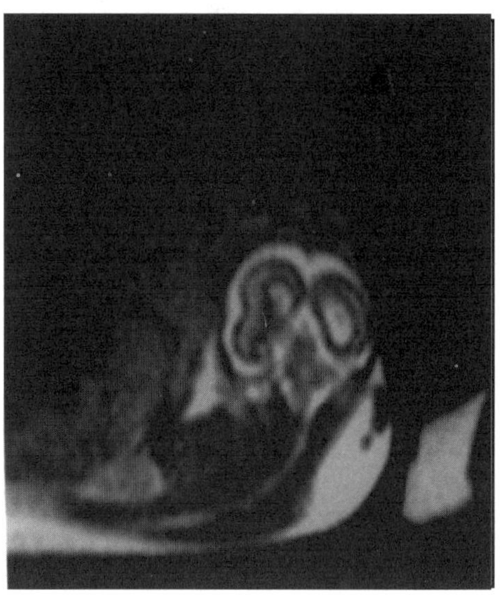

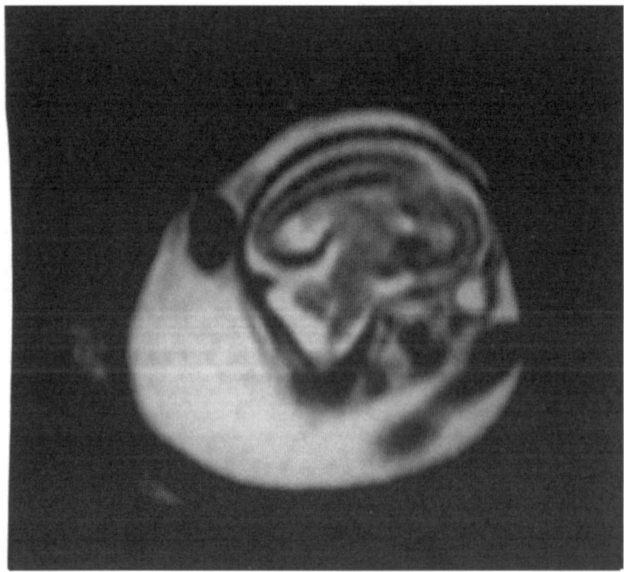

Figure 19i.

References
1. *Levine D, Barnes PD, Sher S, et al. Fetal fast MR imaging: reproducibility, technical quality, and conspicuity of anatomy. Radiology 1998; 206:549*
2. *Vimercati A, Greco P, Vera L, et al. The diagnostic role of ëin uteroï magnetic resonance imaging. J Perinat Med 1999; 27:303*
3. *Liu DPC, Burrowes DM, Qureshi MN. Cyclopia: craniofacial appearance on MR and three-dimensional CT. AJNR 1997; 18:543*

Figure 20 a-d. **Callosal absence in congenital craniopharyngioma.** 10-day-old boy. *a)CT scan, (b, c, and d) T1W MR images.* CT scan shows a huge calcified mass (star) (a). Higher sections showed a cystic component of the lesion. MR images show a huge mass originating from the suprasellar region (T) (b, c), and a cystic component (ct) (c), which was proven to be a craniopharyngioma. Note that the corpus callosum is totally absent, an unusual association of a craniopharyngioma (b, c, d). There is a small interhemispheric lipoma (arrows) (b, d).

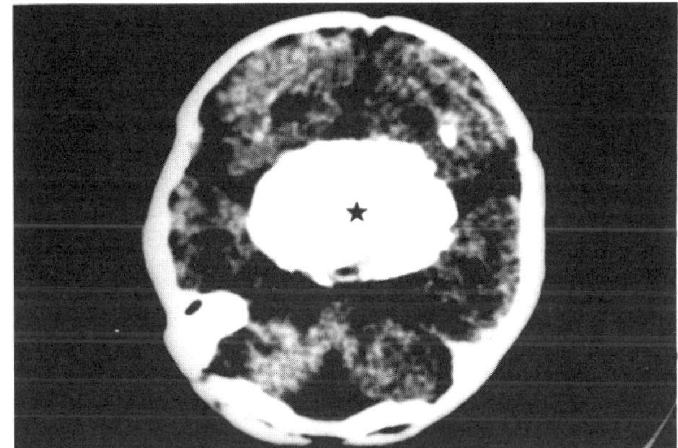

Figure 20a.

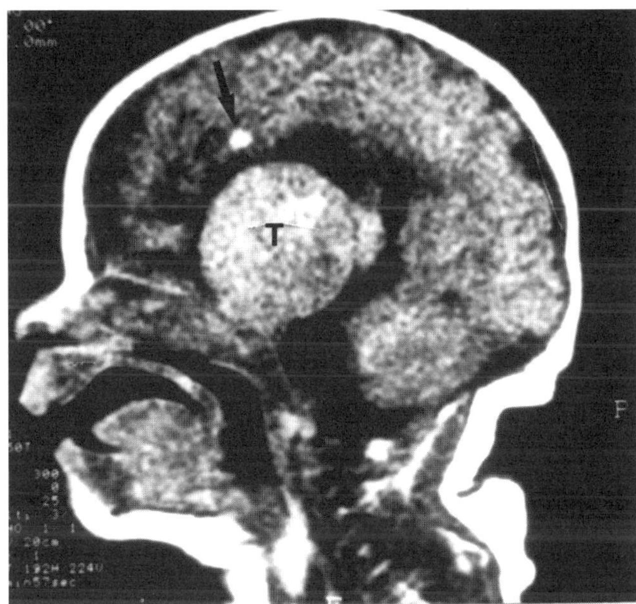

Figure 20b.

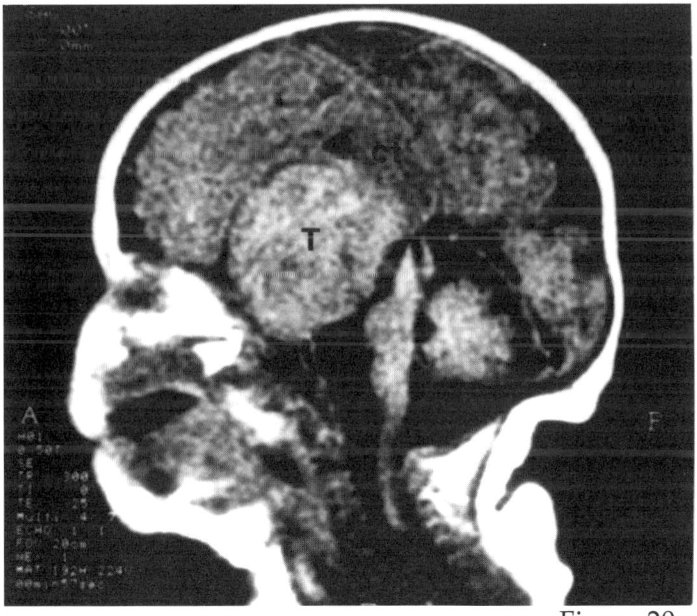

Figure 20c.

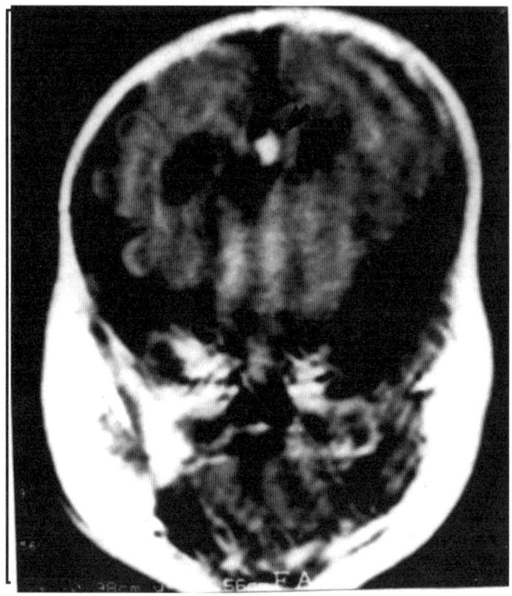

Figure 20d.

References
1.   Hurst RW, McIlheny J, Park TS, et al. Neonatal craniopharyngioma: CT and ultrasonographic features. J Comput Assist Tomogr 1988;12:858

LESIONS DIRECTLY INVOLVING THE CORPUS CALLOSUM

CALLOSAL DYSGENESIS

Figure 21 a-c. **Pericallosal lipoma.** 6-year-old girl. *a, b) SE T1W, and c) SE T2W MR images.* A pericallosal lipoma is seen (arrows), interrupting normal callosal development at the region of the body (a-c). Note peripheral black-white lines on the T2W image (arrows) (c), representing chemical shift artifacts, which is a characteristic feature for a lipoma.

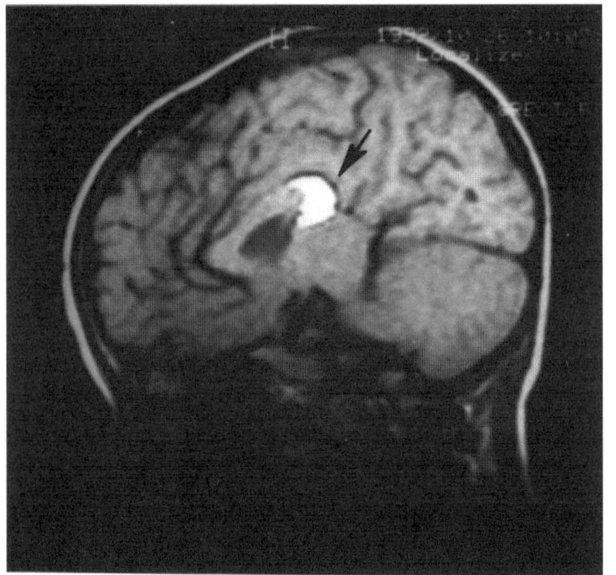
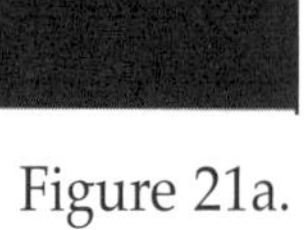

Figure 21a.

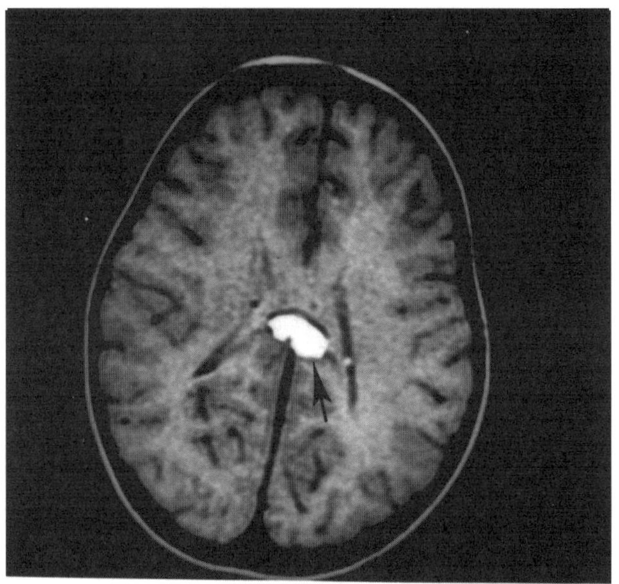

Figure 21b.

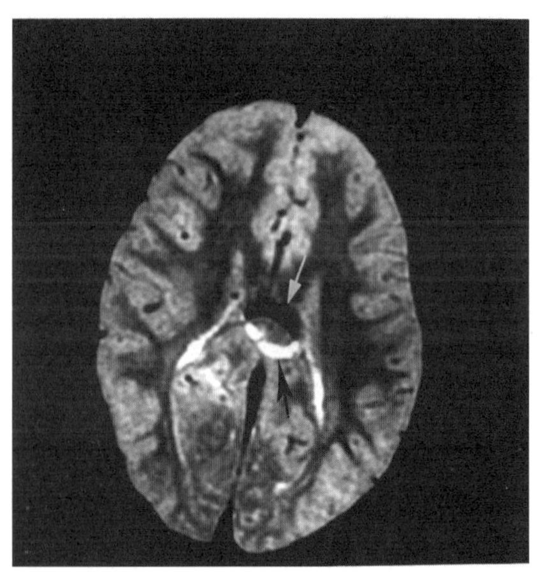

Figure 21c.

References
1. *Tart RP, Quisling RG. Curvilinear and tubulonodular varieties of lipoma of corpus callosum: an MR and CT study. J Comput Assist Tomogr 1991;15:805*
2. *Truwit CL, Barkovic AJ. Pathogenesis of intracranial lipoma: an MR study in 42 patients. AJNR 1990; 11:665*
3. *Truwit CL, Williams G, Armstrong EA, et al. MR imaging of choroid plexus lipomas. AJNR 1990;11:202*
4. *Jinkins JR, Whittemore AR, Bradley WG. MR imaging of callosal and corticocallosal dysgenesis. AJNR 1989;10:339*

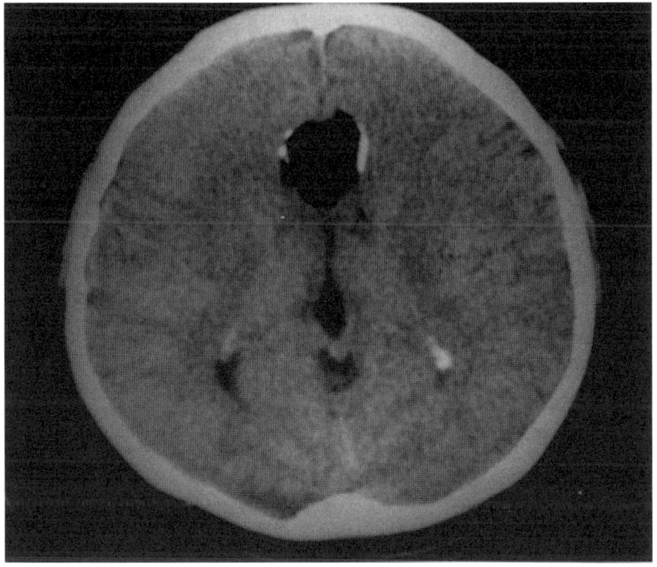

Figure 22a.

Figure 22 a-d. **Pericallosal lipomas.** Two adult cases. CT scan reveals a hypodense (fat density) midline mass with calcified rims, a lipoma (a). Sagittal, T1W MR image reveals the lipoma with high signal. This type of lipoma is referred to as tubulonodular type. A vessel with flow void is entering the lipoma (arrow). Note that, vessels usually pass through lipomas, whereas they are usually displaced by dermoids. The corpus callosum is hypoplastic, and the splenium is absent (b).

Figure 22b.

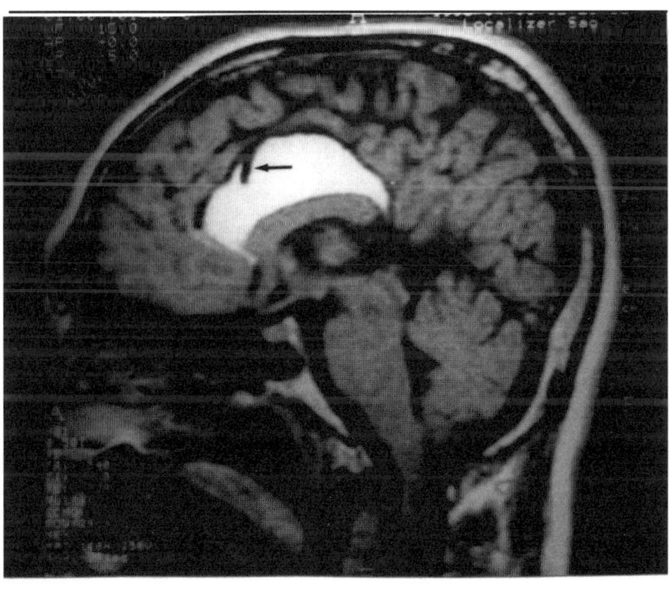

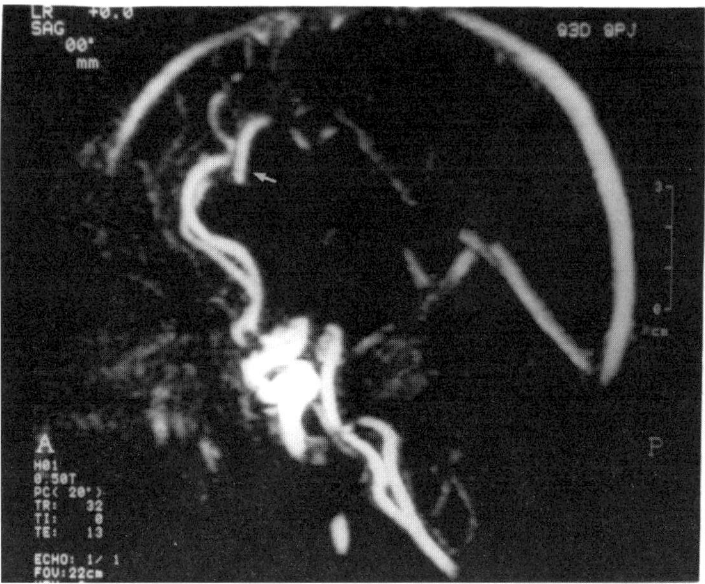

Figure 22c.

MR angiography (3D-PC) identifies the vessel entering the lipoma (arrow) (c). A curvilinear variety of pericallosal lipoma is shown belonging to another patient. Although, the corpus callosum appears to be in normal size, the splenium has been underdeveloped, as the lipoma interferes with its development (d).

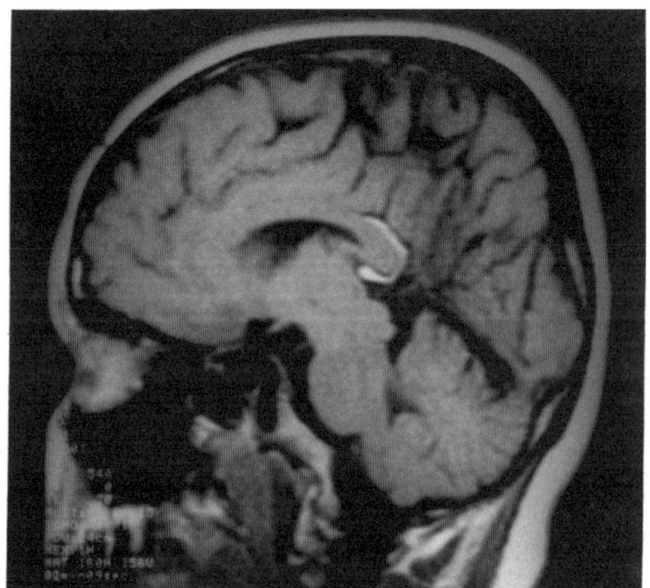

Figure 22d.

Figure 23 a-c. **Interhemispheric-pericallosal lipoma with extensions to the choroid plexuses.** 5-year-old girl. *a, b) SE T1W, and c) SE T2W MR images.* A large interhemispheric-pericallosal lipoma is seen (circles) (a-c) with extensions to the choroid plexuses (large arrows). Associated with this is the corpus callosum is very thin (callosal dysgenesis), (small arrows) (a). Also, posterior growth of the corpus callosum is interrupted by the lipoma (open arrow) (a). (case courtesy of Dr. M. deSilva, Sydney)

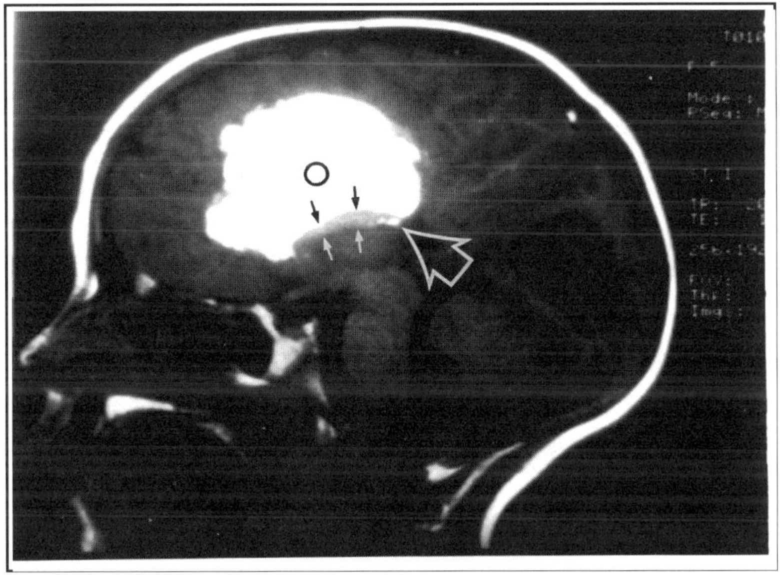

Figure 23a.

References
1.　*Tart RP, Quisling RG. Curvilinear and tubulondular varieties of lipoma of corpus callosum: an MR and CT study. J Comput Assist Tomogr 1991;15:805*
2.　*Truwit CL, Barkovich AJ. Pathogenesis of intracranial lipoma: an MR study in 42 patients. AJNR 1990;11:665*
3.　*Truwit CL, Williams G, Armstrong EA, et al. MR imaging of choroid plexus lipomas. AJNR 1990;11:202*

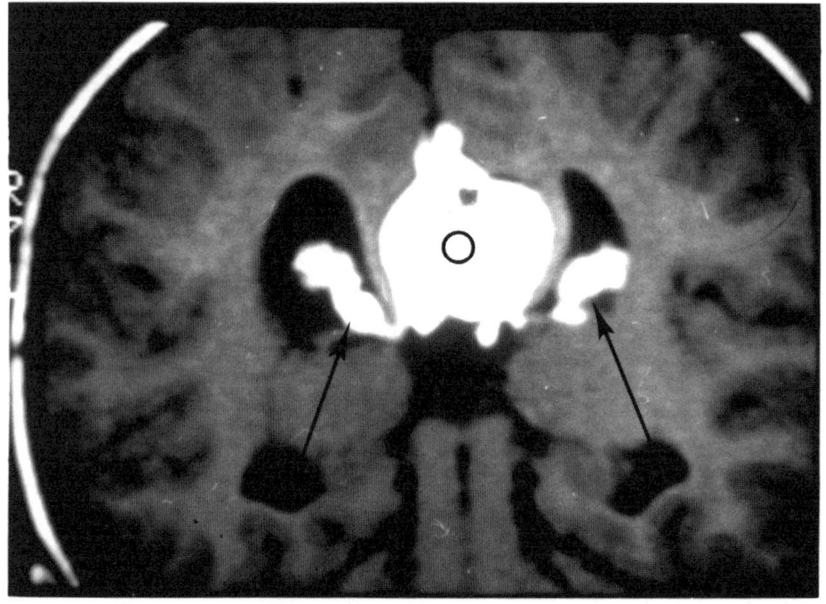

Figure 23b.

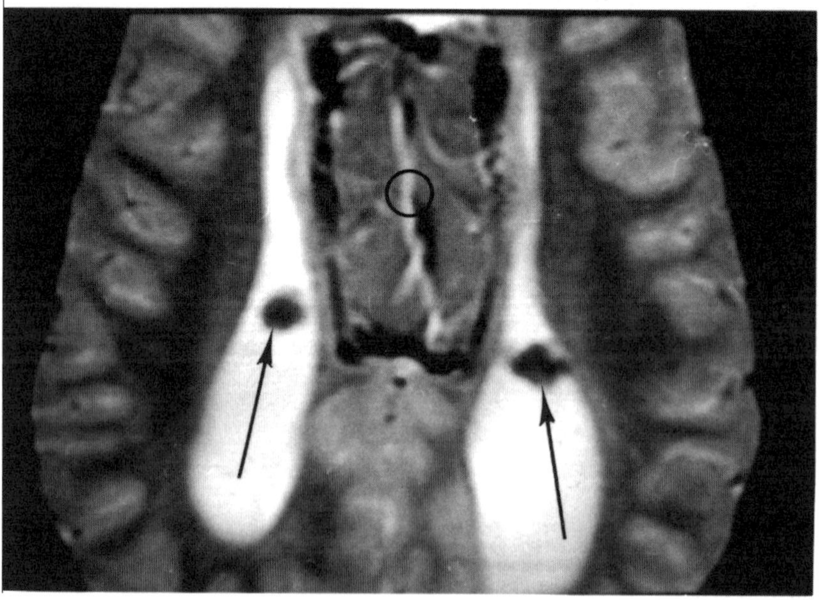

Figure 23c.

Figure 24 a-d. **Pericallosal lipoma on diffusion imaging.** 13-year-old boy. a) FLAIR image, and b-d) echo-planar diffusion images. FLAIR image shows a pericallosal lipoma, causing agenesis of the posterior parts of the corpus callosum (a). b=50T sec/mm^2 (T2-weighted) image has a mean pixel value of 39 (b). b=1000T sec/mm^2 (true diffusion) image has a mean pixel value of 1 (c). (T is trace). The ADC value of this lipoma calculated by Stejskal-Tanner equation: ADC=-(1/b) ln (S/So), is 1.09 x10^{-3} mm2/sec, and is slightly higher than that of normal white matter. (Multiple ADC measurements in this lipoma revealed values ranging from 0.85 to 1.09 X10^{-3} mm^2/sec, most being similar to that of normal white matter).

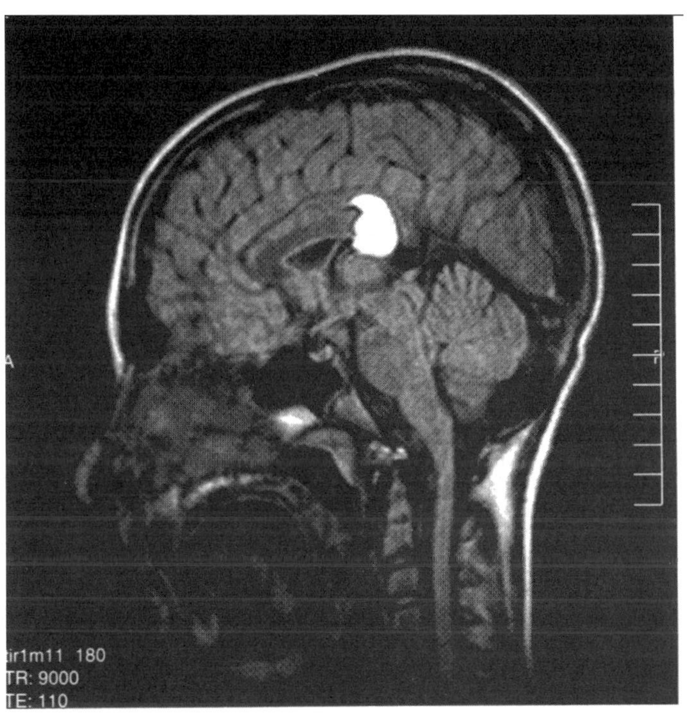

Figure 24a.

Figure 24b.

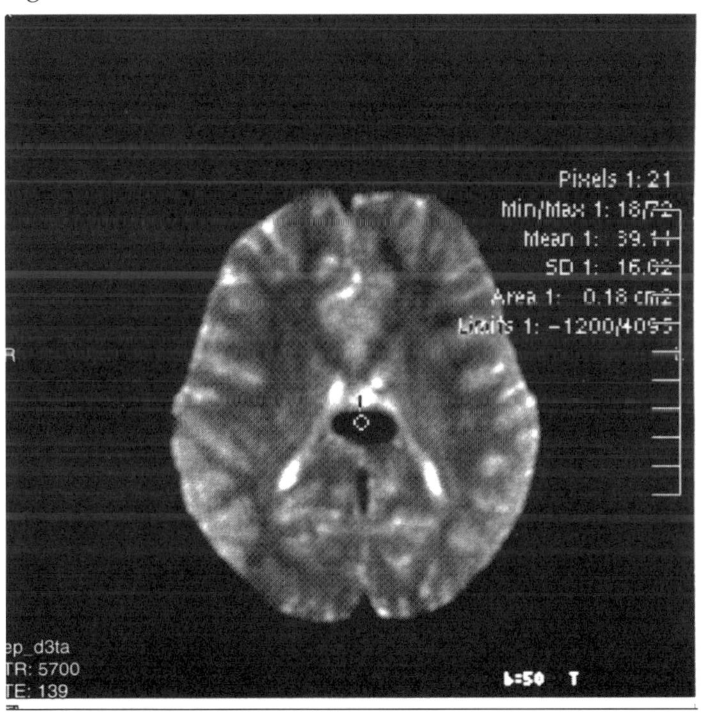

ADC map reveals a value of "zero", which apparently is a misregistration artifact due to chemical-shift effects (d). Therefore the diffusion coefficient of a lipoma is similar to normal brain parenchyma.

Reference
1. *Sener RN. Diffusion MRI: apparent diffusion coefficient (ADC) values in the normal brain, and a classification of brain disorders based on ADC values. Comput Med Imaging Graph 2001; 25:299*

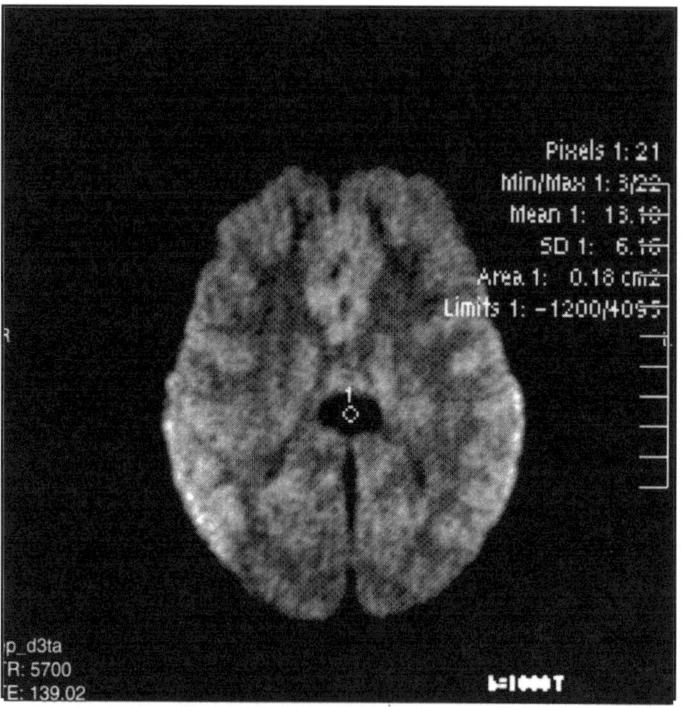

Figure 24c.

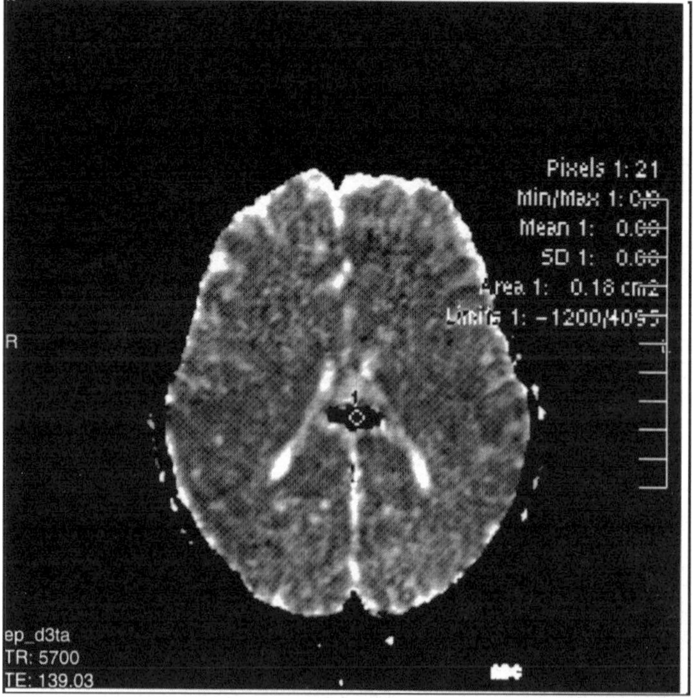

Figure 24d.

Figure 25 a, b **Small lipomatous structure at the tip of the splenium.** 10-month-old girl. *a) SE T1W MR image, and b) water saturation image from a fat-water MR imaging sequence.* A small bright structure is evident at the splenial tip on the SE T1W image (arrow) (a), which is also bright on the water saturation image (arrow) (b). Presence of a bright structure on the water saturation image is considered characteristic for a lipoma. Although this small lipoma does not seem to have interfered with the normal posterior growth of the corpus callosum, there is diffuse thinning of the organ which was associated with moderate cerebral atrophy.

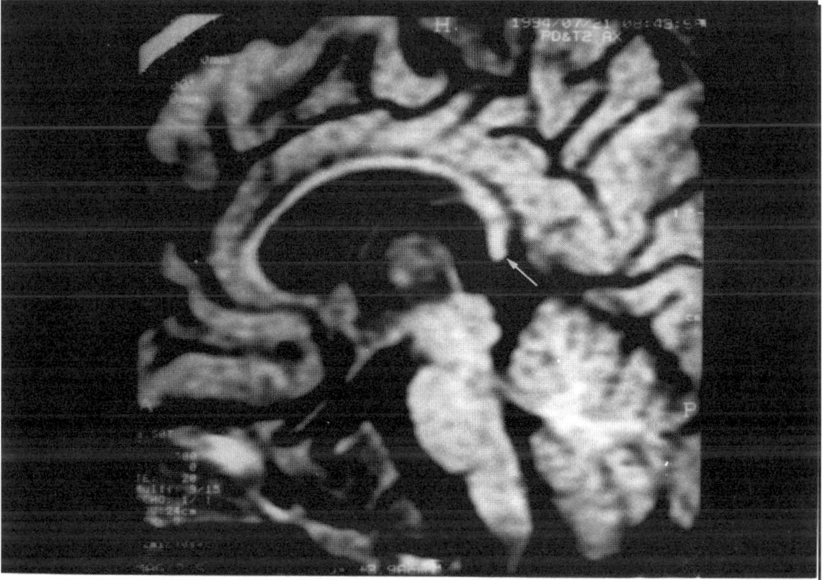

Figure 25a.

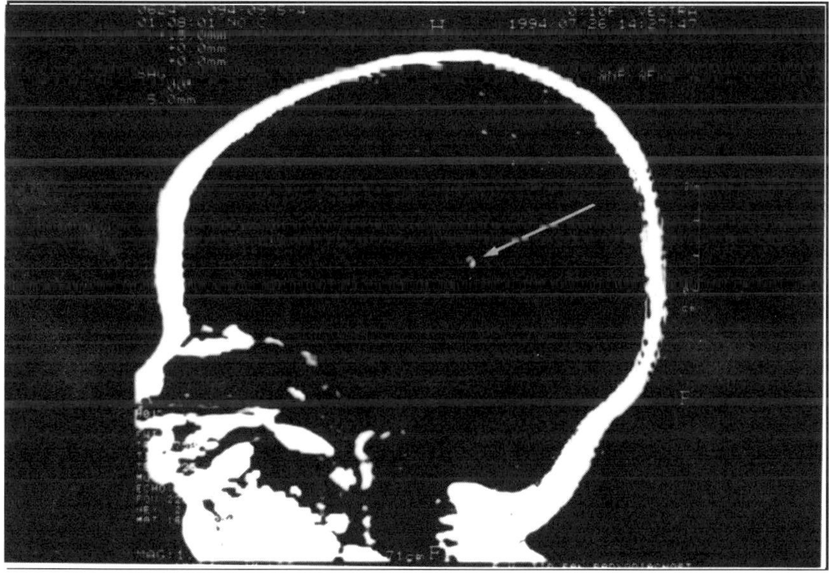

Figure 25b.

Figure 26 a, b. **Callosal dysgenesis associated with an interhemispheric cyst.** 1-year-old boy. *a) SE T1W, and b) IR T1W MR images.* The callosal body shows gradual thinning towards the caudal direction (arrow) (a), and the splenium has not developed (callosal dysgenesis). There is a large interhemispheric cyst (asterisk) (b).

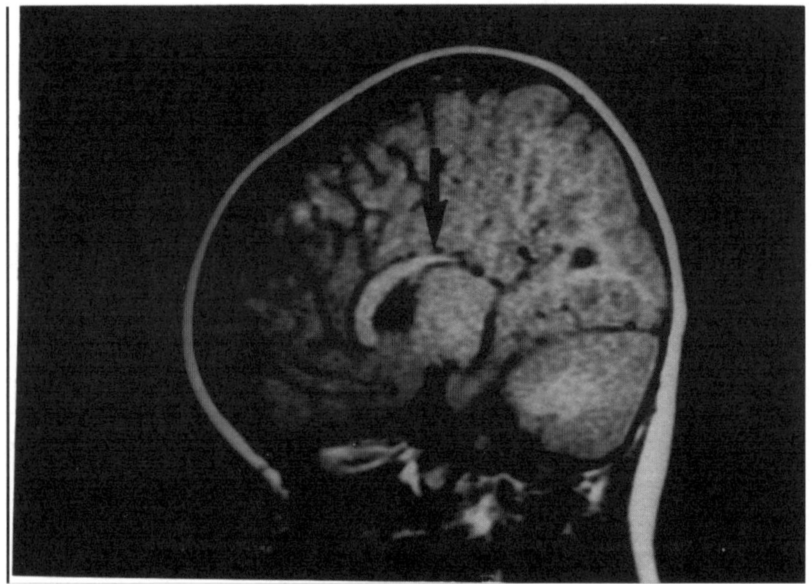

Figure 26a.

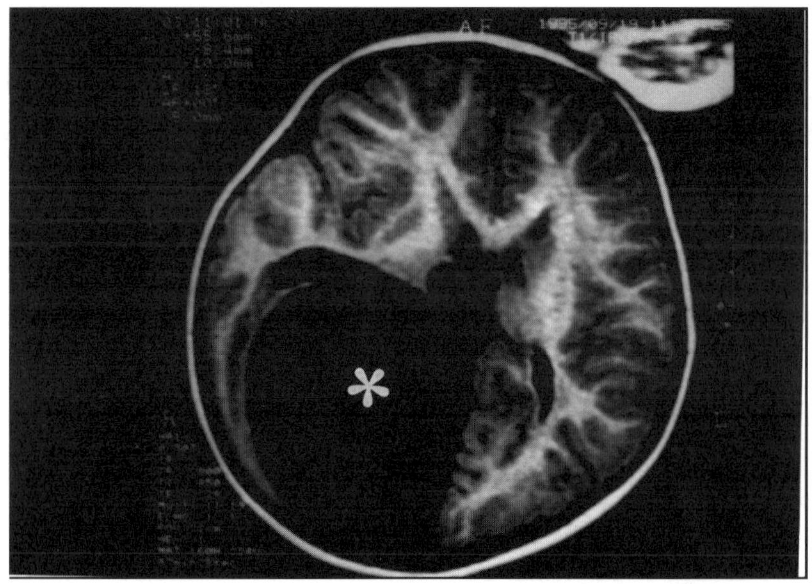

Figure 26b.

References
1. Barkovich AJ, Norman D. Anomalies of the corpus callosum: correlation with further anomalies of the brain. AJNR 1988;9:493
2. Gille M, Jacquemin C, Bachy N, et al. Agenesis of the corpus callsoum, heterotopia of the gray cortex and interhemispheric cyst. Late radiologic diagnosis in an asymptomatic adult. Rev Neurol (Paris) 1994;150:161
3. Inagaki H, Kurosaki M, Hori T, et al. Interhemispheric choroidal epithelial cyst associated with partial agenesis of the corpus callosum: case report and review of the literature. No Shinkei Geka 1992;20:1301
4. Munemoto S, Ishiguro S, Kimura A, et al. Interhemispheric cyst of an adult associated with partial agenesis of the corpus callosum. Rinsho Hoshasen 1990;35:959

Figure 27 a-c. **Interhemispheric cyst (Intrauterine MRI).** 18-week-old fetus. Images with the HASTE (half-fourier single-shot turbo spin eko) sequence reveal a large posterior interhemispheric cyst (a,b). The anterior part of the corpus callosum appears to be intact (a). There is hypoplasia of the cerebellum (c).

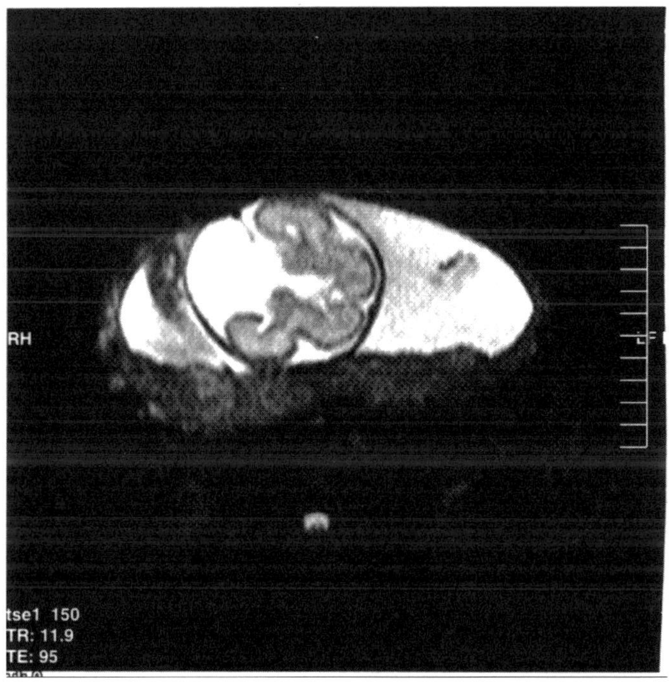

Figure 27a.

Reference
1. Vimercati A, Greco P, Vera L, et al. The diagnostic role of ëin uteroí magnetic resonance imaging. J Perinat Med 1999; 27:303

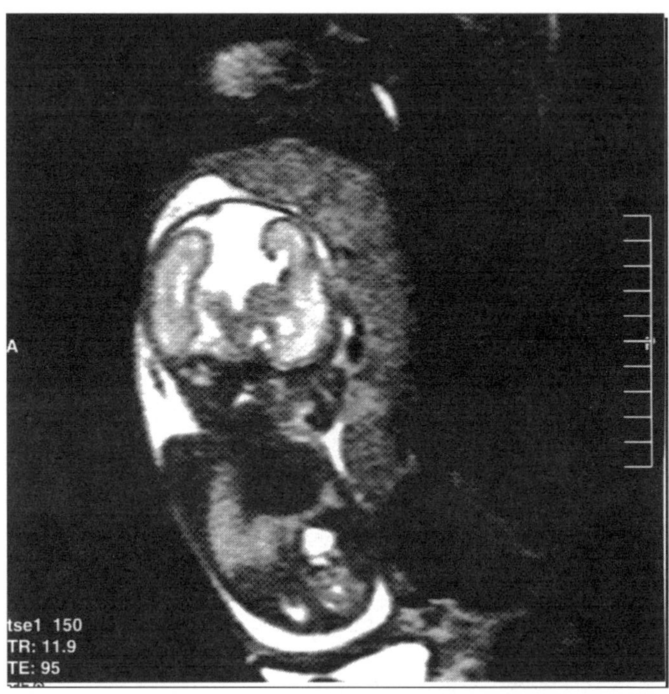

Figure 27b.

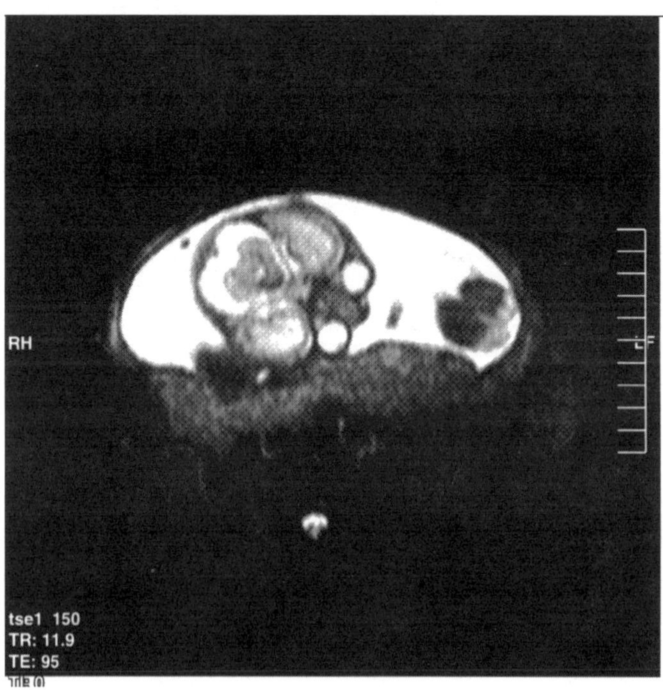

Figure 27c.

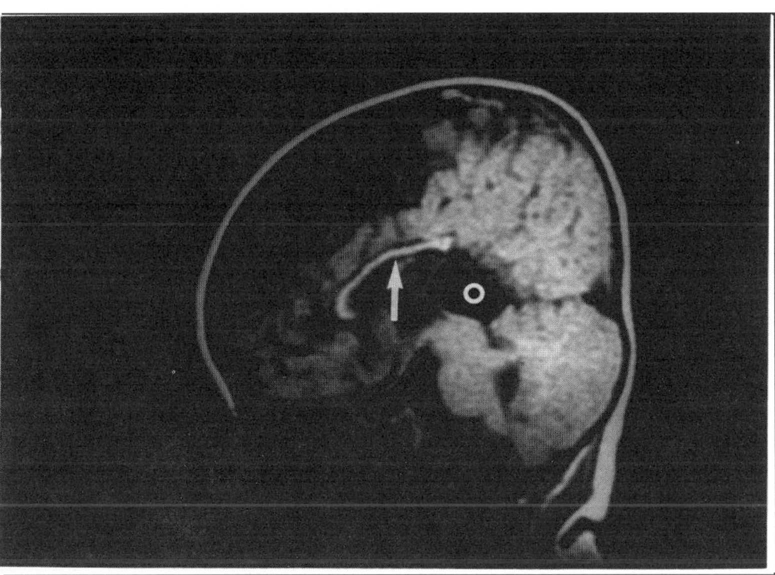

Figure 28a.

Figure 28 a, b. **Callosal dysgenesis associated with Joubert's syndrome.** 9-month-old girl with developmental delay, and with nystagmus and episodes of dyspnea during the neonatal period. *a) SE T1W, and b) IR T1W MR images.* The corpus callosum is diffusely thin (arrow)(a). There is a superior cerebellar cyst in the quadrigeminal cistern (circle) (a) without a compession effect upon the aqueduct. (No sign of hydrocephalus was evident in additional views). A pineal cyst was excluded on additional views. Note a bat-wing appearance of the fourth ventricle, and a characteristic cleft (arrow), lined with heterotopic gray matter, which disconnects the cerebellar hemispheres, representing the typical radiological features for Joubert's syndrome (b). Also not a dysplastic folial pattern of the cerebellar hemispheres (b). The temporal horns of the lateral ventricles appear to be enlarged due to incomplete inversion of the hippocampal formations, but not to hydrocephalus (b).

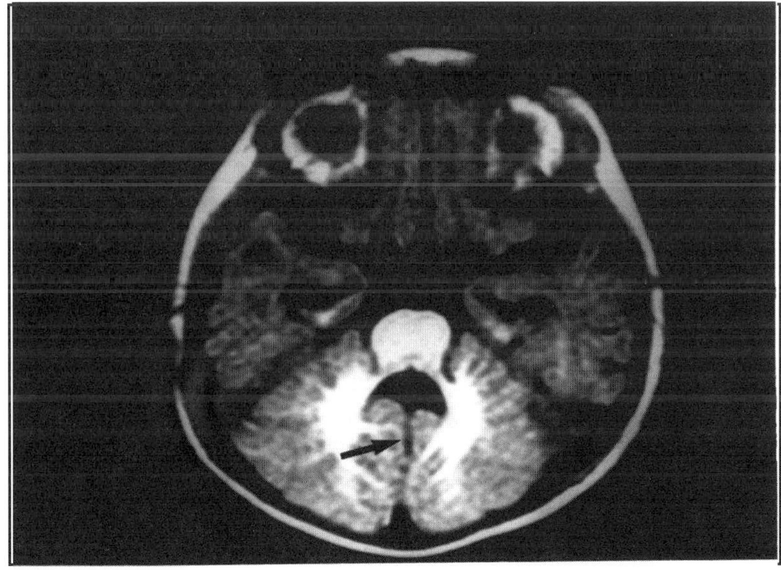

Figure 28b.

Figure 29. **Callosal dysgenesis associated with Joubert's syndrome.** 7-year-old girl with psychomotor retardation and a clinical history of Joubert's syndrome during the neonatal period. Sibling affected? *SE T1W MR image*. Note callosal dysgenesis manifesting as agenesis of the spenium (arrow). Vermian hypoplasia is evident (curved arrow). Callosal dysgenesis is not common in Joubert's syndrome.

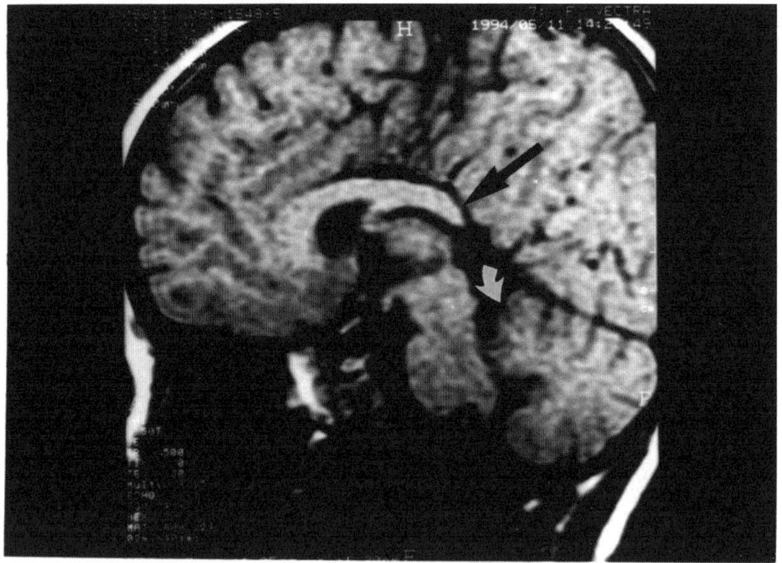

Figure 29.

References
1.   Kendall B, Kingsley D, Lambert SR, et al. Joubert syndrome: a clinico-radiological study. Neuroradiology 1990;31:502-506
2.   Shen W-C, Shian W-J, Chen C-C, et al. MRI of Joubert's syndrome. Eur J Radiol 1994; 18:30

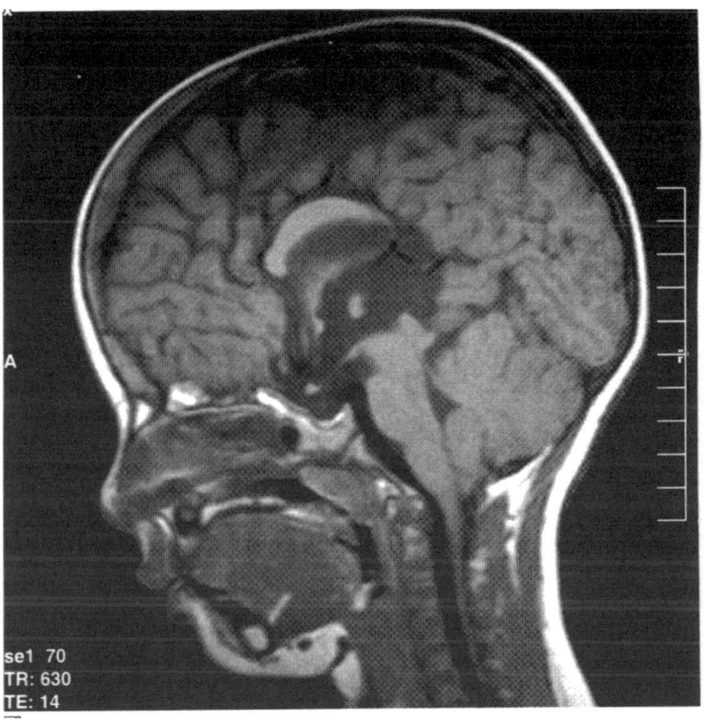

Figure 30a.

Figure 30 a-g. **Callosal dysgenesis associated with rhombencephalosynapsis.** 4-year-old girl. Sagittal, T1W MR image reveals a hypoplastic corpus callosum. Although there is an impression of slight tectal beaking, the posterior fossa has a normal size without tonsillar herniation. There was no lumbar meningomyelocele, excluding Chiari II malformation. Also, note a very thin hypophysis gland (a). T1W (turbo inversion recovery) image reveals abnormal formation of the isthmi of the parahippocampal gyri, and resultant remodeling of the atria of the lateral ventricles (b).

Figure 30b.

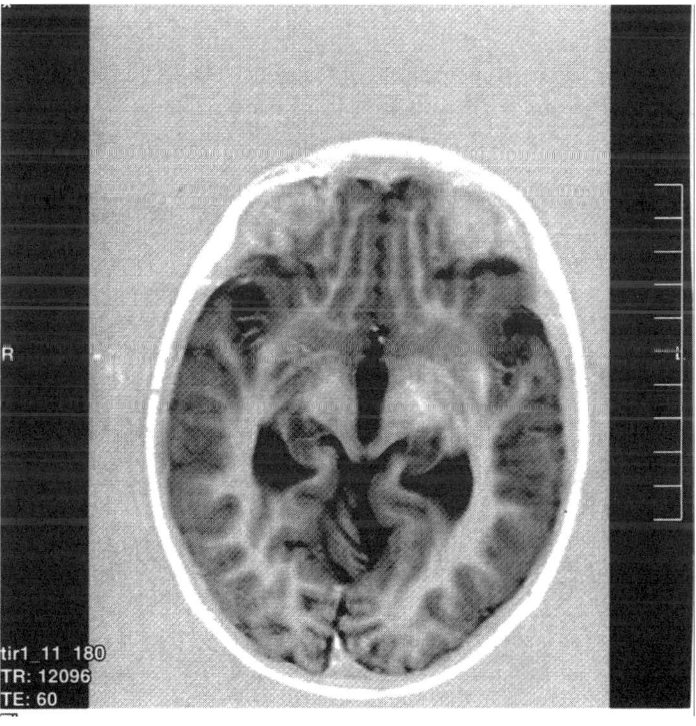

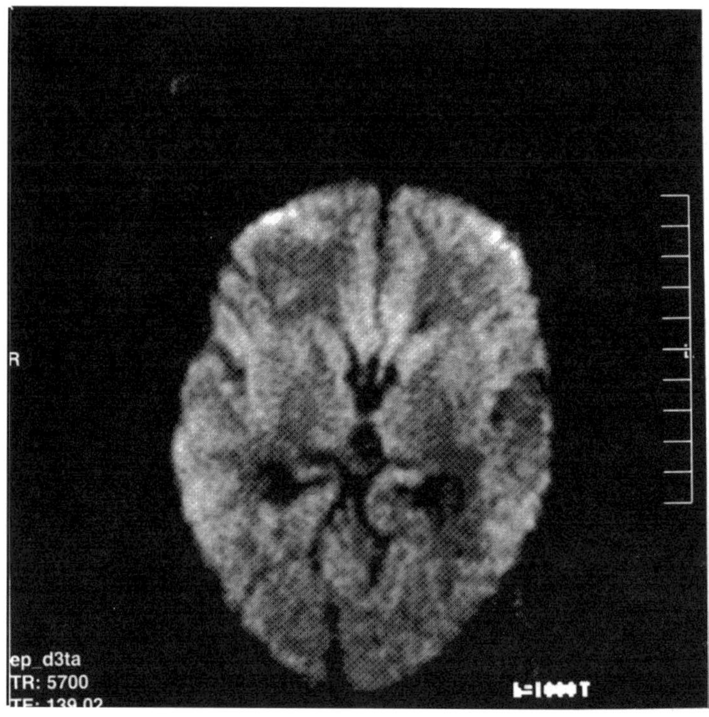

Figure 30c.

True diffusion (b=1000T sec/mm^2) image shows the changes without any signal abnormality (c). T1W (turbo inversion recovery) images reveal vermian aplasia, and fusion of the cerebellar hemispheres (d,e).

Figure 30d.

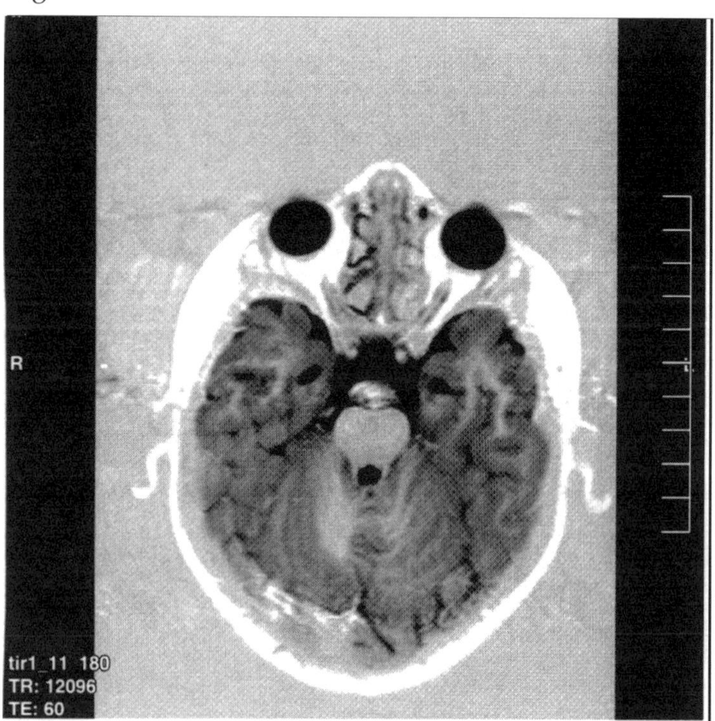

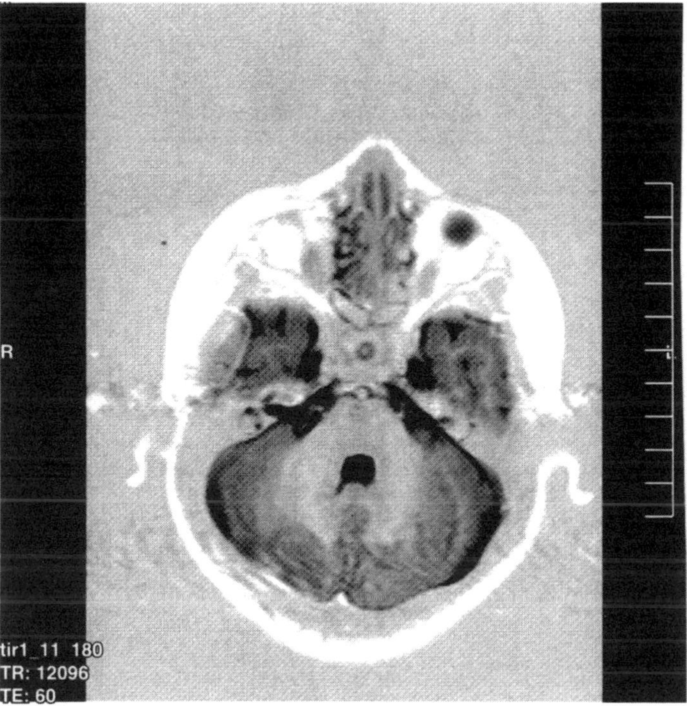

Figure 30e.

Figure 30f.

Vermian aplasia results in a keyhole shaped 4th ventricle (e). The folial pattern of the cerebellar hemispheres appear dysplastic (d-f), and abnormal gray matter nodules are evident in the vicinity of the lower part of the 4th ventricle (f).

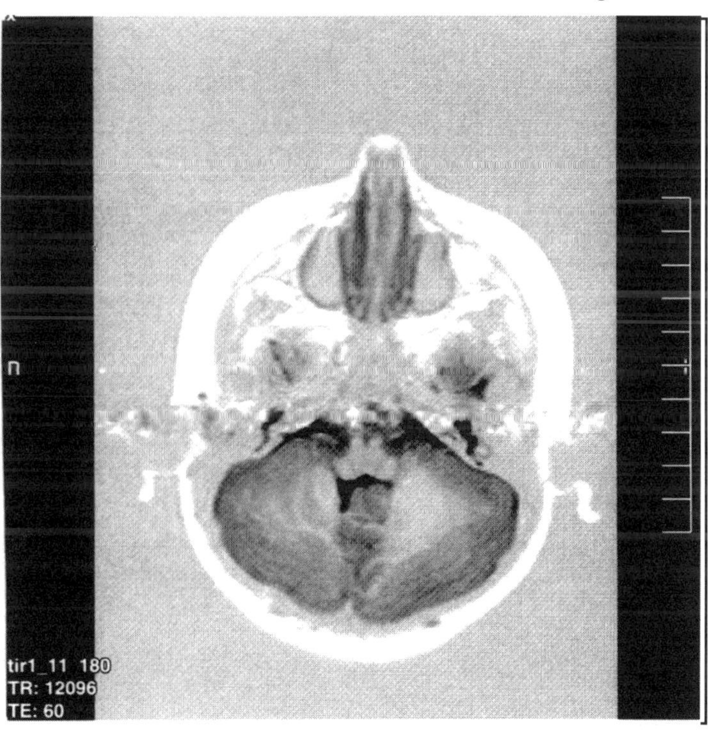

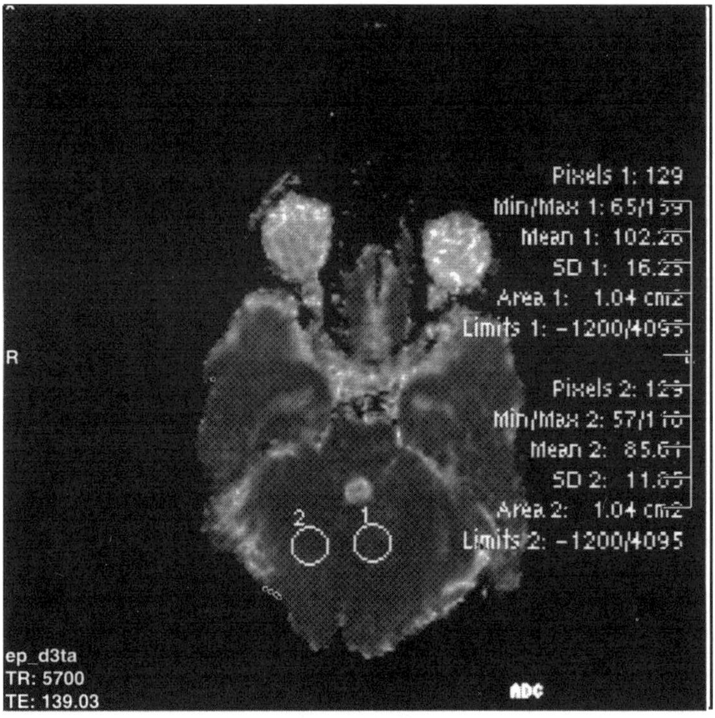

Figure 30g.

ADC map reveals normal cerebellar parenchymal values: 1.02, and 0.85 $X10^{-3}$ mm^2/sec (g).

References
1. *Barkovich AJ. Pediatric neuroimaging. Philadelphia, Lippincott Williams & Wilkins, 2000*
2. *Sener RN. Unusual MRI findings in rhombencephalosynapsis. Comput Med Imaging Graph. 2000; 24:277*

Figure 31 a, b. **Callosal dysgenesis associated with Vein of Galen malformation.** 3-year-old boy. *a) and b) SE T1-weighted MR images.* A dilated Vein of Galen is seen (asterisk). The rostrum and genu (arrow) (a), and the proximal body of the corpus callosum have been formed; however, the caudal part is absent (callosal dysgenesis). Additional MR images, and conventional angiographic studies revealed agenesis of the inferior sagittal sinus, and the pericallosal artery. Callosal dysgenesis is unusual in Vein of Galen malformation (from reference 3).

References
1. *Seidenwurm D, Berenstein A, Hyman A, Kowalski H. Vein of Galen malformation: correlation of clinical presentation, arteriography, and MR imaging. AJNR 1991;12:347*
2. *Quisling RG, Mickle JP. Venous pressure measurements in Vein of Galen aneurysms. AJNR 1989;10:411*
3. *Sener RN. Vein of Galen malformation associated with callosal dysgenesis. IMIR (The International Medical Image Registry) 1995;1:87*

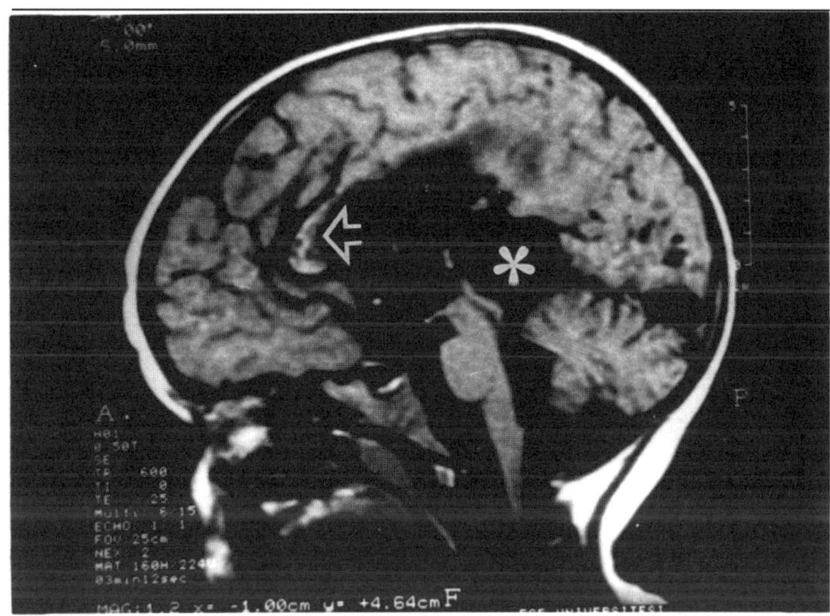

Figure 31a.

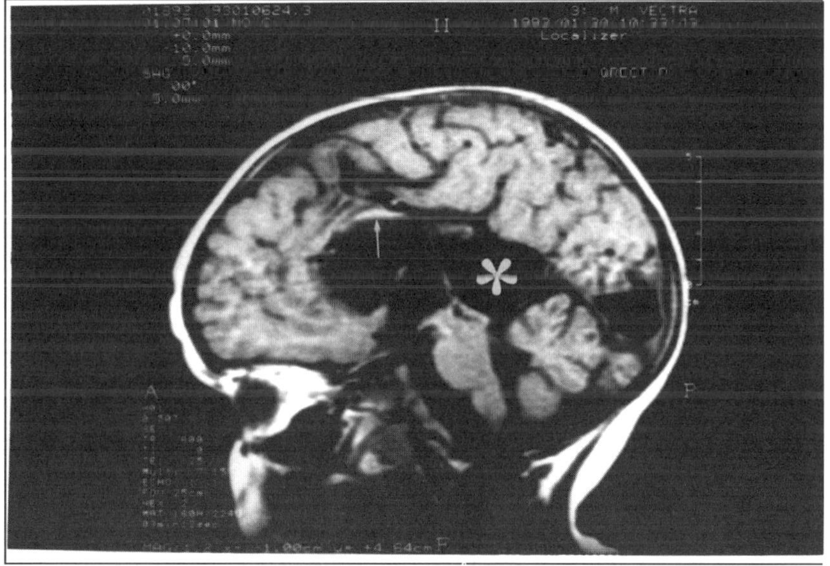

Figure 31b.

Figure 32 a-c. **Atypical callosal dysgenesis in mild, lobar holoprosencephaly**. 6-month-old boy. *a, b and c) SE T1W MR images.* Sagittal image shows the body and the splenium of the corpus callosum have apparently been formed, although thinned (arrows) (a). Coronal image shows the thin body (arrows) (b). Coronal image (anterior to b) shows interhemispheric fusion of the basal frontal lobes (arrow), (c), which is a characteristic feature for holoprosencephaly. This type of callosal dysgenesis (absent rostral parts) is in contrast to the current theories on normal callosal development (from reference 1).

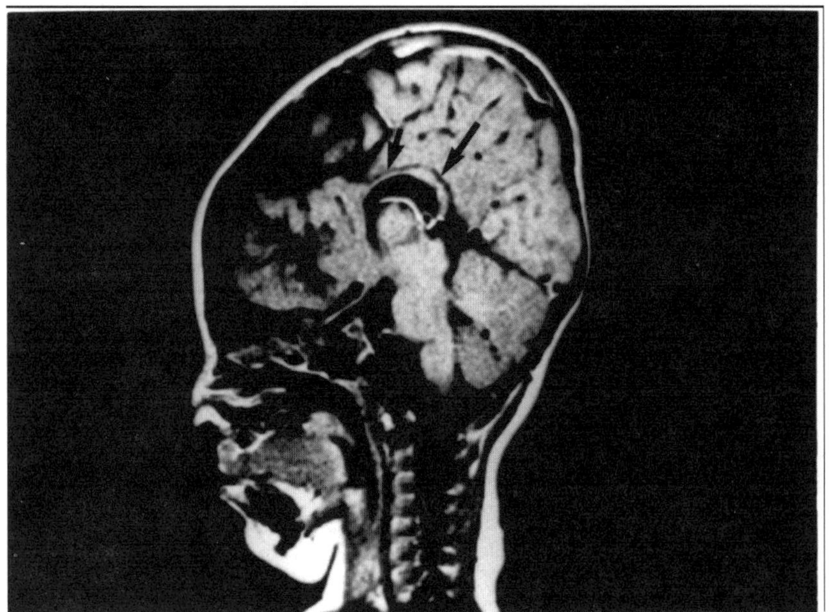

References
1. Sener RN. Anterior callosal agenesis in mild, lobar holoprosencephaly. Pediatr Radiol 1995;25:385
2.. Schaefer GB, Shuman RM, Wilson DA, et al. Partial agenesis of the anterior corpus callosum: correlation between appearance, imaging, and neuropathology. Pediatr Neurol 1991;7:39

Figure 32a.

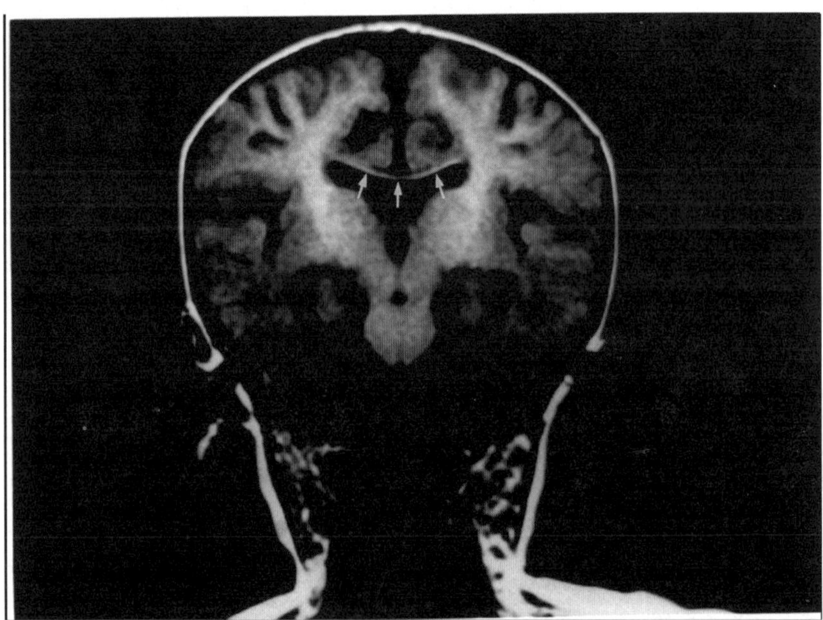

Figure 32b.

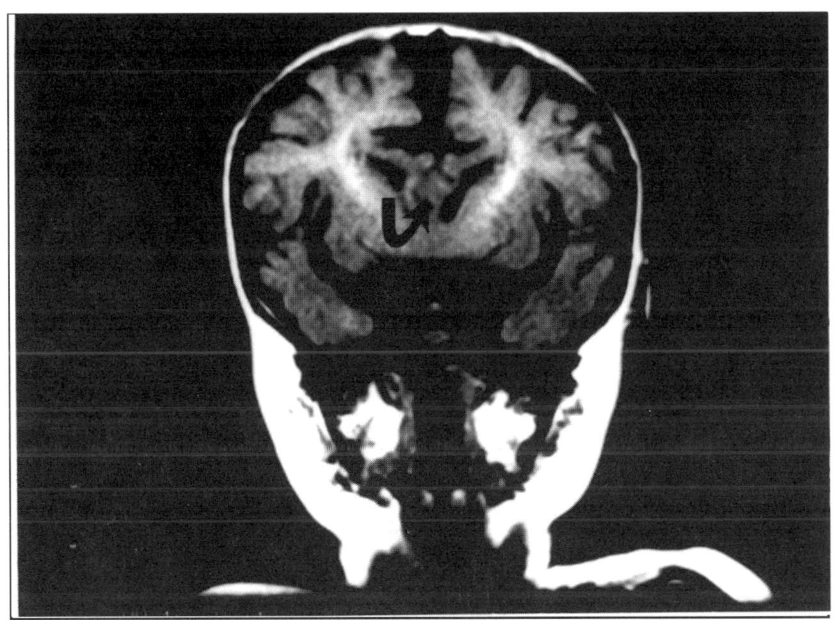

Figure 32c.

Figure 33 a, b. **Atypical callosal dysgenesis in mild, lobar holoprosencephaly.** 3-year-old girl. *a) SE T1W, and b) SE T2W MR images.* The rostral (rostrum and genu), and the caudal (splenium) parts of the corpus callosum are present (arrows) (a); however, the entire body is absent due to interhemispheric fusion (holoprosencephaly). T2W image through the centrum semiovale shows fusion of the white matter (arrows) (b). Additional views revealed several changes consistent with neuronal migrational anomalies. (case courtesy of Dr. M. deSilva, Sydney).

References
1. *Barkovich AJ. Pediatric neuroimaging. New York, Raven Press, 1995;226*
2. *Barkovich AJ, Quint DJ. Midline interhemispheric fusion: an unusual variant of holoprosencephaply. AJNR 1993;14:431*

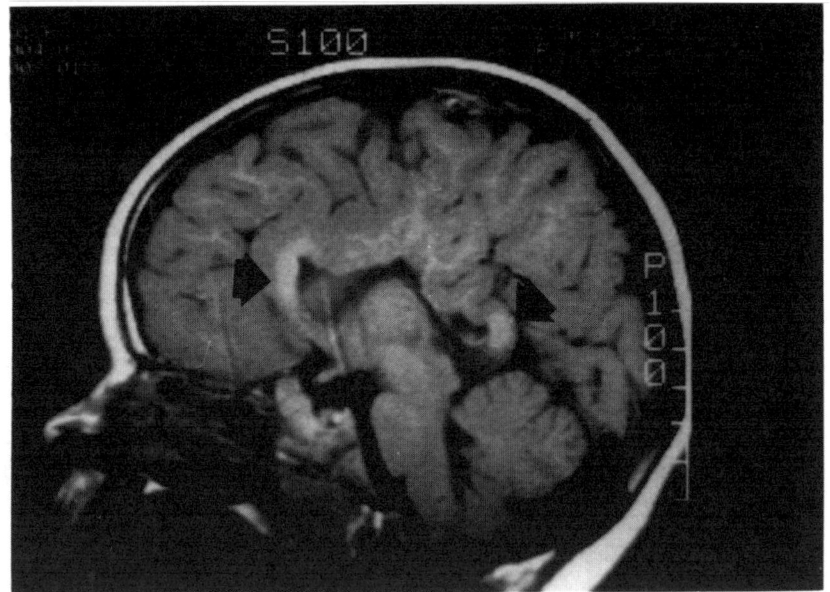

Figure 33a.

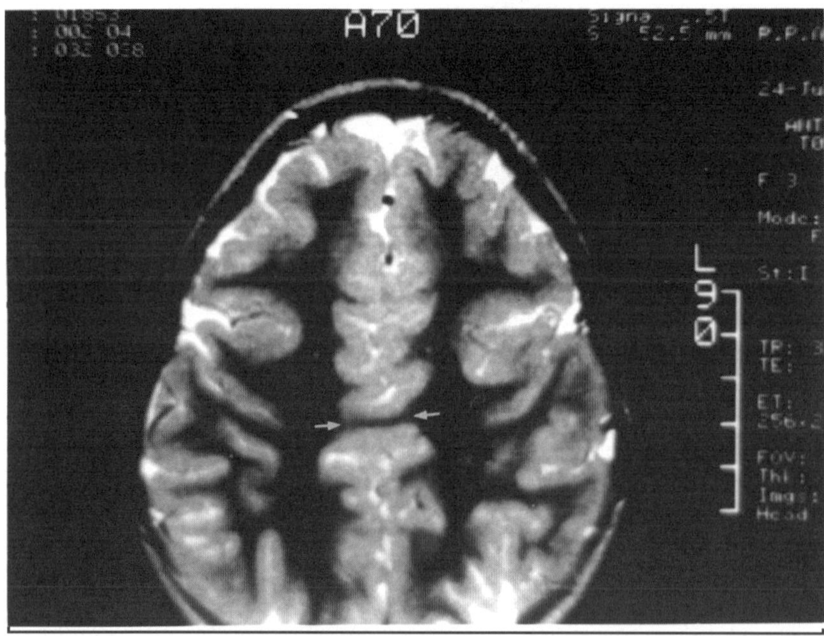

Figure 33b.

Figure 34 a-d. **Thin corpus callosum in lobar holoprosencephaly.** 17-year-old girl. *a, b and c) SE T1W MR images, and d) surface reconstruction image of the face out of the MRI study.* A very thin corpus callosum is identified (arrows) (a, b). A characteristic interhemispheric fusion for holoprosencephaly, distinct from the thin corpus callosum, is noted across the basal frontal lobes (arrow) (c). There is a facial cleft (d), a common feature seen in relatively severe forms of holoprosencephalies. There is a large lipoma (L) in the superior cerebellar region (a). Although the appearance of the lipoma suggests a compression effect upon the aqueduct, clinically no signs and symptoms of increased intracranial pressure was noted, excluding hydrocephalus. Relatively normal-sized temporal horns support this (b). The appearance of the lateral ventricles (monoventricle), and inferior pointing of the frontal horns further support the existence of an anomalous brain rather than hydrocephalus.

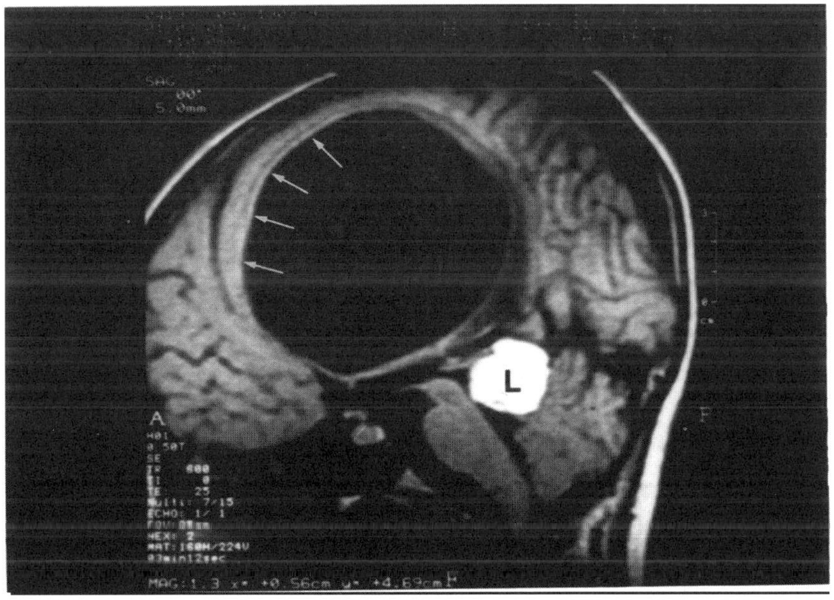

Figure 34a.

References
1. Barkovich AJ, Quint DJ. Midline interhemispheric fusion: an unusual variant of holoprosencephaly. AJNR 1993; 14:431
2. Barkovich AJ. Apparent atypical callosal dysgenesis: analysis of MR findings in six cases and their relationship to holoprosencephaly. AJNR 1990;11:333
3. Filz CR. Holoprosencephaly and related entities. Neuroradiology 1983;25:225

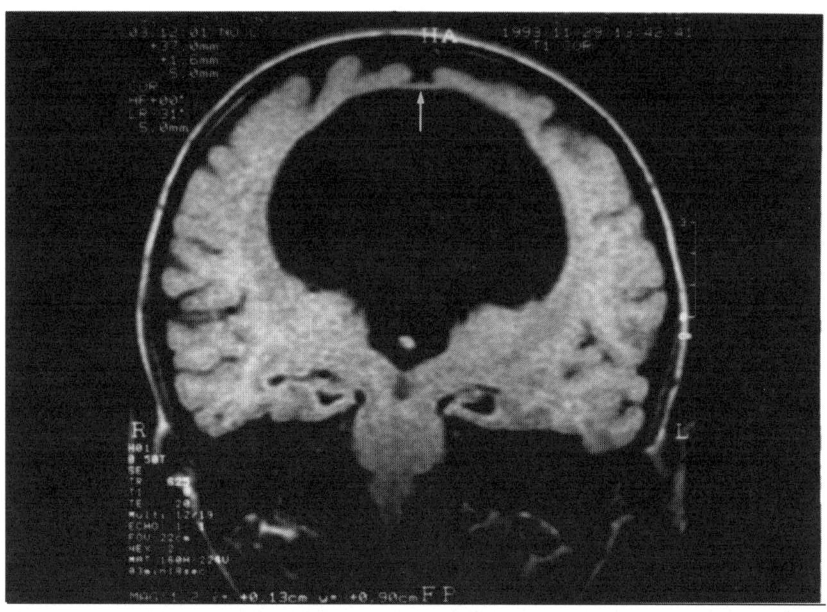

Figure 34b.

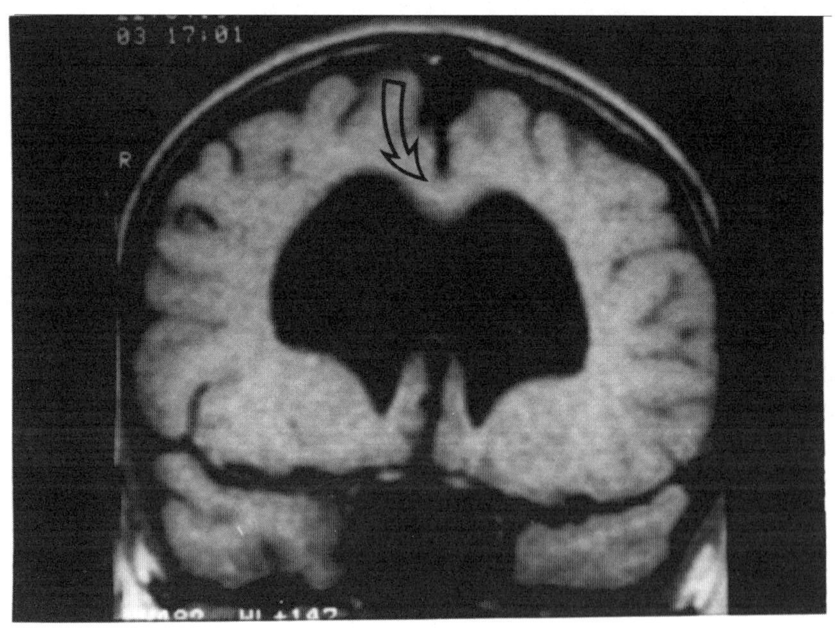

Figure 34c.

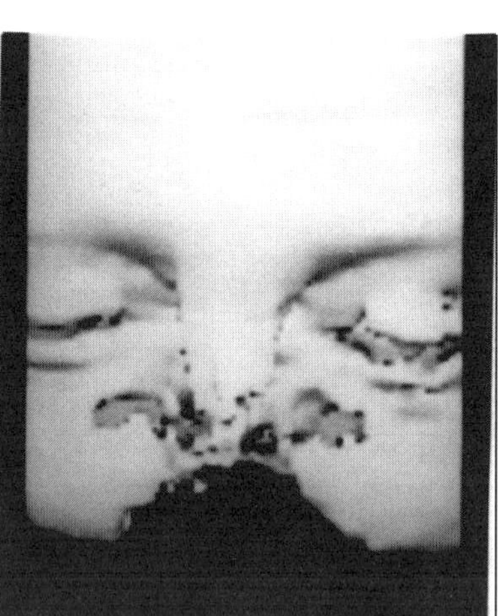

Figure 34d.

Figure 35 a-e. **Atypical callosal dysgenesis in rhombencephalosynapsis.** 1-year-old girl. *a) SE T1W; b and e) IR T1W MR images; c and d) CT scans.* Only the splenium of the corpus callosum is seen (arrow) (a). Absence of the anterior parts of the corpus callosum is confirmed by the axial MR image, which shows direct connection of the anterior parts of the corpus callosum is confirmed by the axial MR image, which shows direct connection of the anterior interhemispheric fissure with the lateral ventricles (arrow) (b). CT scan shows small calcifications at this region (arrow) (c). Periventricular calcifications are noted (d), which was a consequence of a proven cytomegalovirus infection (CMV) the patient had. The dilatation pattern of the third and lateral ventricles suggest hydrocephalus. The dentate nuclei of the cerebellar hemispheres are fused (open arrow), and the fourth ventricle looks like a keyhole (arrow) (e), which are characteristic findings for rhombencephalosynapsis. This patient had signs and symptoms of increased intracranial pressure, and an intraventricular shunt tube was placed with remarkable improvement of hydrocephalus. Coexistence of rhombencephalosynapsis and congenital CMV infection in this patient is unique, and arises the question if the CMV infection might have played a role in the development of rhombencephalosynapsis.

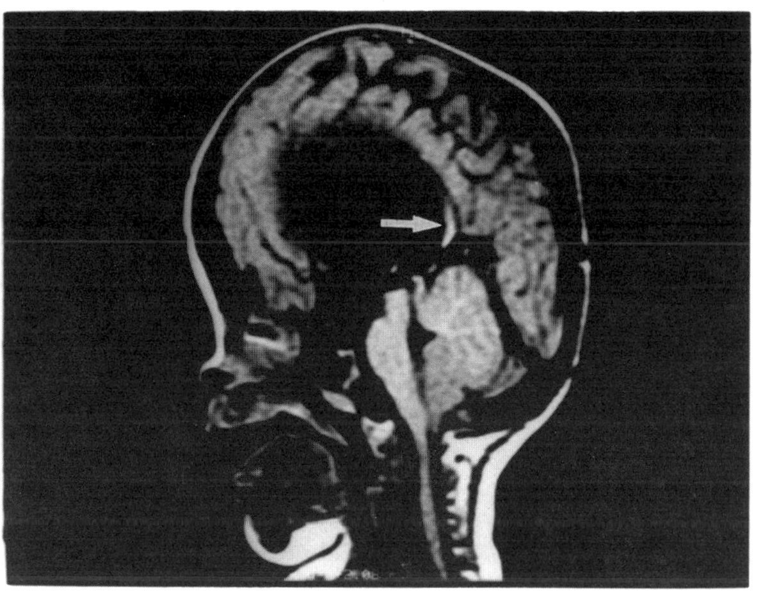

Figure 35a.

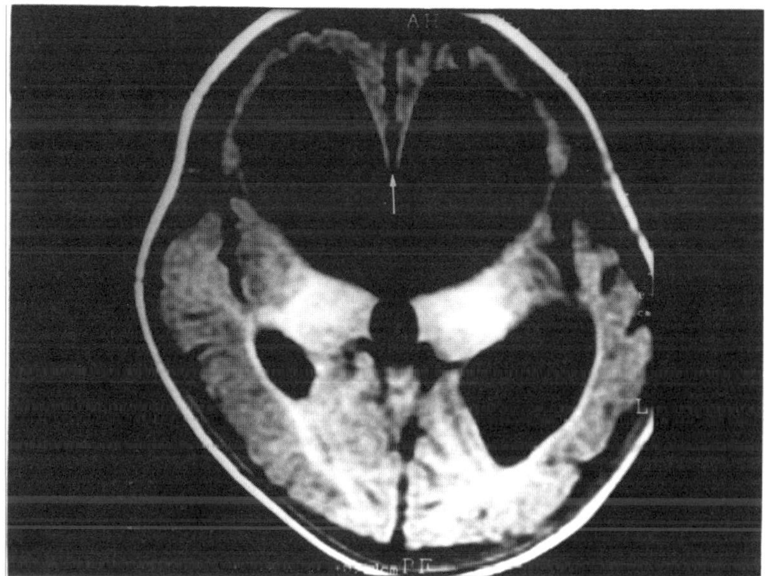

Figure 35b.

References
1. *Simmons G, Damiano TR, Truwit CL. MRI and clinical findings in rhombencephalosynapsis. J Comput Assist Tomogr 1993; 14:211*
2. *Altman NR, Naidich TP, Braffman BH. Posterior fossa malformations. AJNR 1992;13:691*
3. *Minamitani M, Tanaka J, Hasamura M, et al. Cerebral malformations associated with probable intrauterine infection. No To Hattatsu 1993;25:359*

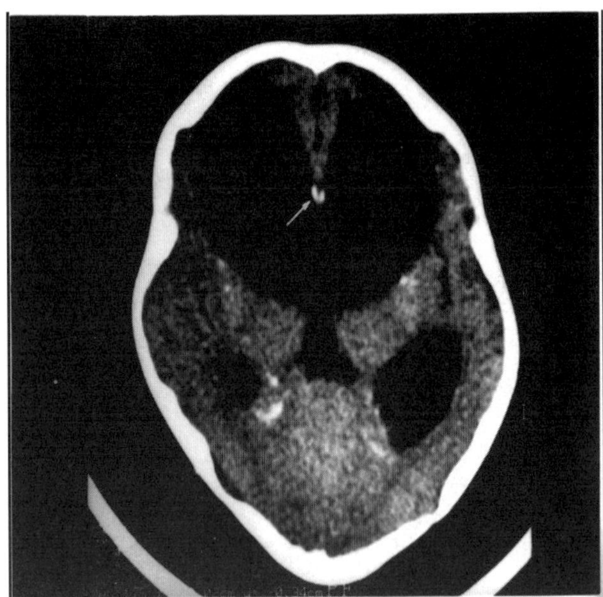

Figure 35c.

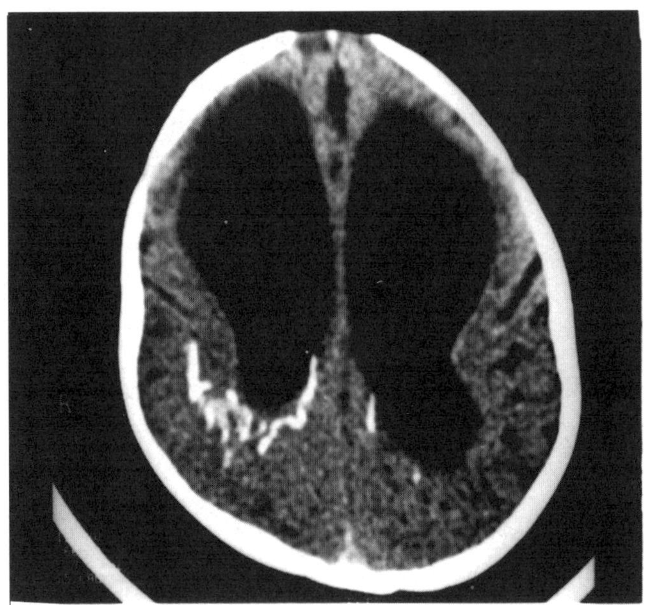

Figure 35d.

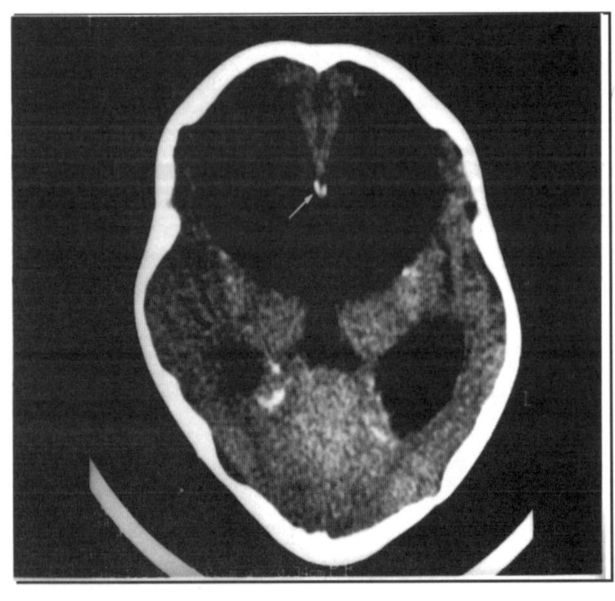

Figure 35e.

Figure 36 a, b. **Callosal dysgenesis in whistling face syndrome (cranio-carpo-tarsal dysplasia or Freeman-Sheldon syndrome).** 7-month-old-girl. *a) SE T1W MR image, and b) surface reconstruction image of the face out of the MRI study.* Gradual thinning of the callosal body and an hypoplastic splenium is noted (callosal dysgenesis), (arrow) (a). The reconstruction image adequately displays the characteristic facies in the whistling face syndrome (b). Note inferior vermian agenesis. Cerebral cortical dysplasia and an abnormal white matter was also noted in this patient (from reference 4)

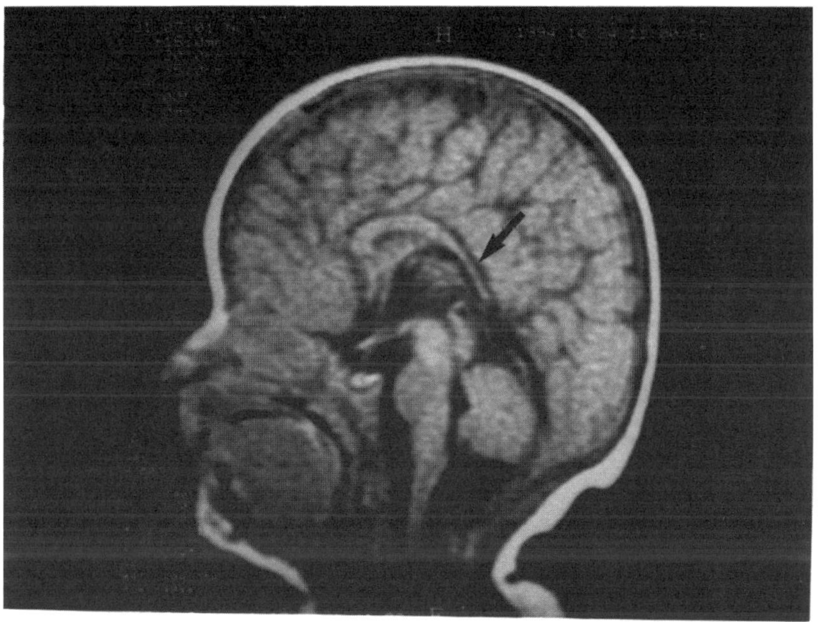

References

1.   *Tamraz JC, Rethore MO, Iba-Zizen MT, et al. Contribution of magnetic resonance imaging to the knowledge of CNS malformations related to chromosomal aberrations. I lum Genet 1987;76:265*

2.   *O'Connel DJ, Hall CM. Cranio-carpo-tarsal dysplasia. A report of seven cases. Radiology 1977; 123:719*

3.   *Parisi G, Molino O, Squadrone NP, et al. Freeman-Sheldon syndrome. Case contribution and review of the literature. Minerva Pediatr 1991;43:653*

4.   *Sener RN. Whistling face syndrome: MR imaging findings in the brain. Eur Radiol 1996;6:102*

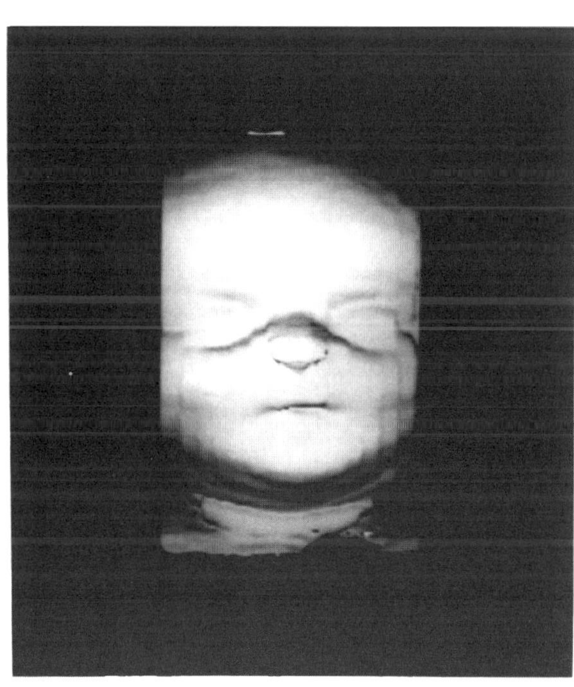

Figure 36b.

Figure 37 a, b. **Callosal dysgenesis in frontal encephalocele.** 5-month-old girl. *a) surface reconstruction image of the face out of an MRI study, and b) SE T1W MR image.* A large frontal encephalocele is displayed in the surface reconstruction image (a). Sagittal MR image shows a very thin corpus callosum (arrows), a large porencephalic cavity and the frontal encephalocele (b).

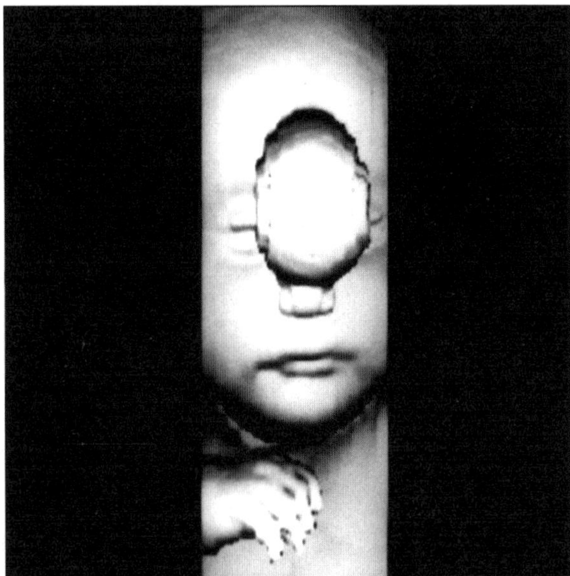

Figure 37a.

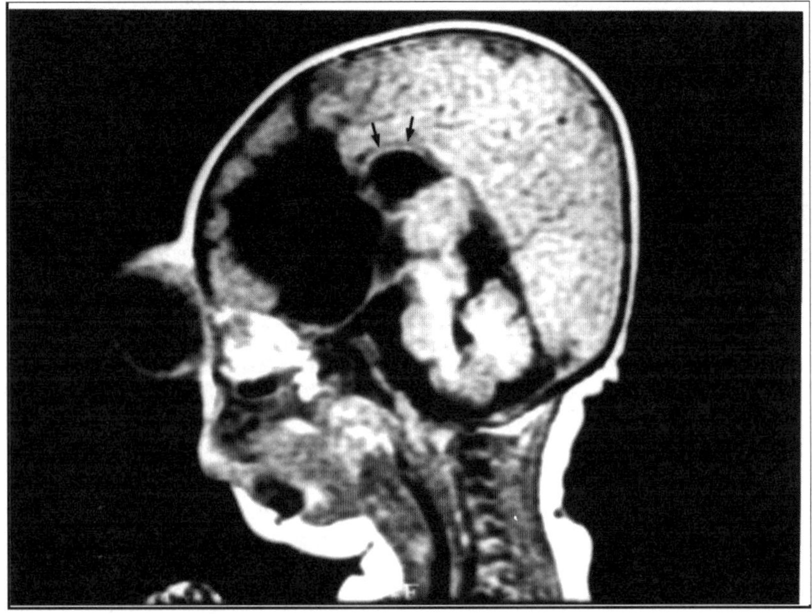

Figure 37b.

Reference
1.   *Barkovich, AJ, Norman D. Anomalies of the corpus callosum: correlation with further anomalies of the brain. AJNR, 1988;9:493*

Figure 38. **Callosal dysgenesis associated with Chiari I malformation and ectopic neurohypophysis.** 11-year-old boy. *SE T1W MR image.* The size of the corpus callosum is well below normal. This was shown by callosal area measurement, which was 340 mm^2, well below the normal ranges for this age group. The rostrum (curved arrow) as well as the splenium (open-closed arrow) are hypoplastic (callosal dysgenesis). An ectopic neurohypophysisis is noted (small arrow). This view, and additional views confirmed the absence of the stalk, which probably accounted for hypophyseal insufficiency present in this patient. The condition is also associated with Chiari I malformation; tonsillar protrusion into the spinal canal (arrow), and a syrinx in the cervical cord (S).

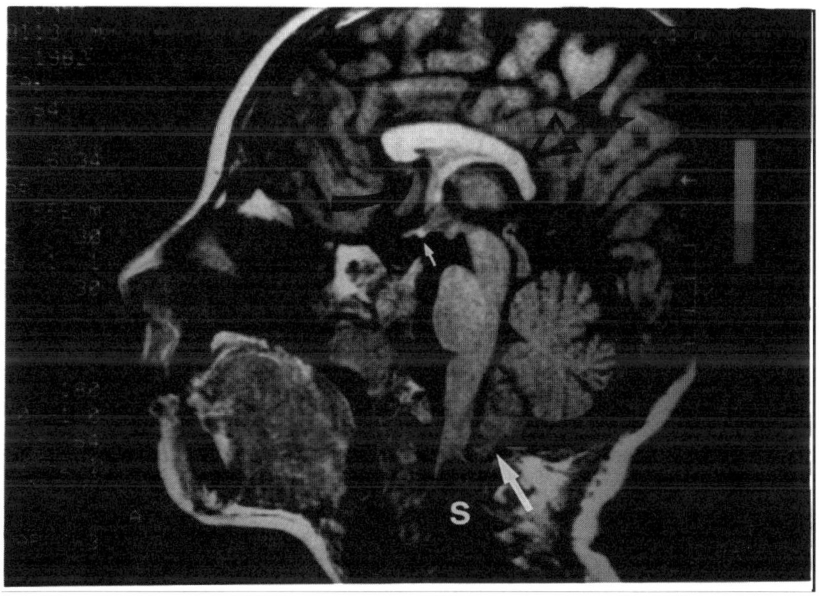

Figure 38.

References
1. *Hunter JV, Youl BD, Moseley IF. MRI demonstration of midbrain deformity in association with Chiari malformation. Neuroradiology 1992;34:399*
2. *Marwaha R, Menon PS, Jena A, et al. Hypothalamo pituitary axis by magnetic resonance imaging in isolated growth hormone deficiency patients born by normal delivery. J Clin Endocrinol Metab 1992;74:654*
3. *Fujita K, Matsuo N, Mori O, et al. The association of hypopituitarism with small pituitary, invisible pituitary stalk, type 1 Arnold-Chiari malformation, and syringomyelia in seven patients born in breech position: a further proof of birth injury theory on the pathogenesis of "idiopathic hypopituitarism.: Eur J Pediatr 1992;151:266*
4. *Maghnie M, Larizza D, Zulani I, et al. Congenital central nervous system abnormalities, idiopathic hypopituitarism and breech delivery: what is the connection? Eur J Pediatr 1993;152:175*
5. *Abrahams JJ, Trefelner E, Boulware SD. Idiopathic growth hormone deficiency: MR findings in 35 patients. AJNR 1991;12:155*

Figure 39 a-d. **Callosal dysgenesis in Dandy-Walker variant.** 2-year-old girl. *a) SE T1W, b) IR T1W, and c) SE, coronal T2W MR images in this patient, and d) SE, coronal T2W MR image in a normal subject.* The appearance of the posterior fossa is consistent with Dandy-Walker variant (a). The corpus callosum is diffusely thin, more prominent in the rostral parts (callosal dysgenesis), probably due to diminished fibers in the forceps minor. There is resultant dilatation of the frontal horns of the lateral ventricles (circles), (b, c). Besides this, it is also noted on the coronal image (c) that the line between the caudate heads and the nuclei lentiformi has become more horizontal (arrows), (c) compared to that seen in a normal individual (arrows), (d) which reflects an interesting consequence of callosal dysgenesis.

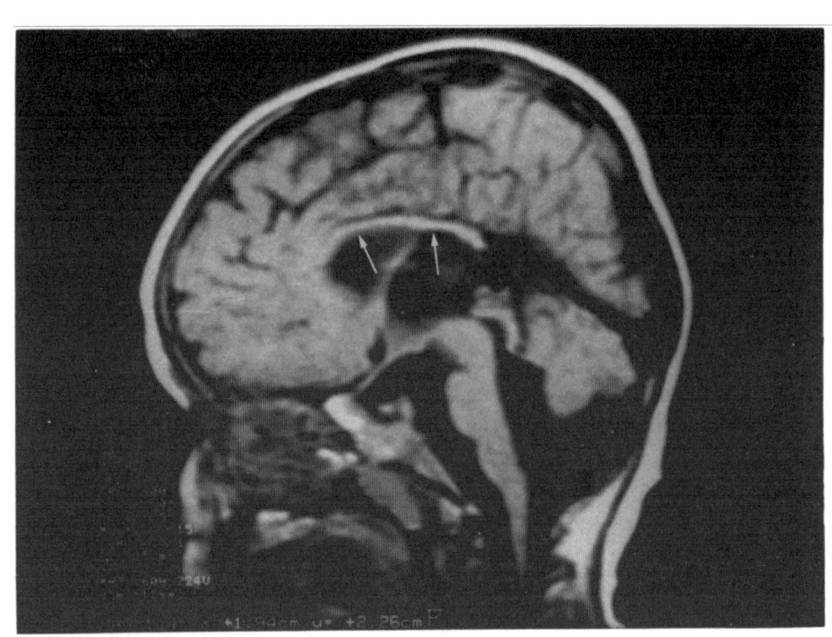

Figure 39a.

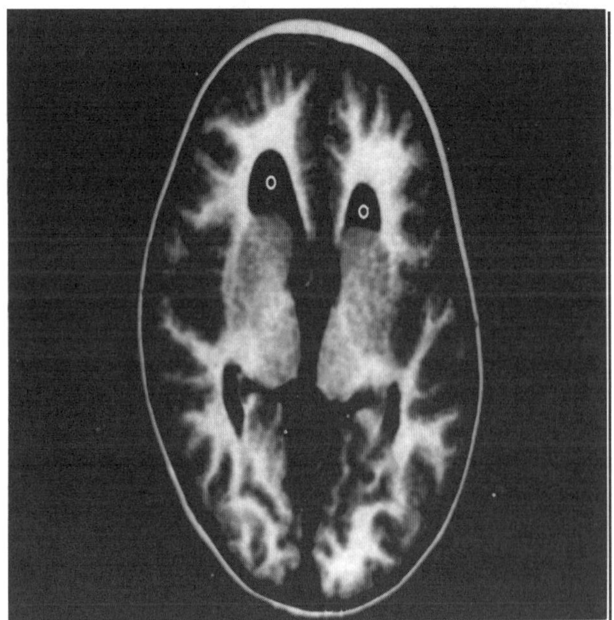

Figure 39b.

Reference
1.   Barkovich AJ, Norman D. Anomalies of the corpus callosum: correlation with further anomalies of the brain. AJNR 1988;9:493

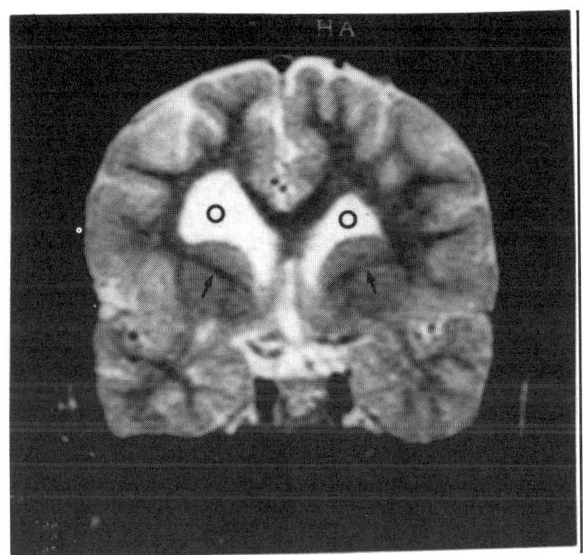

Figure 39c.

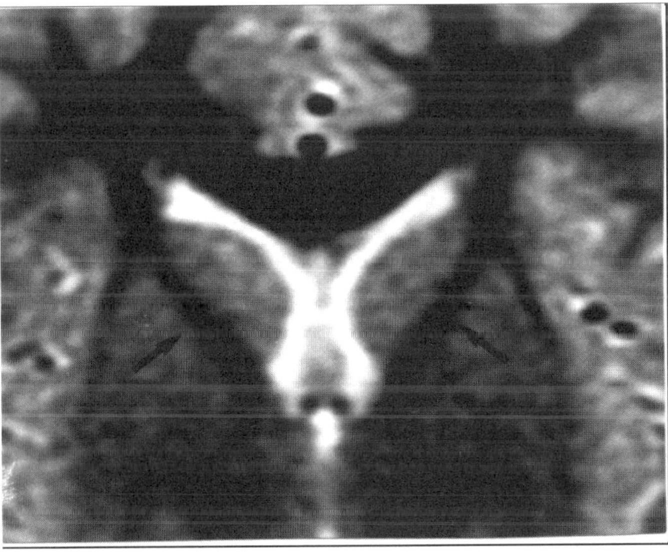

Figure 39d.

Figure 40 a, b. **Callosal dysgenesis in tuberous sclerosis.** 5-year old boy. *a) CT scan, and b) SE T1W MR image.* Subependymal calcified nodules (small arrows) of tuberous sclerosis are seen as well as a nodule at the right foramen of Monro (large arrow), a characteristic location. There is a calcified tuber in left frontal lobe (square) (a). MR image demonstrates diffuse callosal thinning (callosal dysgenesis), (straight arrow) (b). Callosal dysgenesisis is not a common finding in tuberous sclerosis. Note the appearance of the calcified left frontal lobe (curved arrow) (b).

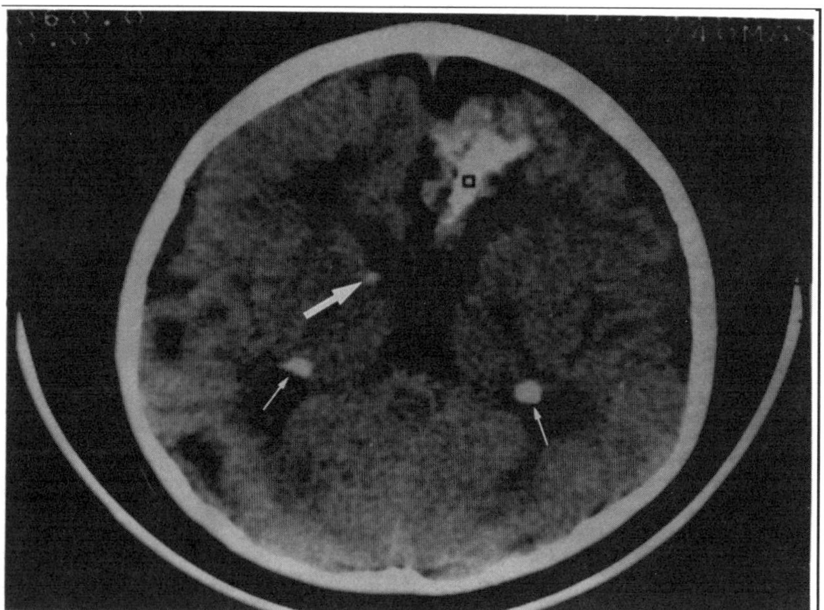

Figure 40a.

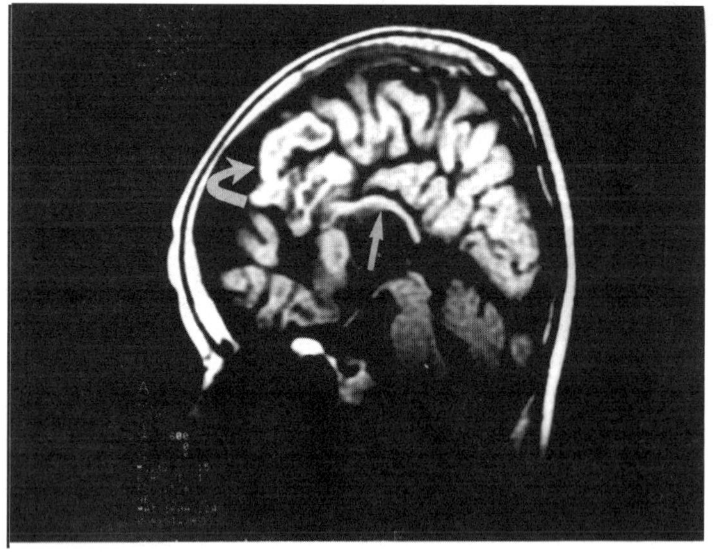

References
1. Barkovich AJ: Pediatric neuroimaging. New York, Raven Press, 1995;296
2. De Marco P. Tuberous sclerosis, agenesis of the corpus callosum and Lennox-Gastaut syndrome: mere chance or a new syndrome? Clin Electroencephalogr 1992;23:7

Figure 40b.

Figure 41 a, b. **Callosal dysgenesis in tuberous sclerosis.** 3-year-old boy. *a) SE T1W MR image, and b) SE T1W MR image after administration of contrast medium.* The corpus callosum is diffusely thin (callosal dysgenesis) (arrow) (a). The characteristic subependymal nodules of tuberous sclerosis that are located at the region of the foramina of Monro are demonstrated (arrows). Contrast-enhancement of these nodules on MRI is commonly seen, and does not necessarily reflect a tumoral involvement. However, there is an enhancing parenchymal lesion (open arrow) which was due to an infiltrating giant cell astrocytoma. Also note multiple, hypointense, parenchymal tubers.

References

1. *Barkovich AJ: Pediatric neuroimaging. New York, Raven Press, 1995;296*
2. *De Marco P. Tuberous sclerosis, agenesis of the corpus callosum and Lennox-Gastaut syndrome: mere chance or a new syndrome? Clin Electroencephalogr 1992;23:7*

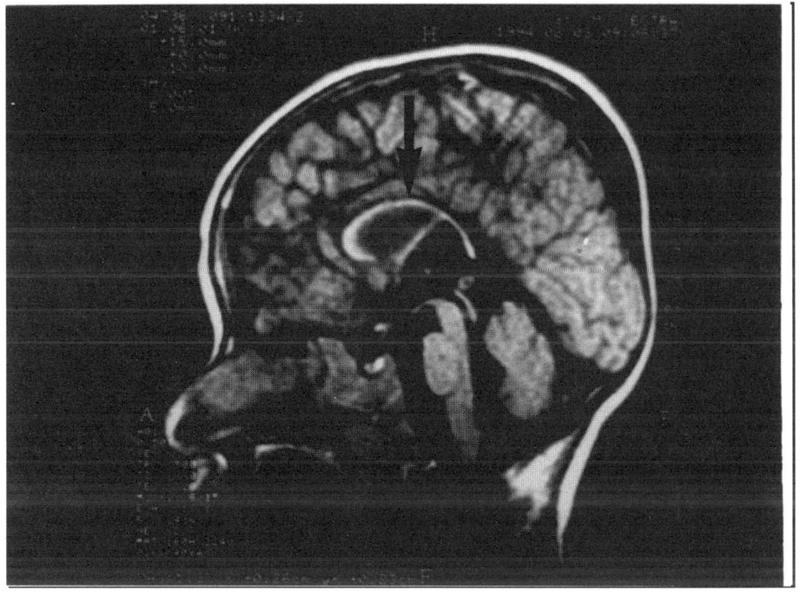

Figure 41a.

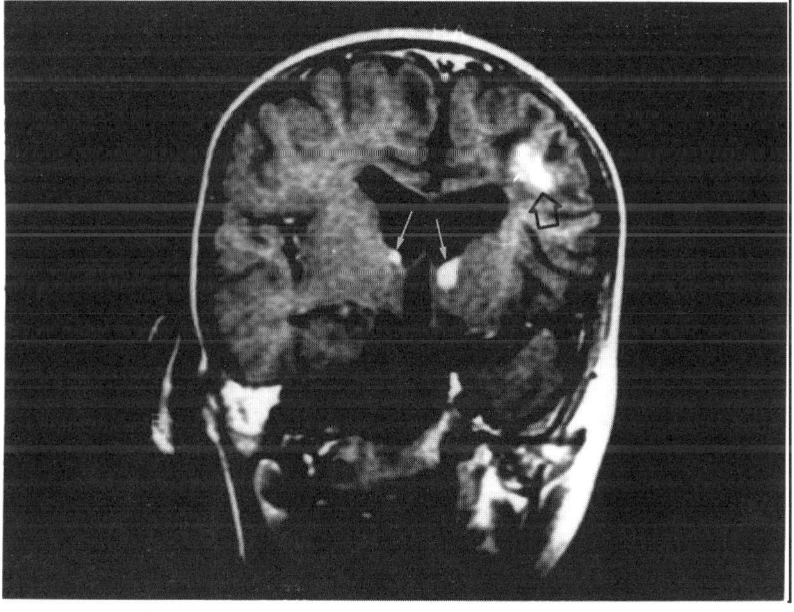

Figure 41b.

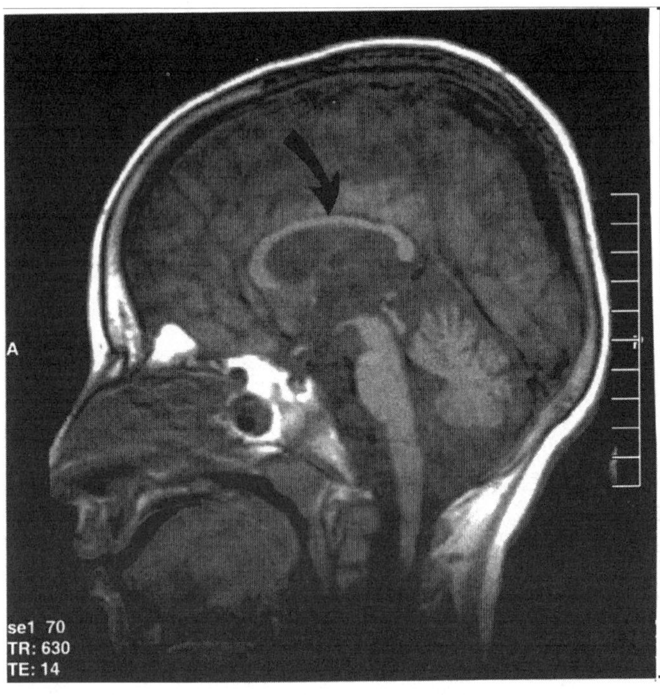

Figure 42a.

Figure 42 a-c. **Callosal dysgenesis in tuberous sclerosis.** 8-year-old boy. Sagittal T1W MR image reveals a diffusely thinned corpus callosum, a relatively common finding in tuberous sclerosis (arrow) (a).

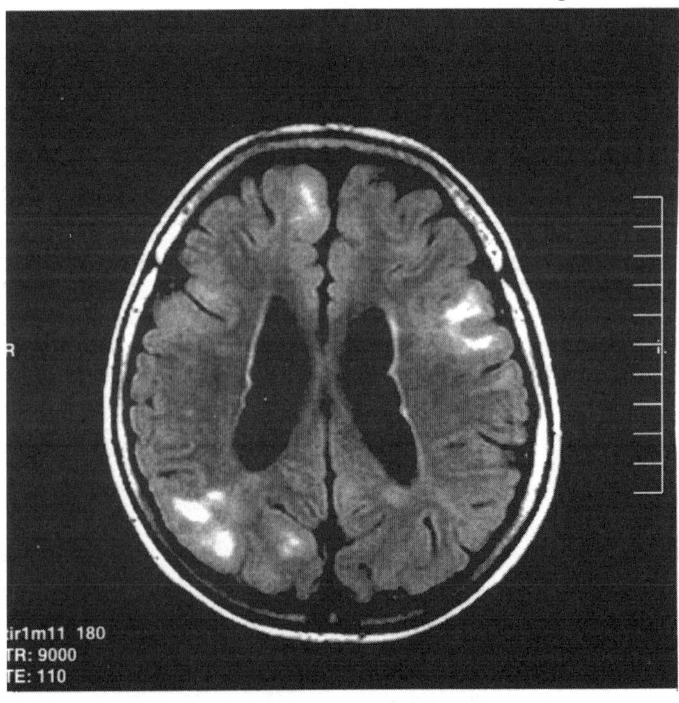

FLAIR image reveals multiple high-signal parenchymal hamartomas (b). ADC map reveals high ADC values of parenchymal hamartomas: 1.70, 1.73, 1.91, and 1.40 $\times 10^{-3}$ mm^2/sec. These indicate existence of relatively free molecular movement of water in the hamartomas (corresponding to relatively loose tissue structure of hamartomas), compared to the normal white matter (c).

Reference
1. Barkovich AJ. Pediatric neuroimaging.
    Philadelphia, Lippincott Williams & Wilkins, 2000

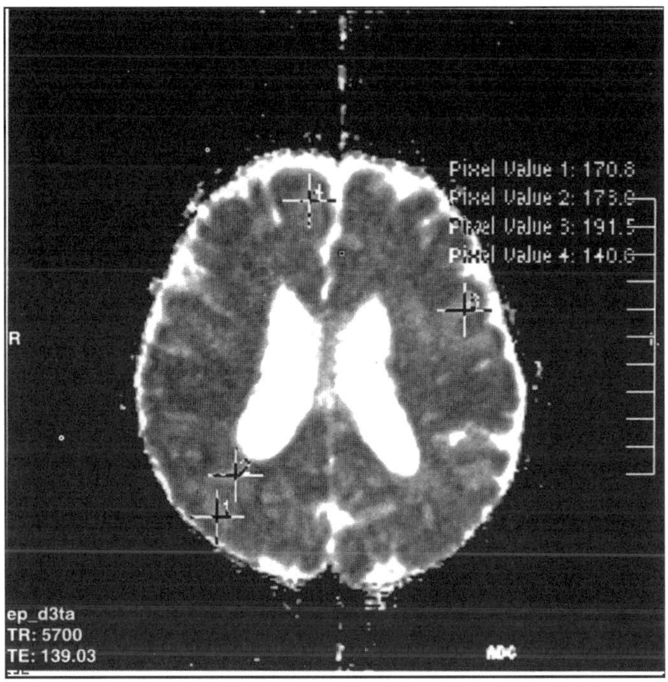

Figure 42c.

Figure 43 a-c. **Callosal dysgenesis associated with total hemimegalencephaly.** 8-year-old boy. T1W MR image reveals a hypoplastic corpus callosum with absence of the posterior parts (arrow) (a). T1W (inversion recovery) images reveal enlargement of the right hemisphere of the cerebrum, and that of the cerebellum as well (b,c). Therefore, this patient represents a total form of hemimegalencephaly affecting the cerebrum and cerebellum together. Usually, one cerebral hemisphere is involved in hemimegalencephaly.

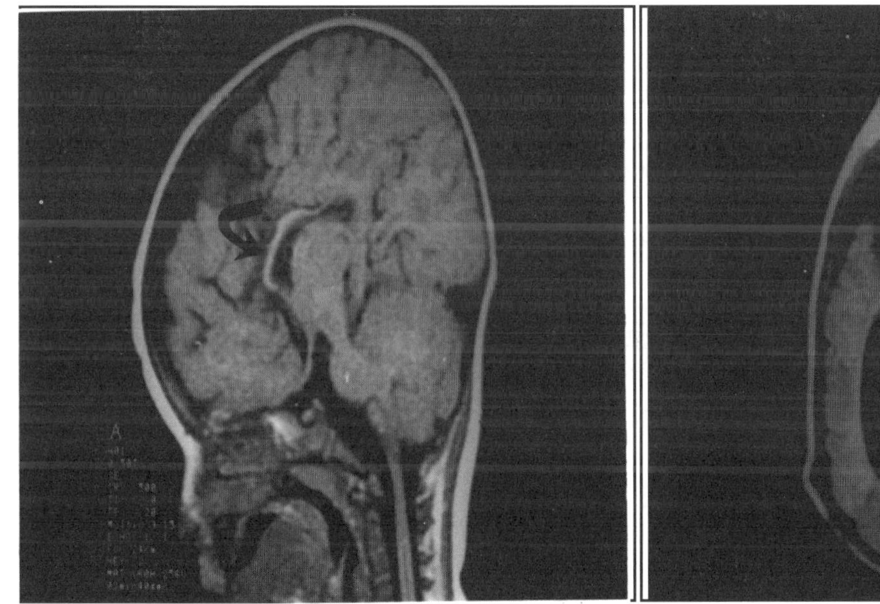

Figure 43a.

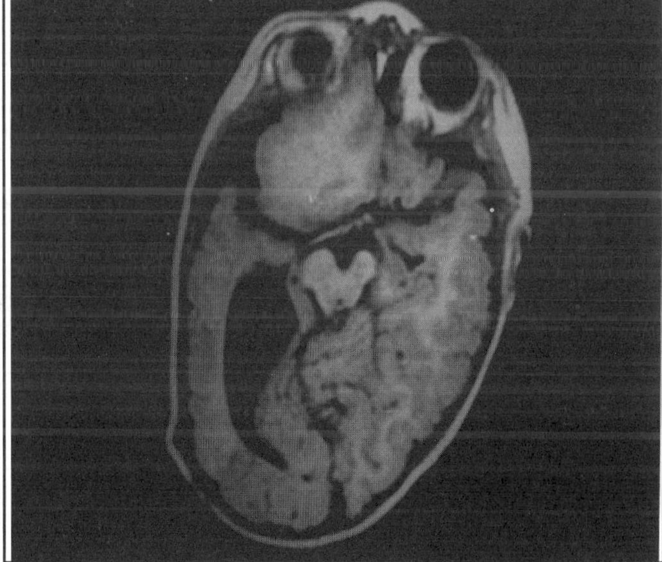

Figure 43b.

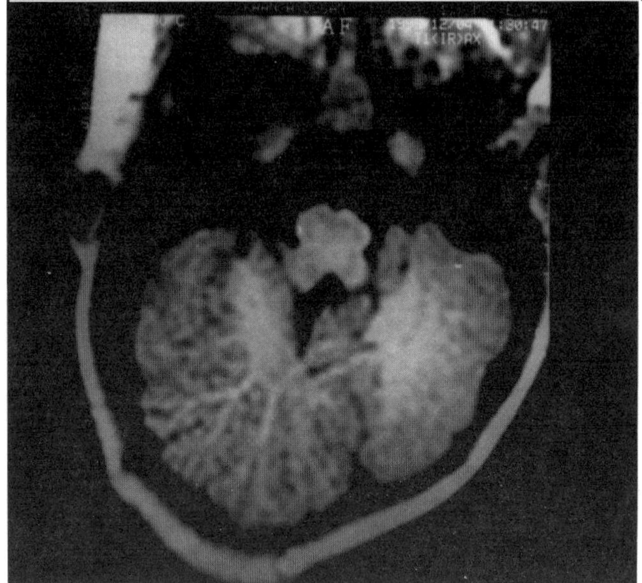

Figure 43c.

References
1. *Sener RN. MR demonstration of cerebral hemimegalencephaly associated with cerebellar involvement (total hemimegalencephaly). Comput Med Imaging Graph 1997;21:201*
2. *Barkovich AJ. Pediatric neuroimaging. Philadelphia, Lippincott Williams & Wilkins, 2000*

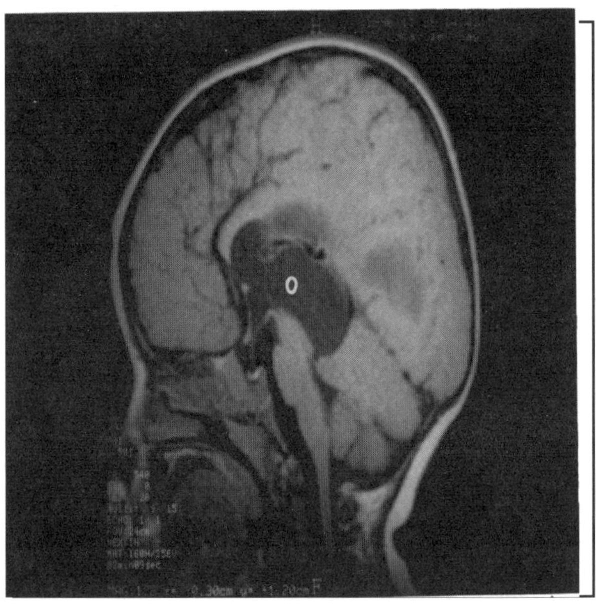

Figure 44.

Figure 44. **Callosal dysgenesis associated with transtentorial arachnoid cyst.** 2-year-old boy. T1W MR image reveals a hypoplastic corpus callosum with absence of its posterior portions. Transtentorial cyst (circle) compresses the aqueduct, displaces the 3rd venrticle upwards. Also, it compresses the vermis.

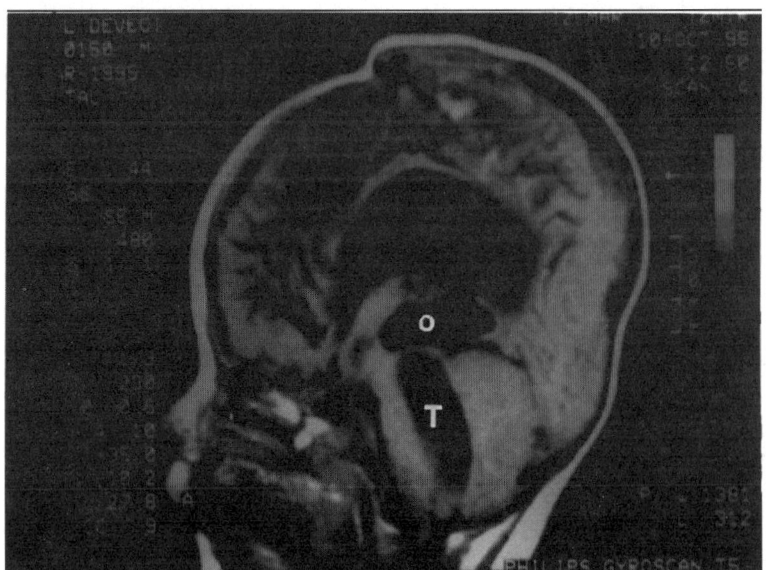

Figure 45.

Figure 45. **Callosal dysgenesis associated with transtentorial arachnoid cyst, and isolated fourth ventricle.** 7-month-old boy. T1W MR image reveals a hypoplastic corpus callosum with absence of the posterior parts. Transtentorial cyst (circle) causes prominent hydrocephalus, and extends posteriorly over the tentorium. The 4th ventricle is isolated, trapped (T) by occlusion of the aqueduct and 4th ventricular outlet foramina, Magendi, and Luskhas. The condition was associated with rhombencephalosynapsis.

Figure 46. **Callosal dysgenesis in a normal individual.** 11-year-old girl. *SE T1W MR image.* The splenium of the corpus callosum appears as if it has been cut off (arrow), an atypical appearance for splenial dysgenesis.

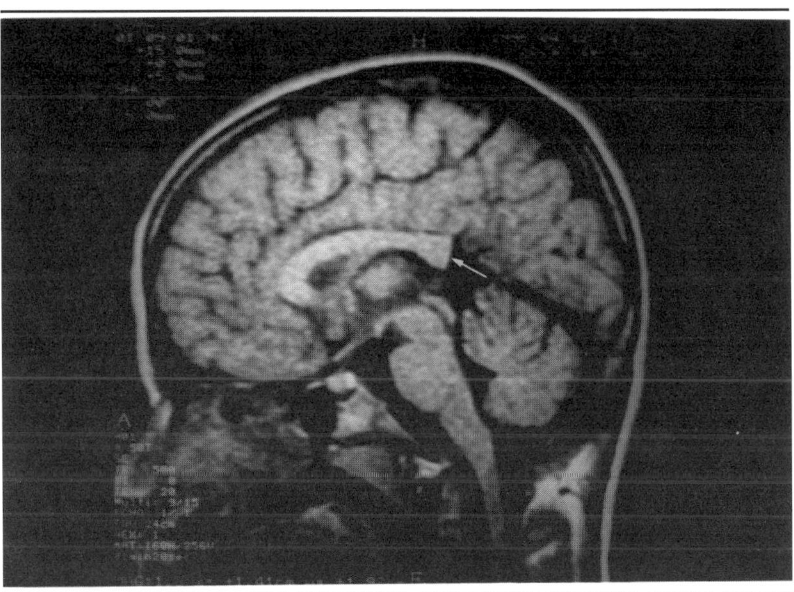

Figure 46.

Figure 47. **An unusual type of callosal dysgenesis in a normal individual.** *SE T1W MR image.* 14-year-old boy. The genu appears as if it has been cut off (arrow), otherwise the corpus callosum has developed normally. This condition is very unusual, and is in contrast to the current theories on callosal development. The currently favoured theories suggest that the corpus callosum develops in an anterior to posterior direction, a process that is completed by approximately 20 weeks gestational age. The genu forms first followed by posterior growth to form the body and splenium, and the rostrum forms latest of all.

Reference
1. *Schaefer GB, Shuman RM, Wilson DA, et al. Partial agenesis of the anterior corpus callosum: correlation between appearance, imaging, and neuropathology. Pediatr Neurol 1991;7:39*

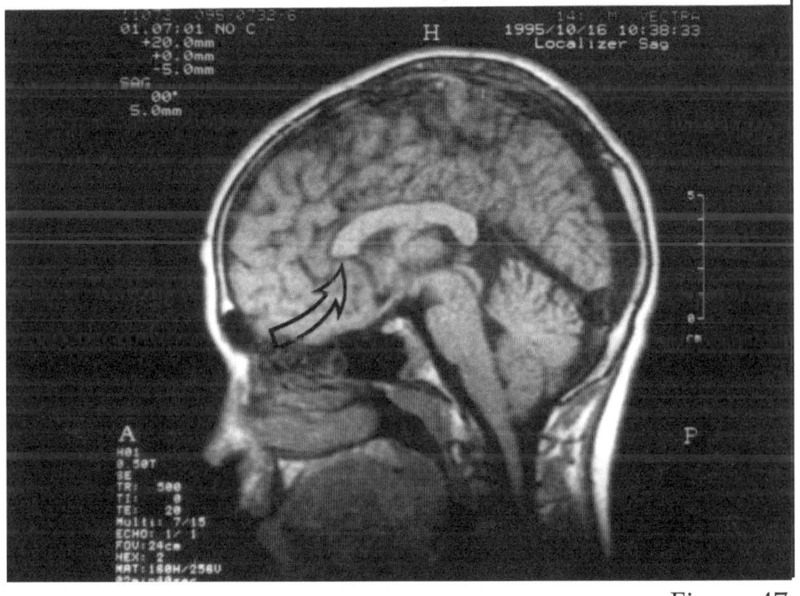

Figure 47.

Figure 48 a-c. **Atypical callosal dysgenesis.**
71-year-old woman. Sagittal, T1W MR image
reveals pinpointing of the anterior part of the
body of the corpus callosum (arrow). Therefore, the rostrum and genu are absent (a).
The patient has diffuse white matter changes
manifested with high signal, consistent with
leukoariasis as shown by a T2-weighted image (b), and by an ADC map from an echo-
planar diffusion imaging study (c).

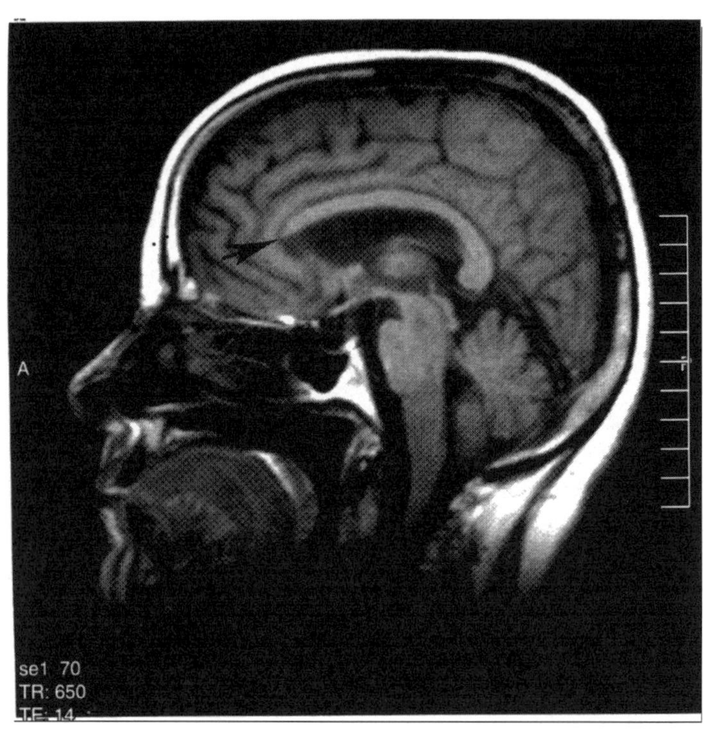

Figure 48a.

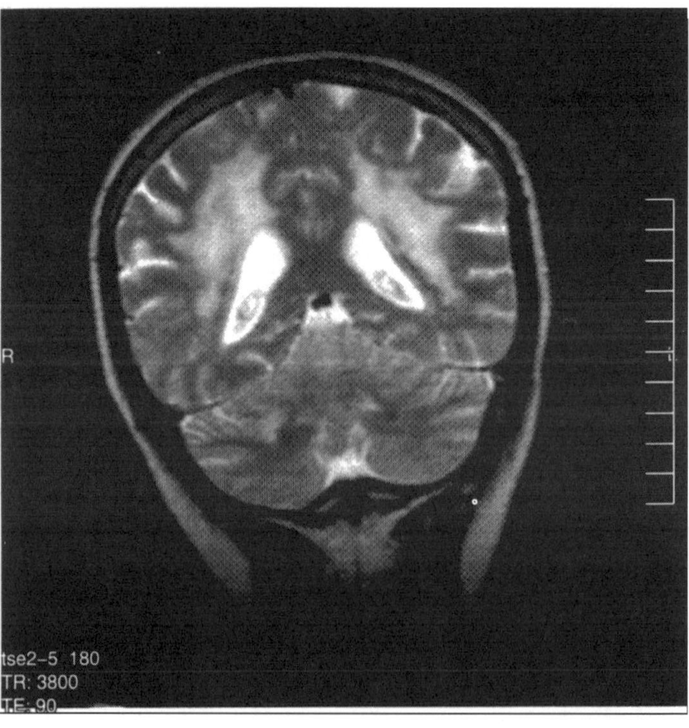

Figure 48b.

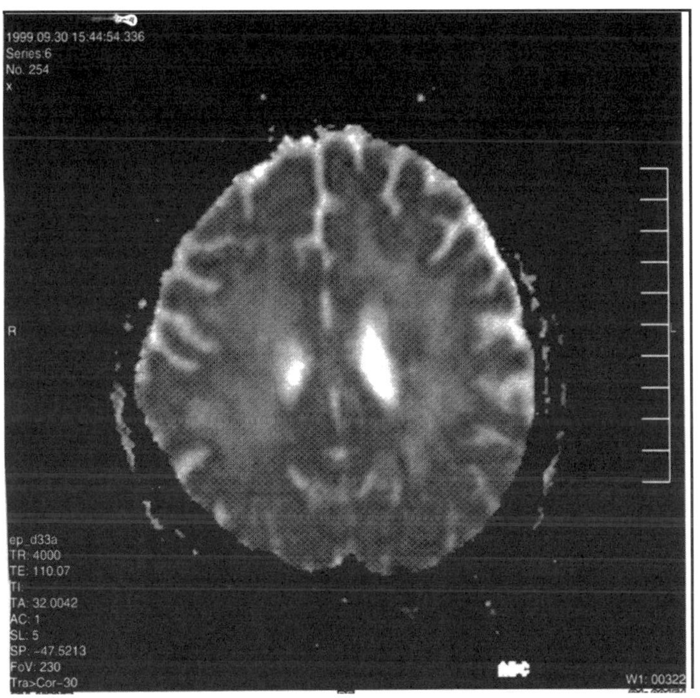

Figure 48c.

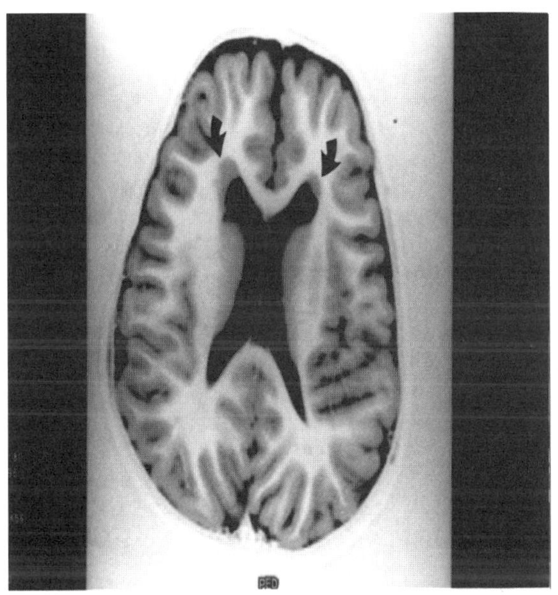

Figure 49a.

Figure 49 a,b **Atypical callosal dysgenesis associated with heterotopia.** 7-year-old girl. T1W (turbo inversion recovery) image reveals nodular heterotopic gray matter at the tips of the frontal horns (arrows) (a). The anterior part of the corpus callosum is absent, probably due to presence of another heterotopic nodule at that region (arrow) (b).

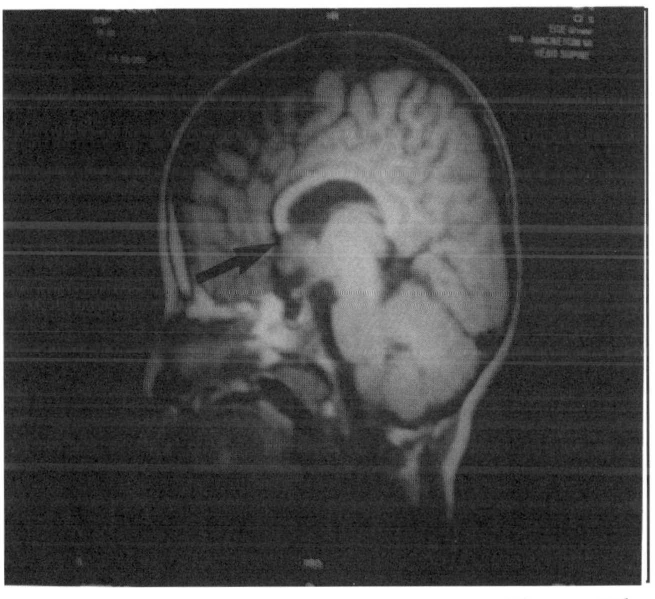

Figure 49b.

Figure 50 a-d. **Atypical callosal dysgenesis.** 47-year-old man. Sagittal, T1W MR image reveals an unusual kinking, and a bump in the body of the corpus callosum (a). The patient has a developmental venous anomaly located in the right temporal lobe as shown by T1W images (b,c), and TOF (time of flight) MR angiography (d).

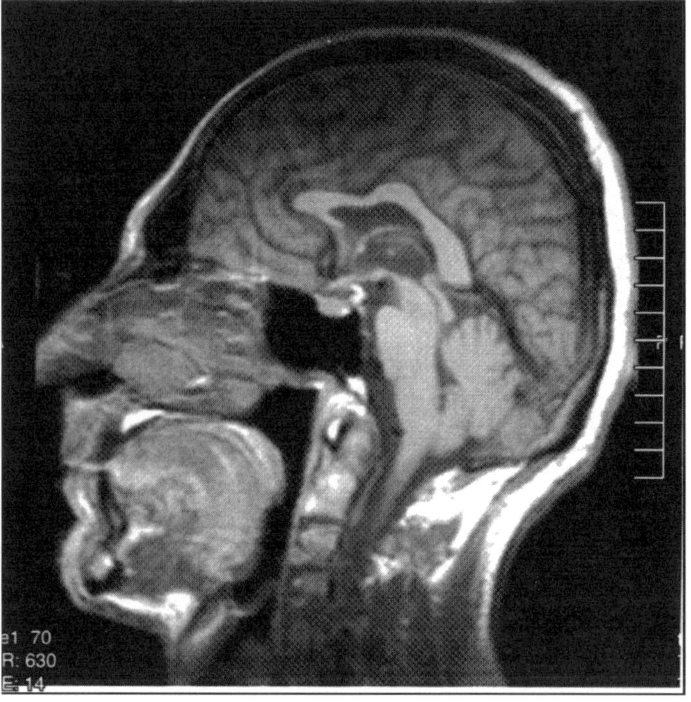

Figure 50a.

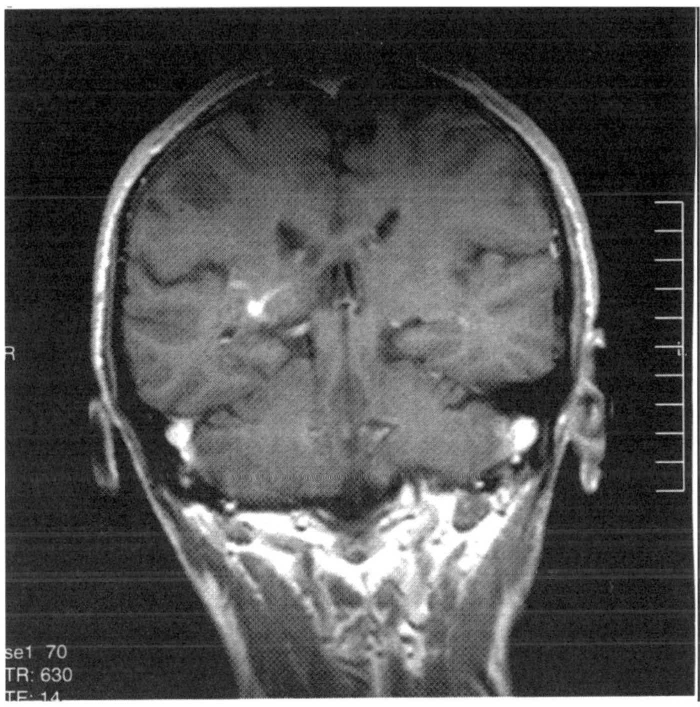

Figure 50b.

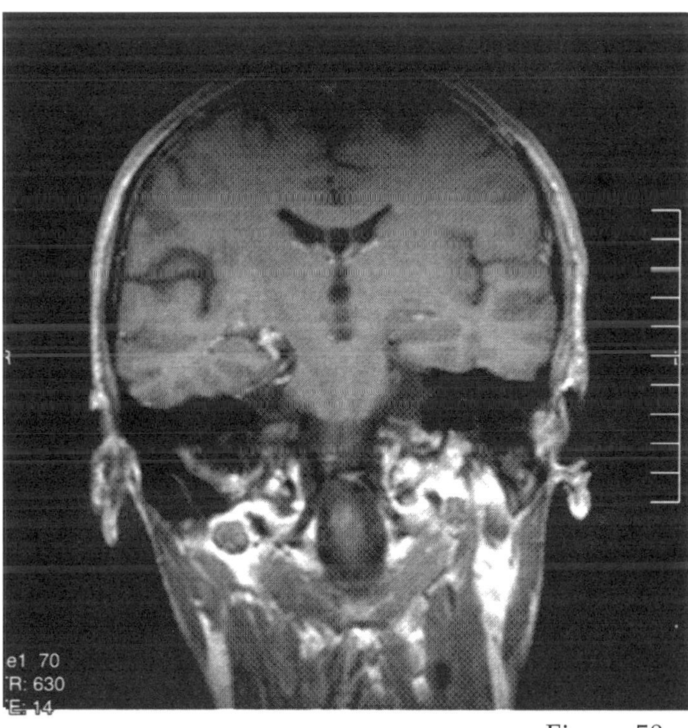

Figure 50c.

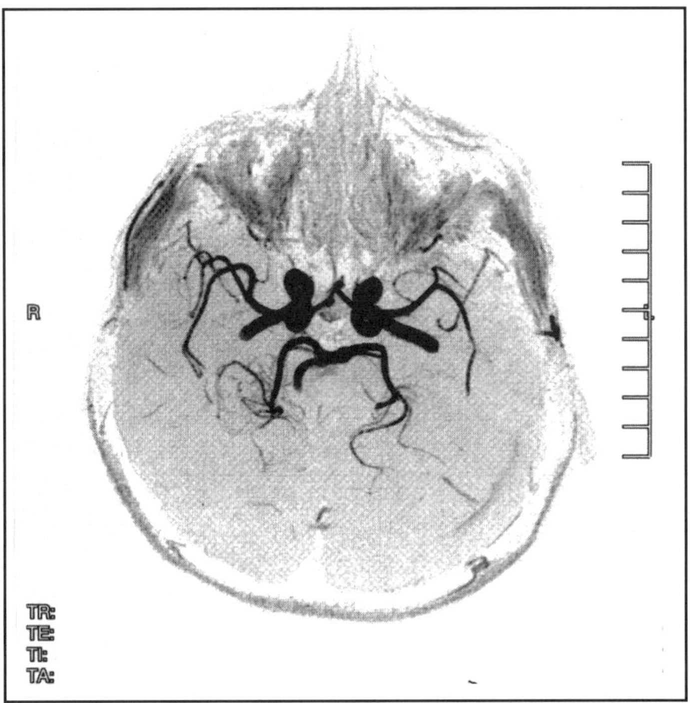

Figure 50d.

LESIONS DIRECTLY INVOLVING THE CORPUS CALLOSUM

THE CORPUS CALLOSUM IN DISORDERS OF NEURONAL MIGRATION AND ORGANIZATION

Figure 51 a, b. **Pachygyria. 5-month-old boy.** *a) SE T1W MR image, and b) SE T1W MR image after administration of contrast medium.* There is microcephaly. The corpus callosum has a dome-like appearance (shows an arc-like upward bulging) (arrowhead) (a). Note thickened cortex, broad gyri with a few sulci throughout both cerebral hemispheres, that is consistent with pachygyria (b).

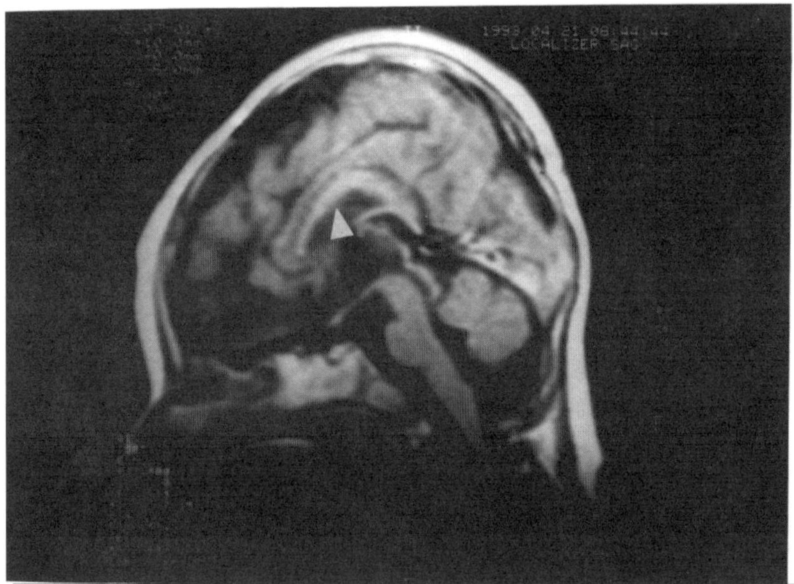

Figure 51a.

References
1. Barkovich AJ. Pediatric neuroimaging. New York, Raven Press, 1995;202
2. Gabrielli O, Salvolini U, Bonifazi V, et al. Morphological studies of the corpus callosum by MRI in children with malformative syndromes. Neuroradiology 1993;35:109

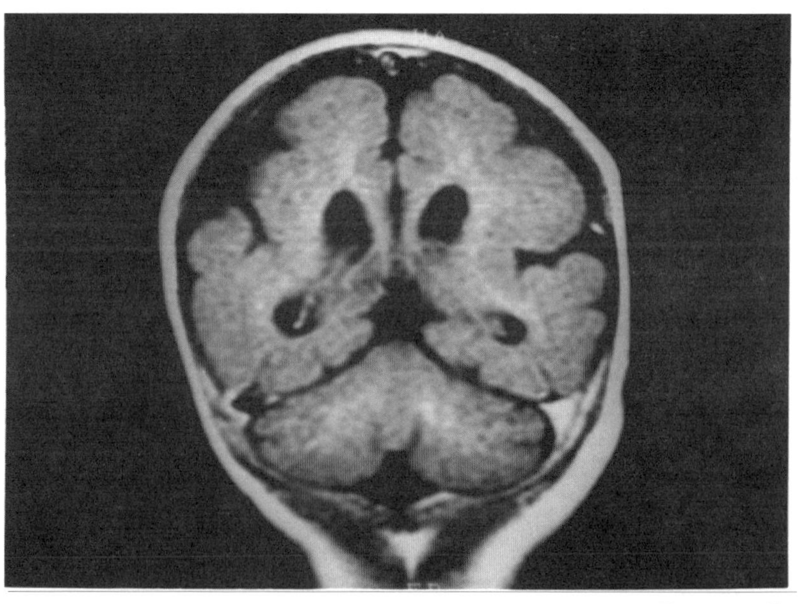

Figure 51b.

Figure 52a, b. **Unilateral cortical dysplasia.** 1-year-old boy. *a) SE T1W, and b) SE T2W MR images.* Note a dome-like corpus callosum (arrowhead). There is cortical dysplasia in the right hemisphere (star), manifesting as a thickened cortex with diminished underlying white matter.

References

1. *Barkovich AJ. Pediatric neuroimaging. New York, Raven Press, 1995;202*
2. *Barkovich, AJ, Kjos BO. Nonlissencephalic cortical dysplasias, correlation of imaging findings with clinical deficits. AJNR 1992;13:95*
3. *Kuzniecky R, Andermann F, CBPS study group. The congenital bilateral perisylvian syndrome: imaging findings in a multicenter study. AJNR 1994;15:139*
4. *Jinkins JR, Whittemore AR, Bradley WG. MR imaging of callosal and cortico-callosal dysgenesis. AJNR 1989;10:339*
5. *Sener RN. Unilateral cortical dysplasia associated with contralateral hyperplasia of the brainstem. Pediatr Radiol 1995;25:440*
6. *Gabrielli O, Salvolini U, Bonifazi V, et al. Morphological studies of the corpus callosum by MRI in children with malformative syndromes. Neuroradiology 1993;35:109.*

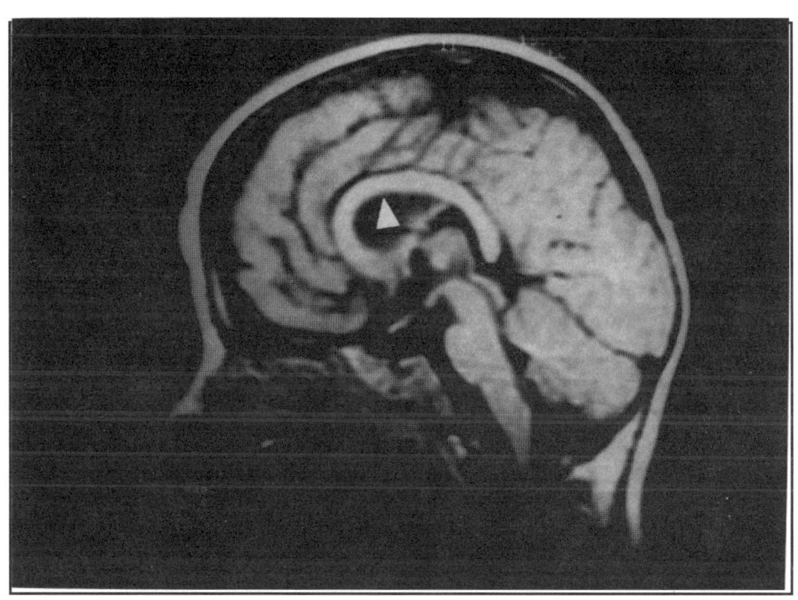

Figure 52a.

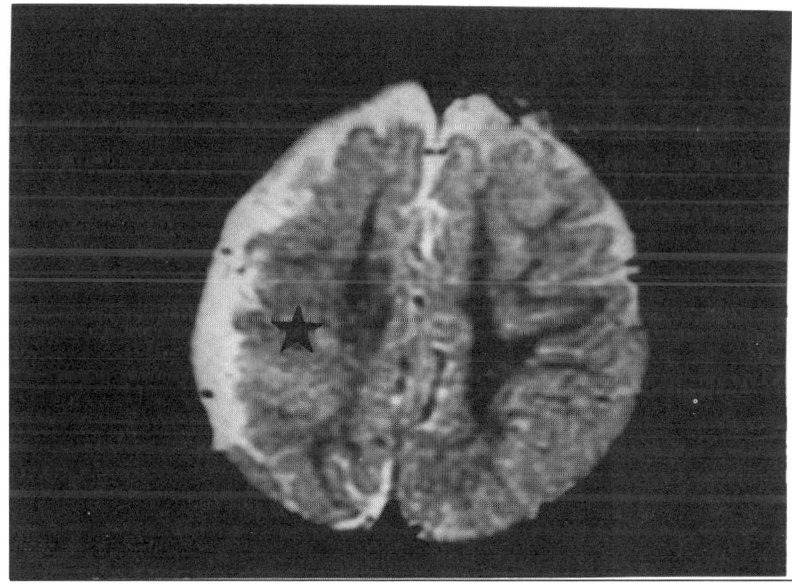

Figure 52b.

Figure 53 a-c. **Schizencephaly.** 3-year-old boy. *a, b) SE T1W, and c) SE T2W MR images.* The corpus callosum is dome-like (arrowhead) (a). An open-lip schizencephalic cleft, lined with heterotopic gray matter, is seen in the right hemisphere (arrows) (b, c). There is a small cleft in the left hemisphere (small arrow) (c).

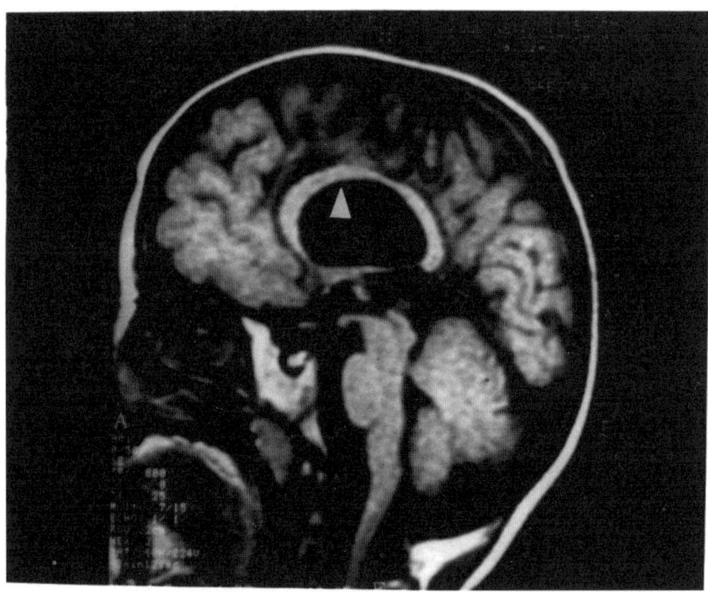

Figure 53a.

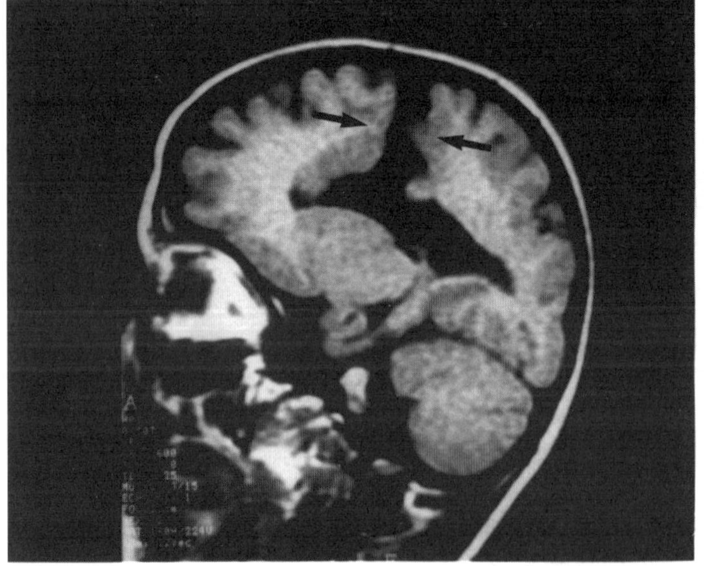

Figure 53b.

Figure 53c.

References
1. *Barkovich AJ, Kjos BO. Schizencephaly: correlation of clinical findings with MR characteristics. AJNR 1992;13:85*
2. *Gabrielli O, Salvolini U, Bonifazi V, et al. Morphological studies of the corpus callosum by MRI in children with malformative syndromes. Neuroradiology 1993;35:109.*

Figure 54 a, b. **Schizencephaly.** 3-year-old boy. *a) SE T1W, and b) IR T1W MR images.* A dome-like corpus callosum is seen (arrowhead) (a). Note a closed-lip schizencephalic cleft (arrow) in the left hemisphere (b). The condition was associated with septo-optic dysplasia.

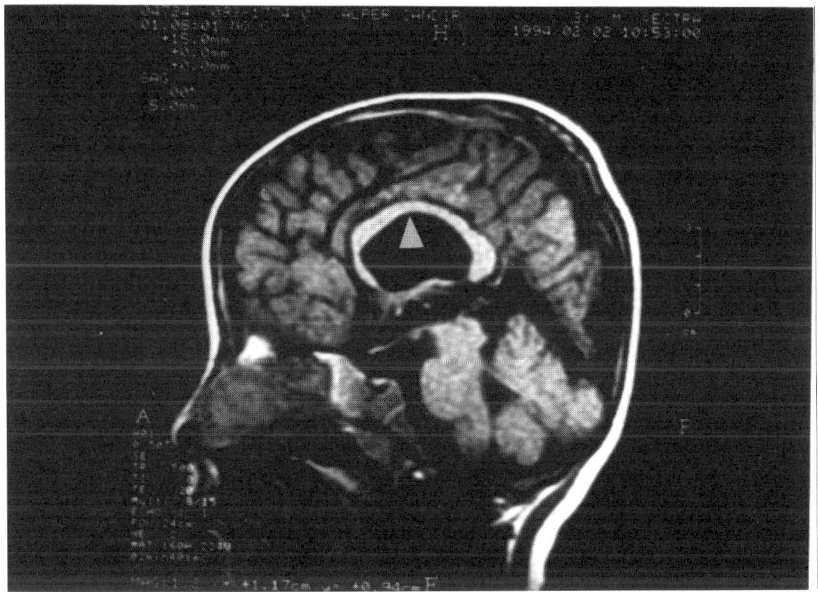

Figure 54a.

References
1   Barkovich AJ, Kjos BO. Schizencephaly: correlation of clinical findings with MR characteristics. AJNR 1992;13:85
2. Gabrielli O, Salvolini U, Bonifazi V, et al. Morphological studies of the corpus callosum by MRI in children with malformative syndromes. Neuroradiology 1993;35:109

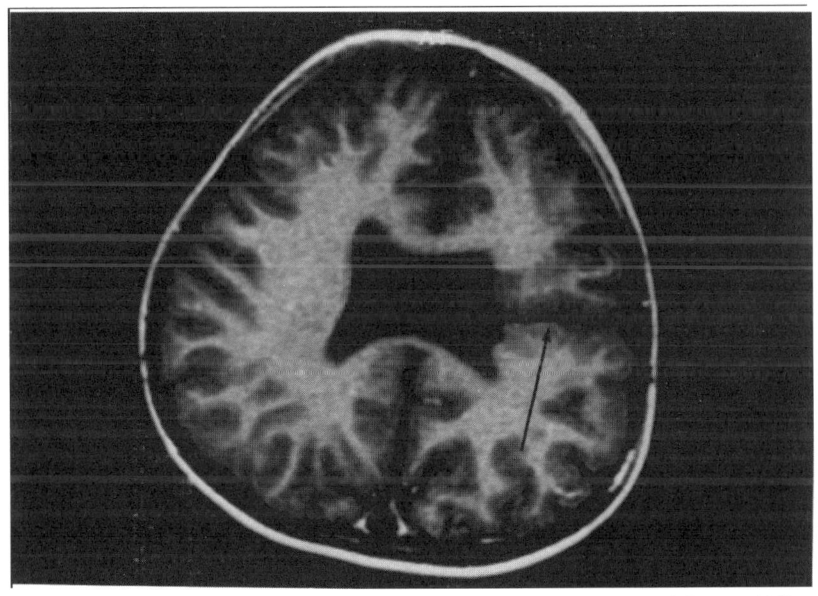

Figure 54b.

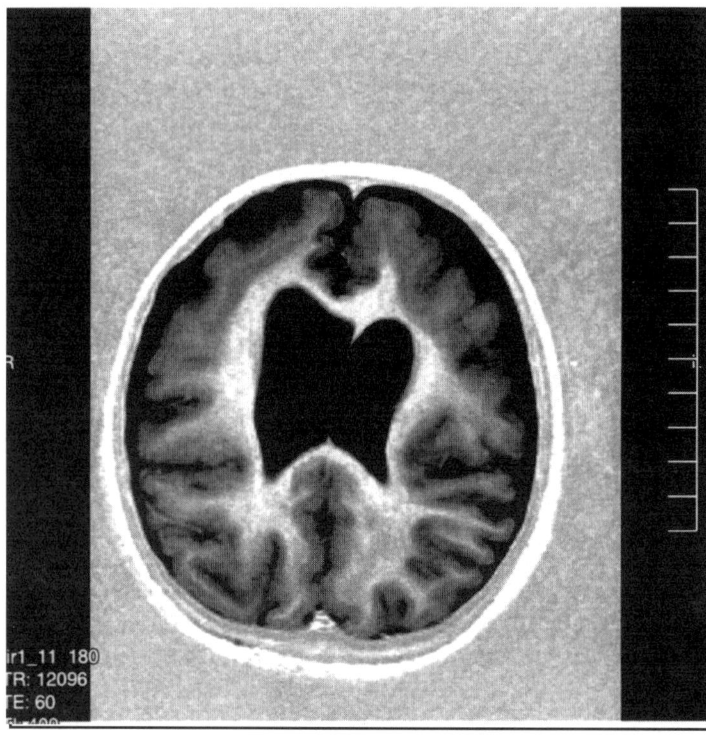

Figure 55a.

Figure 55 a-d. **Pachygyria.** 14-year-old girl. T1W (turbo inversion recovery) images show abnormal cortices, mainly in the frontal lobes including the sylvian regions. Thin bands of heterotopic gray matter are also evident at the frontal regions (band heterotopia) (a,b).

Figure 55b.

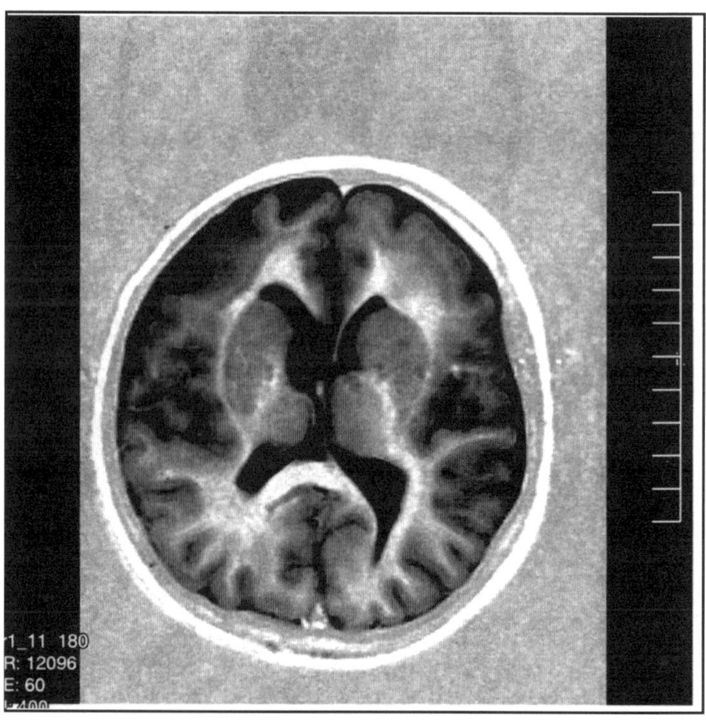

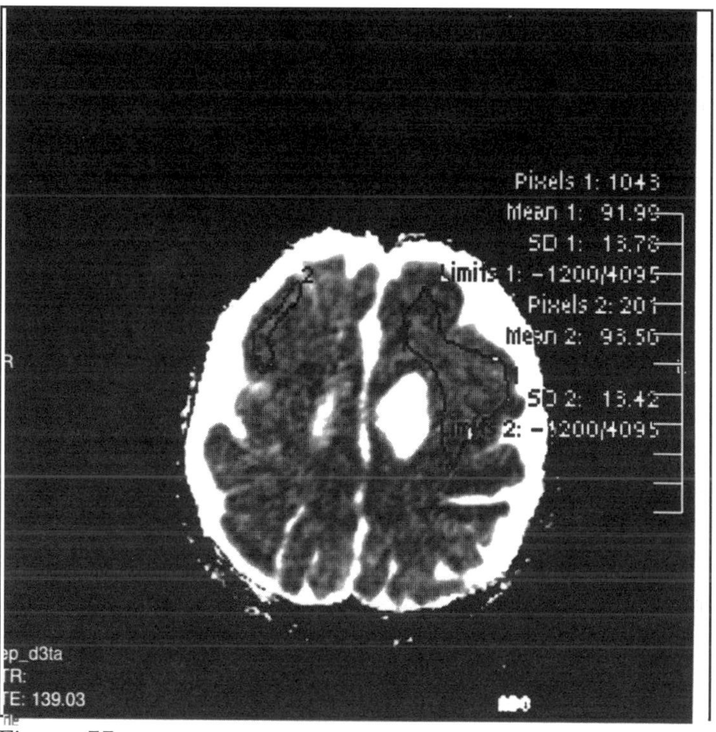

Figure 55c.

ADC map from an echo-planar diffusion MRI sequence reveal normal parenchymal ADC values: 0.91 and 0.93 X10^{-3} mm^2/sec. In most of the neuronal migrational disorders, diffusion MRI, hence ADC map findings are normal, unless there is abnormal signal in the subcortical white matter. In normal individuals the ADC value ranges of the brain parenchyma are 0.60 to 1.05 X10^{-3} mm^2/sec (c). T1W image reveals a dome-like appearance of the corpus callosum with abnormal margins (d).

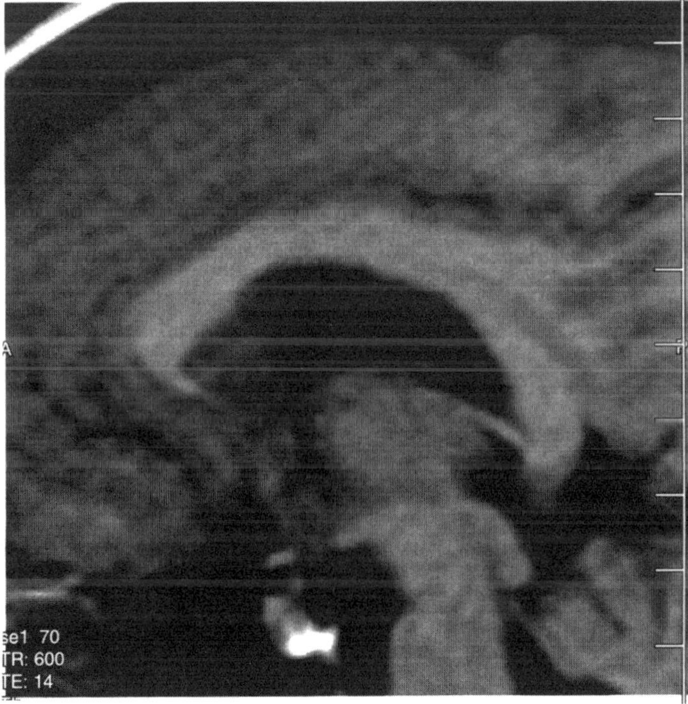

Figure 55d.

References

1. *Barkovich AJ. Pediatric neuroimaging. Philadelphia, Lippincott Williams & Wilkins, 2000*

2. *Sener RN. Diffusion MRI: apparent diffusion coefficient (ADC) values in the normal brain, and a classification of brain disorders based on ADC values. Comput Med Imaging Graph 2001; 25:299*

Figure 56a.

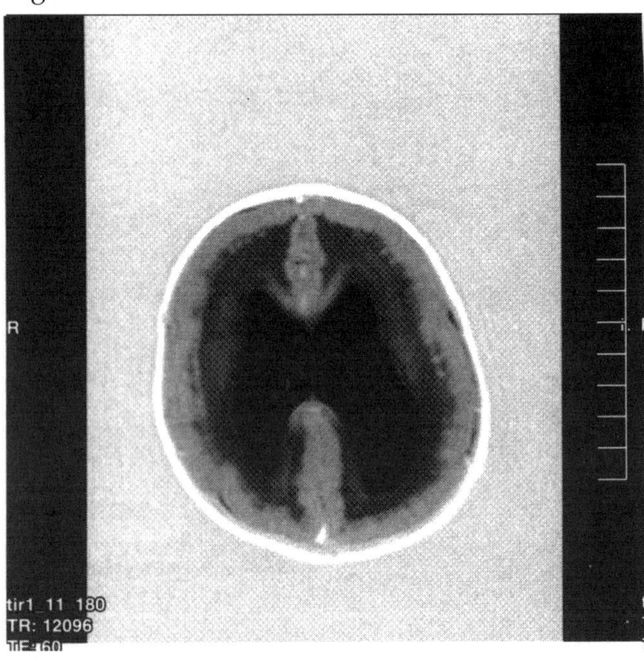

Figure 56 a-g. **Callosal dysgenesis associated with Walker-Warburg syndrome.** 5-month-old boy. T1W (turbo inversion recovery) image reveals thickened cortex without gyri, and with an inner cobblestone appearance. The white matter is hypointense due to lack of myelination. Ventricular dilatation is secondary to callosal dysgenesis, and associated Dandy-Walker variant (a). Sagittal, T1W image reveals an abnormal configuration, a dome-like appearance of the corpus callosum (curved arrow) There is a characteristic kink in the medulla oblongata for Walker-Warburg syndrome (arrow). Also, changes consistent with Dandy-Walker variant are evident (b). ADC map reveals low values from the cortex 0.48, 0.48, and 0.64 X10^{-3} mm^2/ sec.

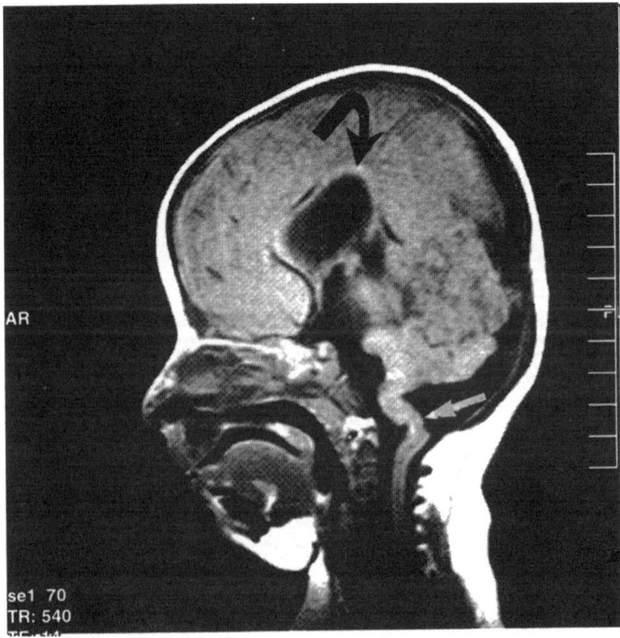

Figure 56b.

High values from the white matter are: 1.59, and 2.01 $X10^{-3}$ mm^2/sec, representing increased molecular motion of water, consistent with lack of myelination (c). ADC map from a lower section reveals normal cortical ADC values: 0.99, and 1.00 $X10^{-3}$ mm^2/sec, and a very high white matter value: 2.10 $X10^{-3}$ mm^2/sec (d) Associated subretinal hemorrhages are shown on transverse, and sagittal T1W images (e-g).

Figure 56c.

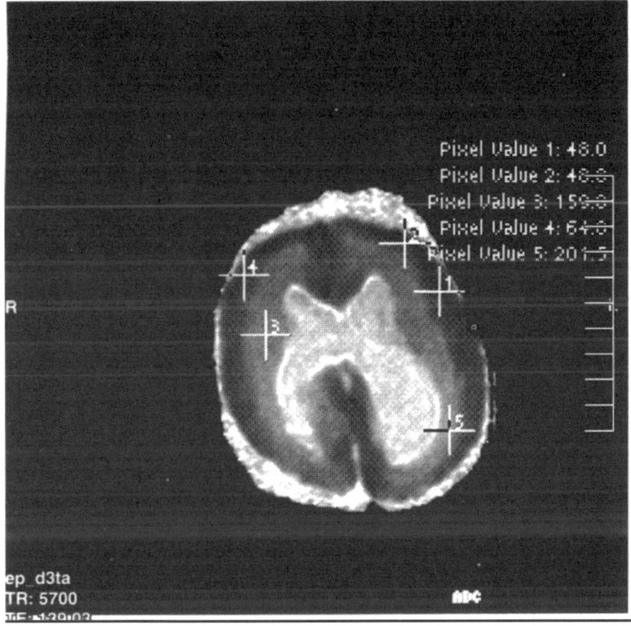

Figure 56d.

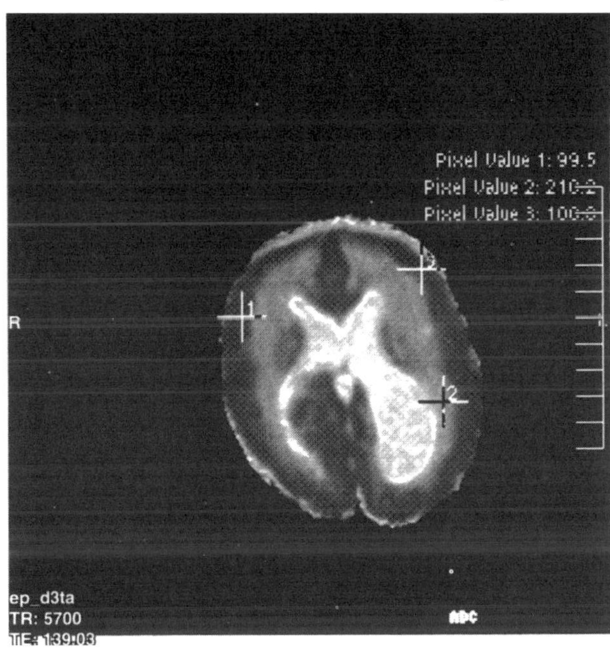

Figure 56e.

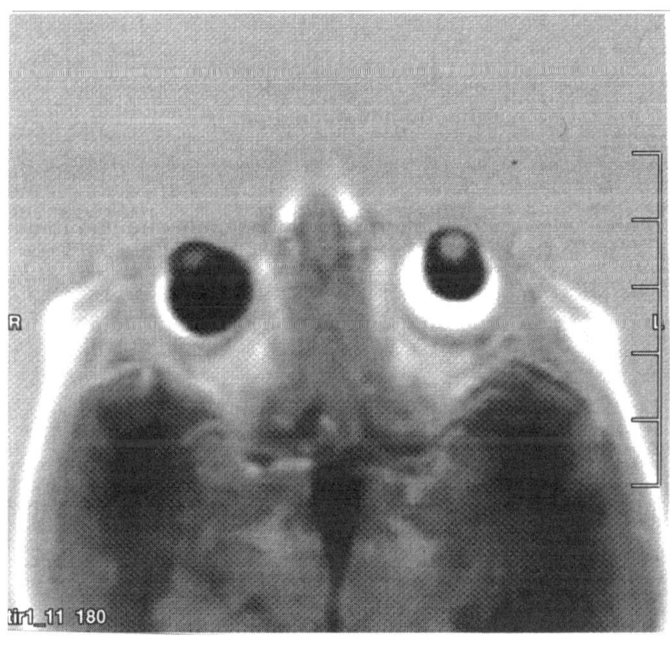

References
1. *Barkovich AJ. Pediatric neuroimaging. Philadelphia, Lippincott Williams & Wilkins, 2000*
2. *Sener RN. Diffusion MRI: apparent diffusion coefficient (ADC) values in the normal brain, and a classification of brain disorders based on ADC values. Comput Med Imaging Graph 2001; 25:299*

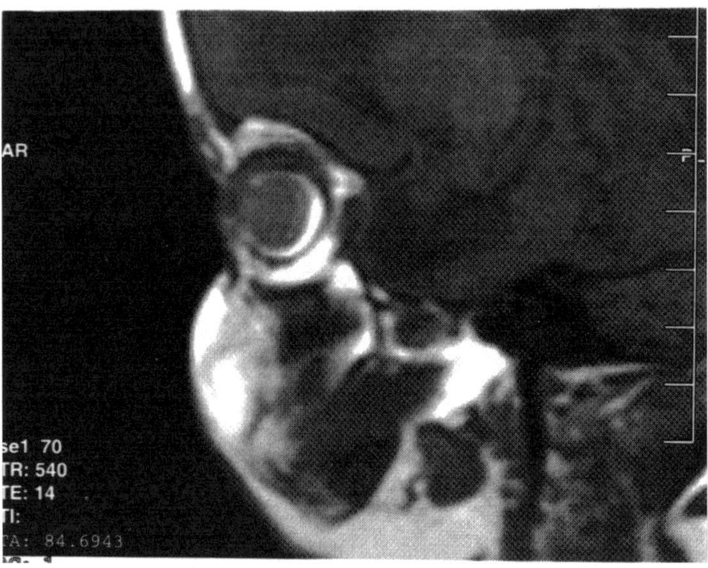

Figure 56f.

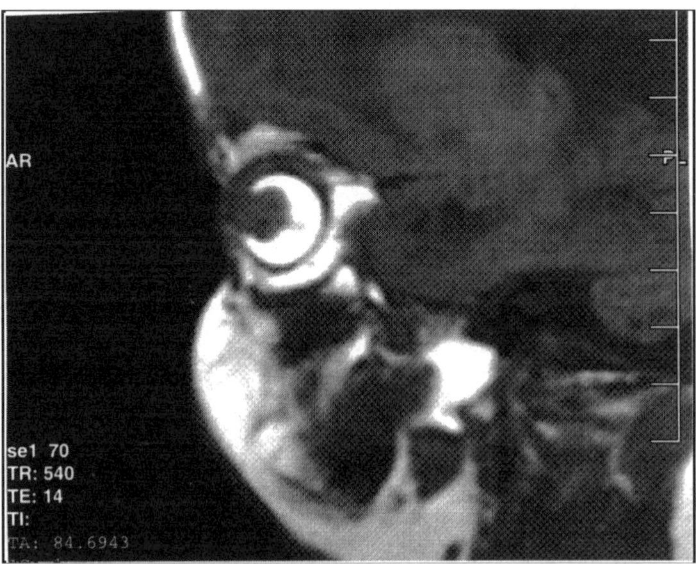

Figure 56g.

LESIONS DIRECTLY INVOLVING THE CORPUS CALLOSUM

THE CORPUS CALLOSUM IN PERINATAL ISCHEMIC BRAIN LESIONS

Figure 57 a, b. **Bilateral periventricular leukomalacia.** 3-year-old boy. *a) SE T1W, and b) SE T2W MR images*. The corpus callosum has been very thinned at the region of the isthmus (arrow) (a). T2W image shows hyperintense gliotic changes in both hemispheres due to periventricular leukomalacia. Involvement of the corpus callosum in perinatal ischemic brain lesions is a common finding.

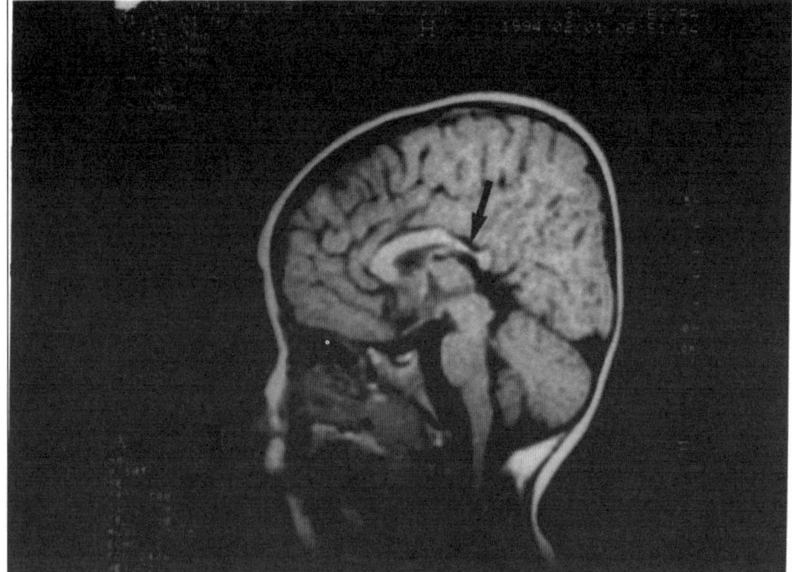

Figure 57a.

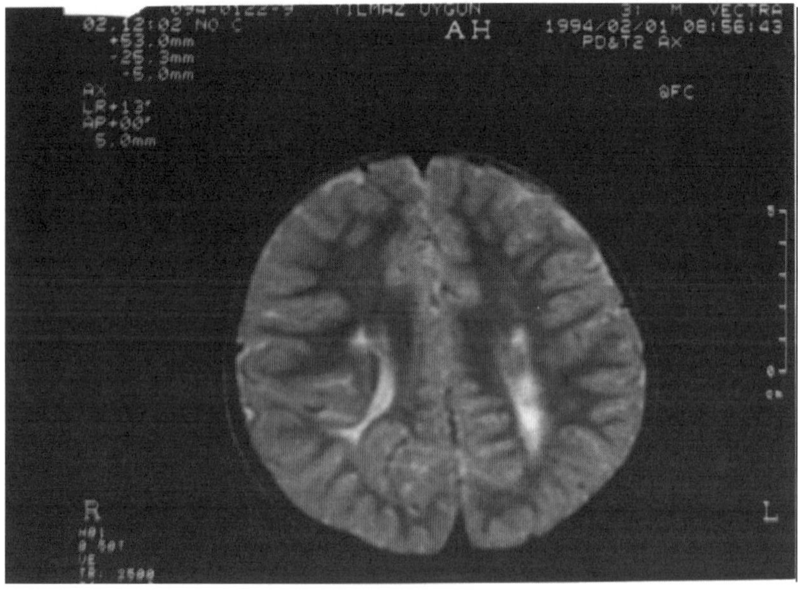

Figure 57b.

Reference
1.   *Truwit CL, Barkovich AJ, Koch TK, et al. Cerebral palsy: MR findings in 40 patients. AJNR 1992; 13:67*

Figure 58 a, b. **Unilateral periventricular leukomalacia.** 5-year-old boy. *a) SE T1W, and b) SE T2W MR images.* The isthmus of the corpus callosum is very thin (large arrow) (a). Gliotic changes due to periventricular leukomalacia is noted in the right hemisphere (large arrow), (b). There is an incidental lipoma in the superior cerebellar cistern (small arrows) (a, b).

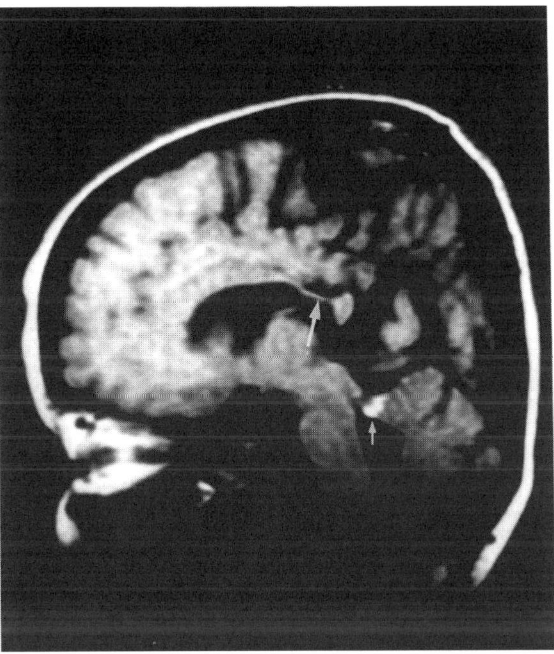

Figure 58a.

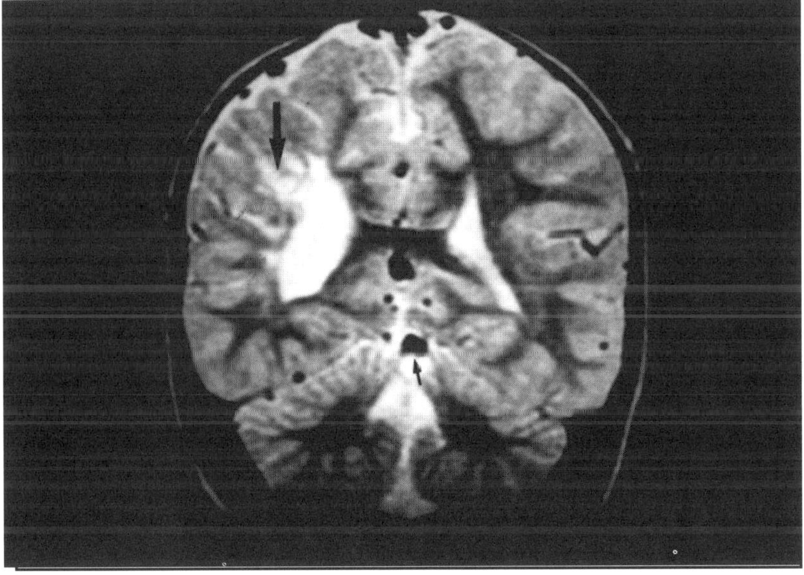

Figure 58b.

Reference
1.   Truwit CL, Barkovich AJ, Koch TK, et al. Cerebral palsy: MR findings in 40 patients. AJNR 1992;13:67

Figure 59 a, b. **Bilateral periventricular leukomalacia.** 2-year-old boy. *a) SE T1W, and b) SE proton density-weighted (PDW) MR images.* The corpus callosum has been diffusely affected, and the caudal part has a straight configuration (arrow) (a). The condition is secondary to bilateral periventricular leukomalacia (b).

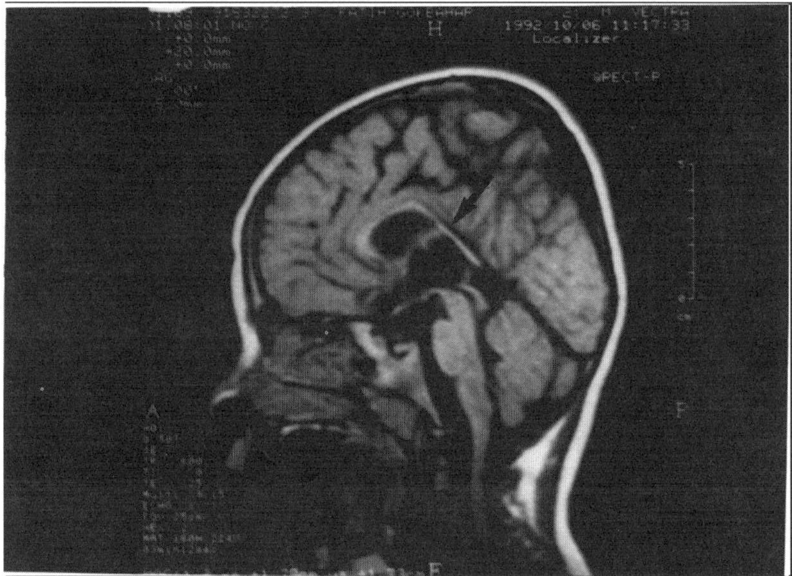

Figure 59a.

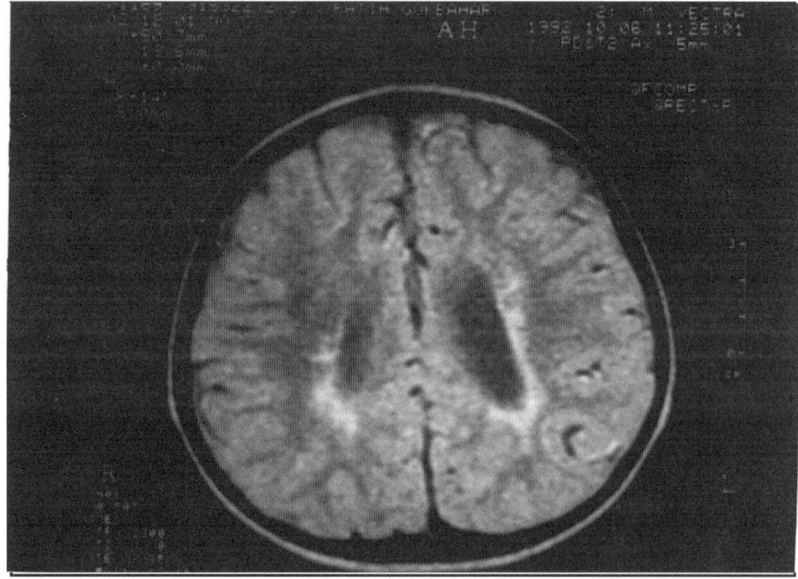

Figure 59b.

Reference
1. *Truwit CL, Barkovich AJ, Koch TK, et al. Cerebral palsy: MR findings in 40 patients. AJNR 1992; 13:67*

Figure 60 a, b. **Bilateral periventricular leukomalacia.** 7-year-old girl. *a) SE T1W, and b) SE T2W MR images.* The anterior parts of the corpus callosum has been destroyed (arrow)(a) by the ischemic process causing periventricular leukomalacia. Note that the lesions due to periventricular leukomalacia are more prominent in the vicinity of the frontal horns (arrow) (b).

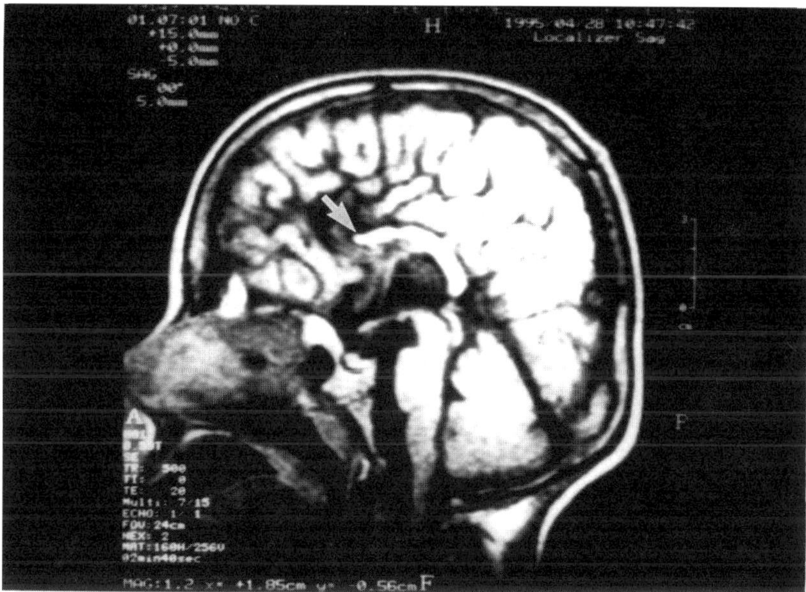

Figure 60a.

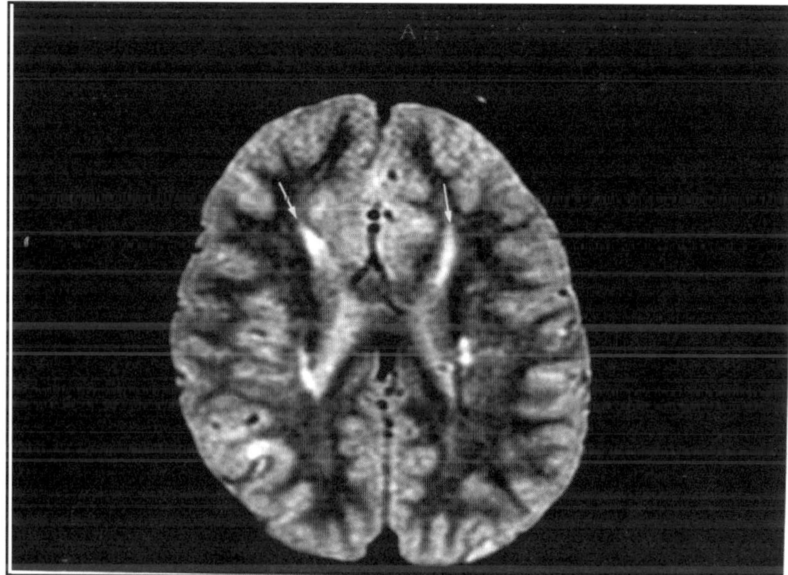

Figure 60b.

Reference
1.   Truwit CL, Barkovich AJ, Koch TK, et al. Cerebral palsy: MR findings in 40 patients. AJNR 1992; 13:67

Figure 61 a-c. **Unilateral periventricular leukomalacia.** 13-year-old girl. *a) SE T1W, b) SE PDW, and c) SE T2W MR images*. The anterior part of the body has been destroyed (white arrow), and the isthmus has been thinned (black arrow) (a). Accordingly, the lesions due to periventricular leukomalacia is extensive in the left frontal region. Also note an occipital lesion (c).

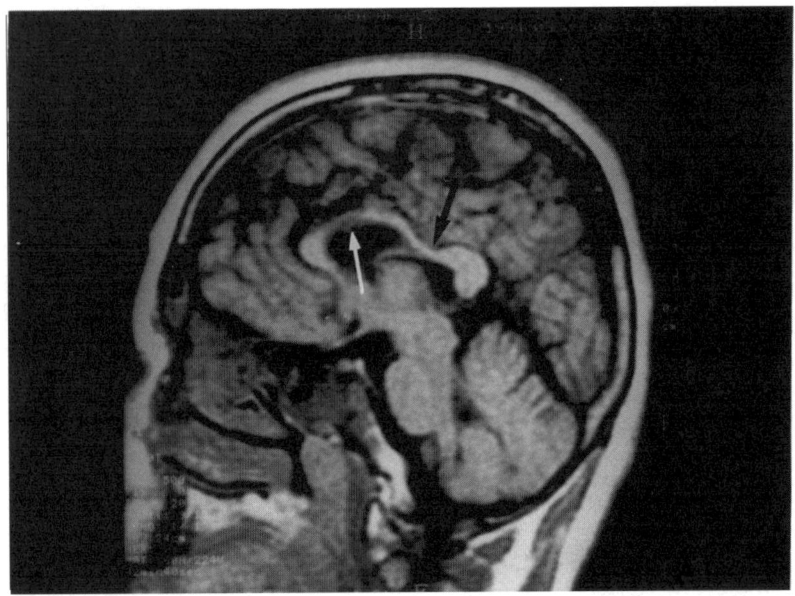

Figure 61a.

Reference
1.   *Truwit CL, Barkovich AJ, Koch TK, et al. Cerebral palsy: MR findings in 40 patients. AJNR 1992;13:67*

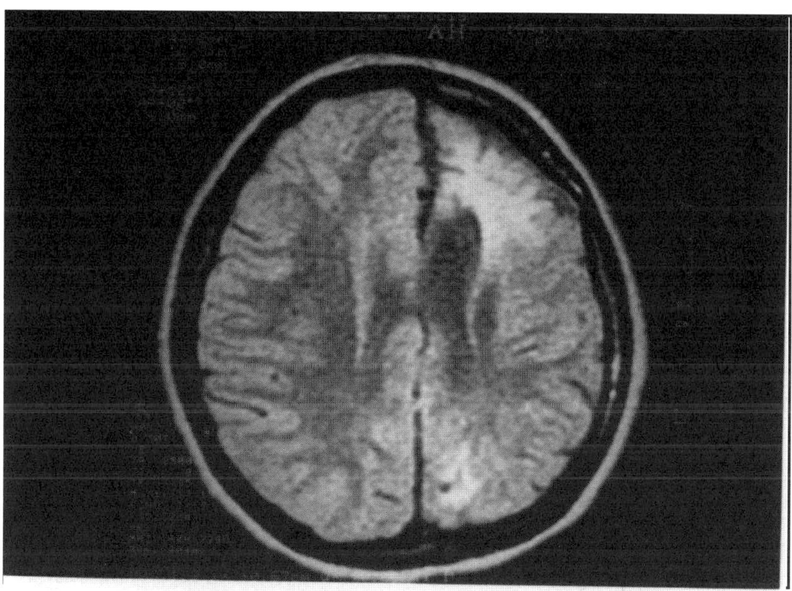

Figure 61b.

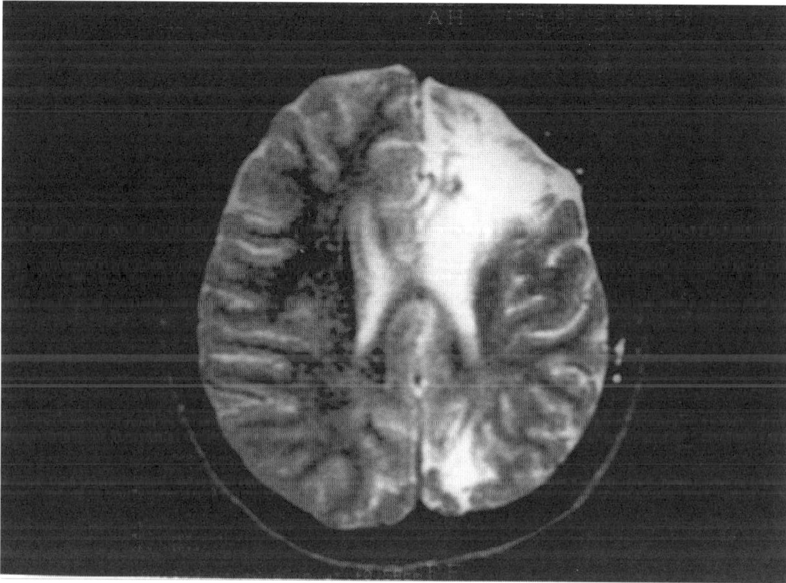

Figure 61c.

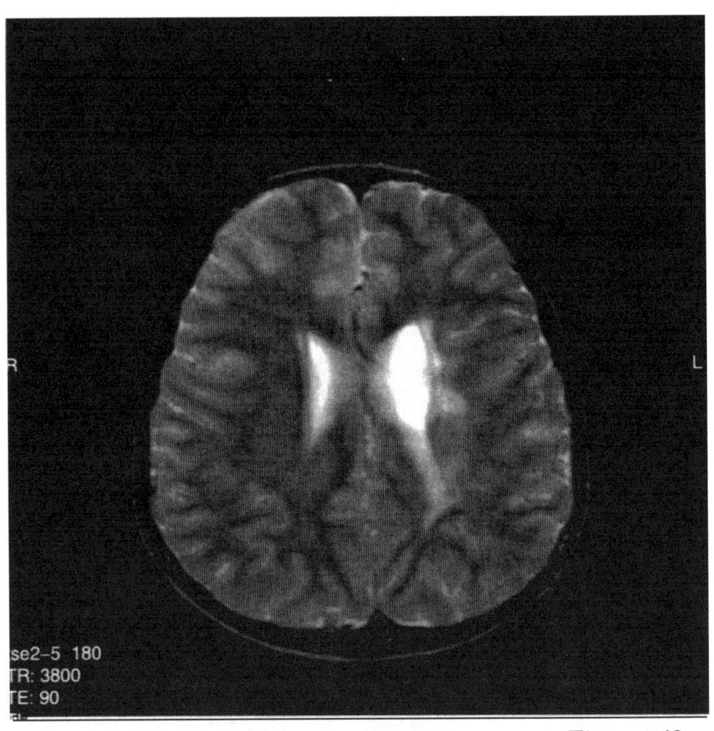

Figure 62a.

Figure 62 a-d. **Unilateral periventricular leukomalacia.** 10-year-old boy. T2W MR image reveals high-signal gliotic changes next to the slightly dilated left lateral ventricle (a). Sagittal, FLAIR image reveals gliosis to better advantage (b). The middle part of the body of corpus callosum is thinned due to the ischemic process leading to periventricular leukomalacia (c). ADC map reveals high ADC values: 2.02 and 1.69 $X10^{-3}$ mm^2/sec from the gliotic areas, compared to the normal contralateral periventricular region: 0.74 $X10^{-3}$ mm^2/sec. This suggests that tissue integrity is loosened in gliotic tissue associated with increased motion of water molecules, compared to normal parenchyma. ADC value of CSF is shown: 3.05 $X10^{-3}$ mm^2/sec (d).

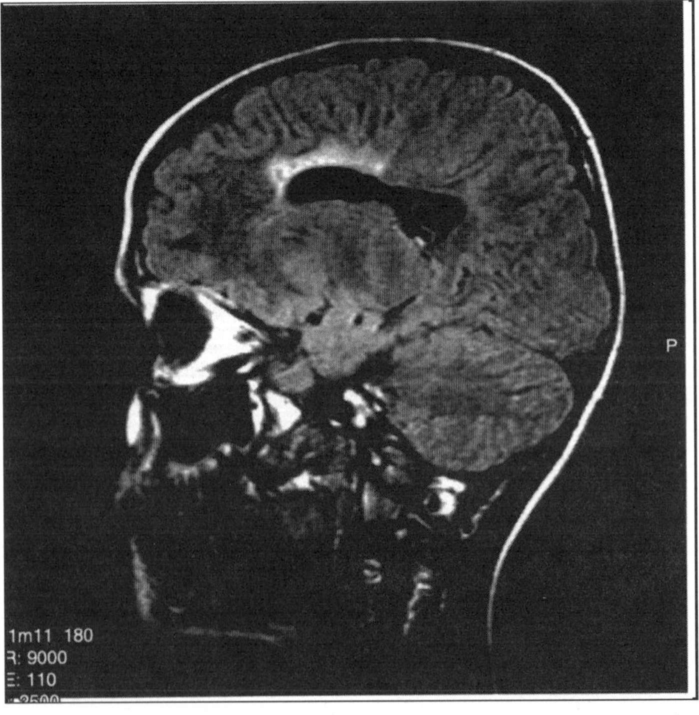

Figure 62b.

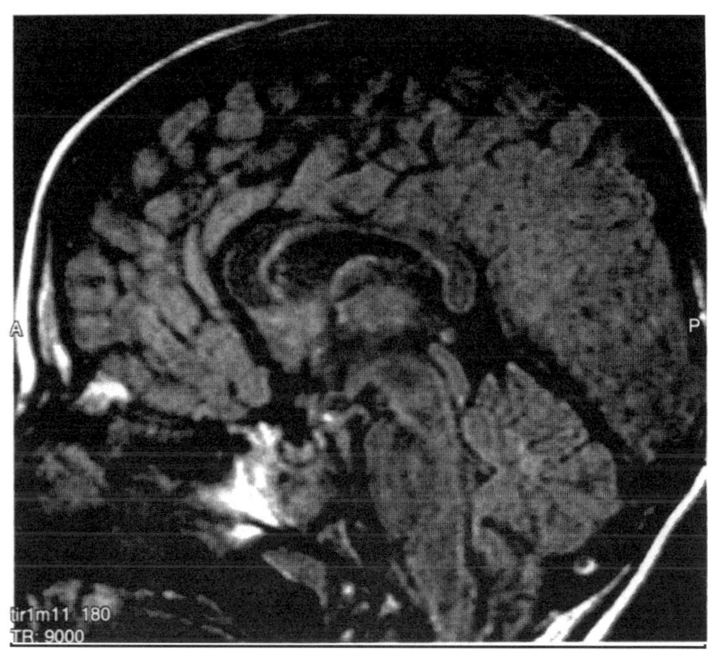

Figure 62c.

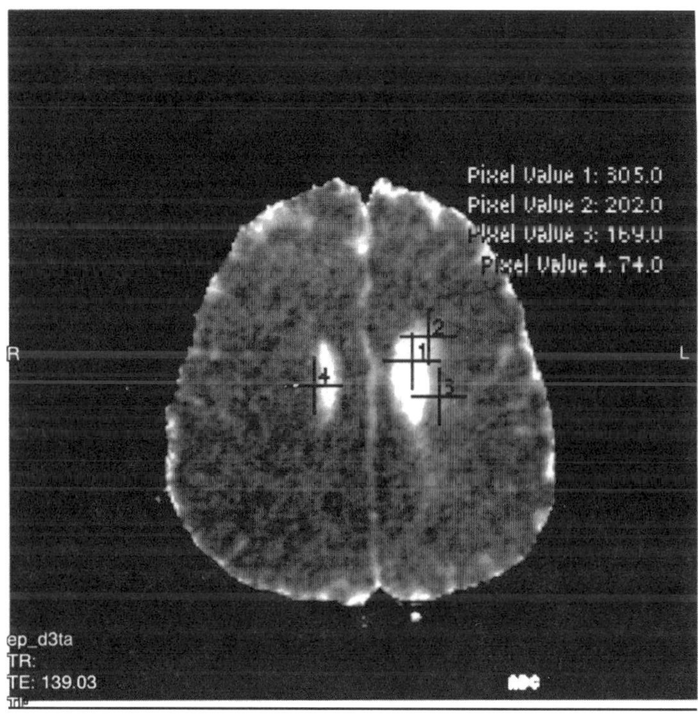

Figure 62d.

Figure 63 a, b. **Unilateral periventricular leukomalacia.** 15-year-old girl. *a) SE T1W, and b) SE PDW MR images.* A small region approximately at the junction of the genu and body has been thinned (arrow) (a). Accordingly, there is a subtle lesion in the left hemisphere due to periventricular leukomalacia (arrow) (b).

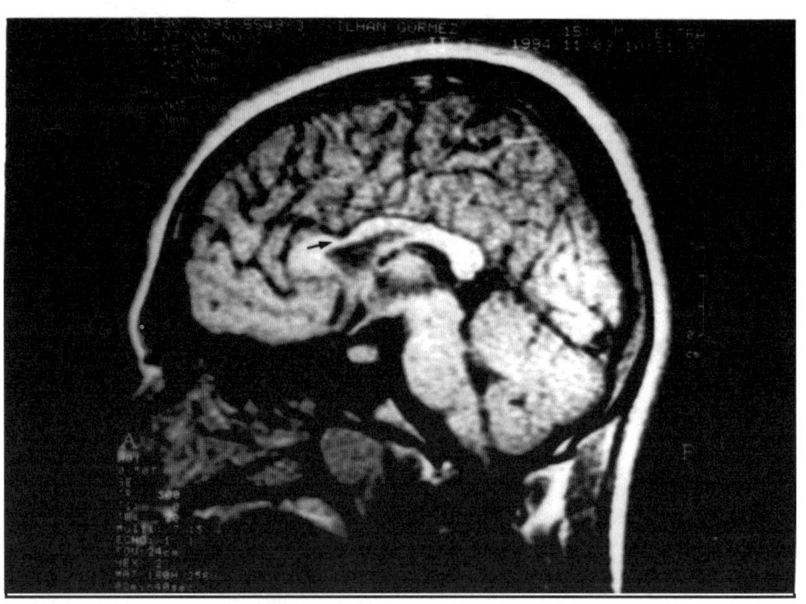

Figure 63a.

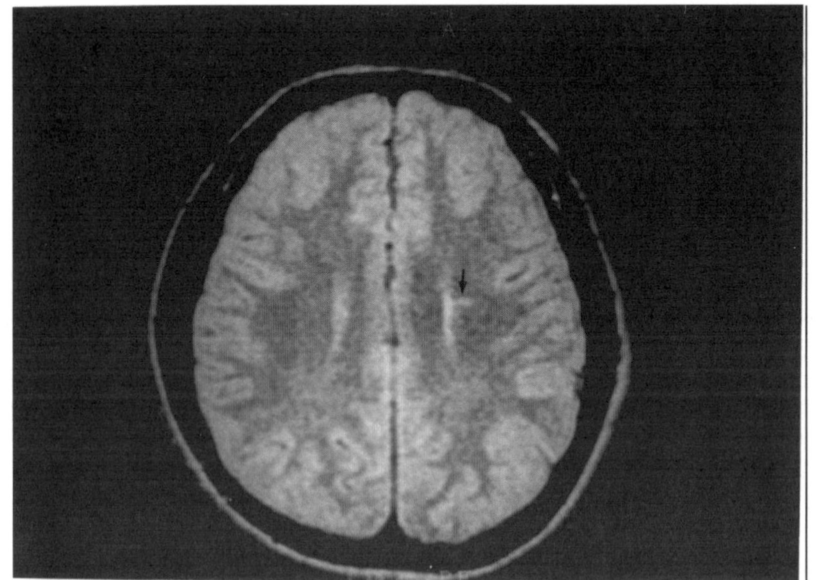

Figure 63b.

Reference
1. Truwit CL, Barkovich AJ, Koch TK, et al. Cerebral palsy: MR findings in 40 patients. AJNR 1992;13:67

Figure 64 a, b. **Bilateral periventricular leukomalacia.** 3-year-old girl. *a) SE T1W, and b) IR T1W MR images.* The corpus callosum has diffusely been destroyed (arrow) (a), and there is extensive parenchymal changes due to periventricular leukomalacia (b). Note a lipoma in the superior cerebellar cistern (a).

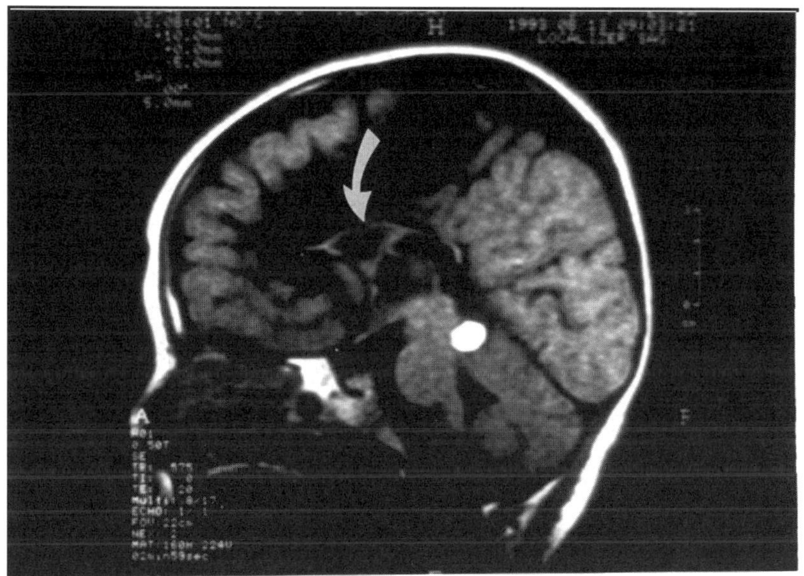

Figure 64a.

Reference
*1.   Truwit CL, Barkovich AJ, Koch TK, et al.
      Cerebral palsy: MR findings in 40
      patients. AJNR 1992;13:67*

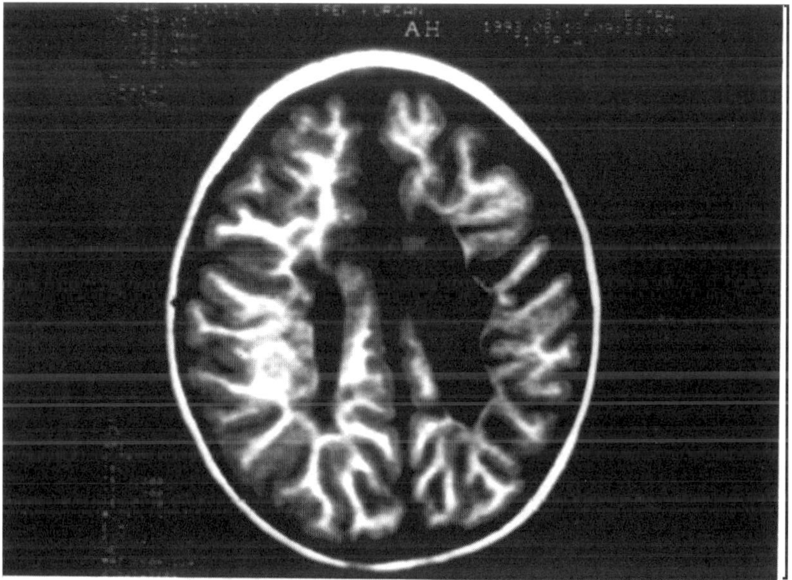

Figure 64b.

Figure 65a.

Figure 65 a-c. **Callosal thinning associated with periatrial gliosis.** 5-year-old boy. T1W image reveals apparent thinning of the posterior parts of the corpus callosum (a).

FLAIR image reveals bilateral high-signal changes in the periatrial regions. These could represent normally hypomyelinated regions of the white matter. However, in the setting of callosal changes and clinical correspondence (spasticity), these likely represent gliosis due to a perinatal ischemic lesion (b).

ADC map reveals high values in the gliotic regions: 1.20 and 1.16 X10^{-3} mm^2/sec. ADC values of the normal parenchyma are shown: 0.97 and 0.87 X10^{-3} mm^2/sec (c).

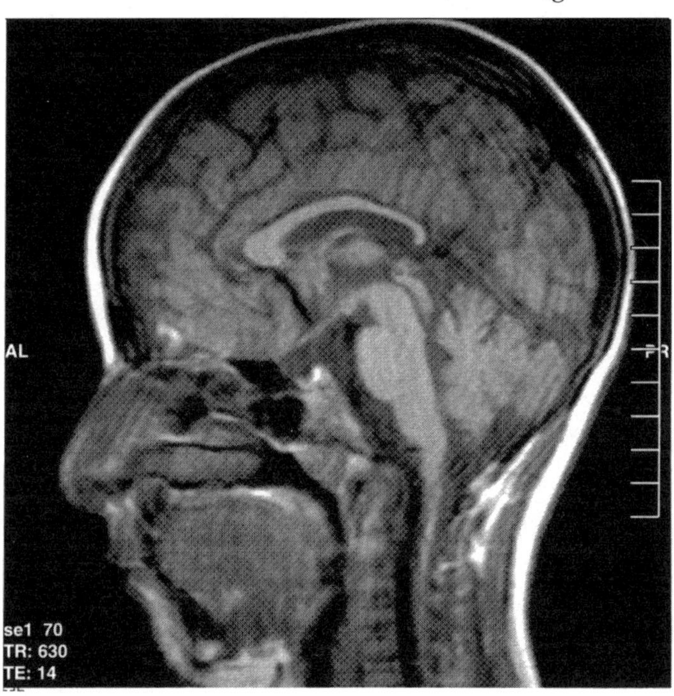

Figure 65b.

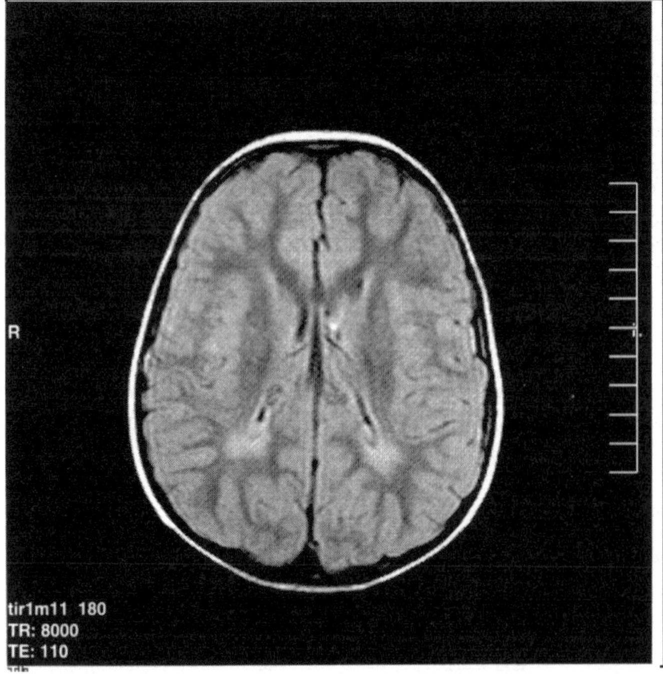

Figure 65c.

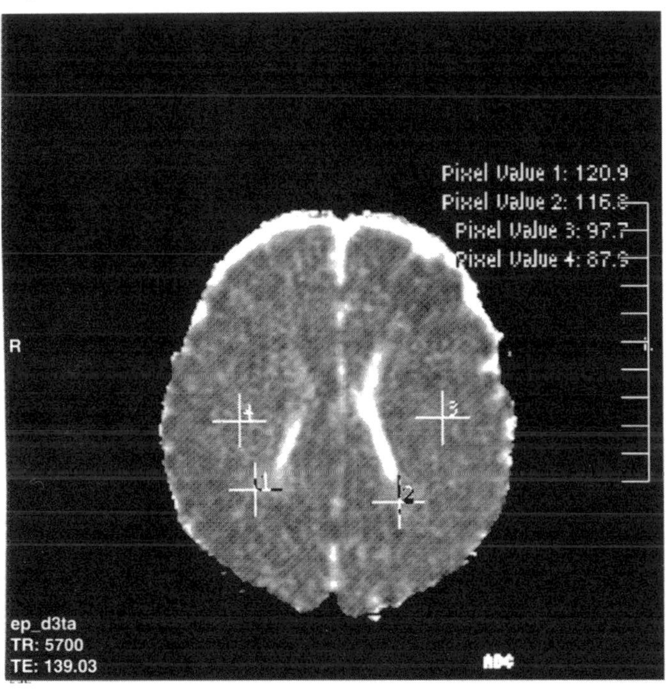

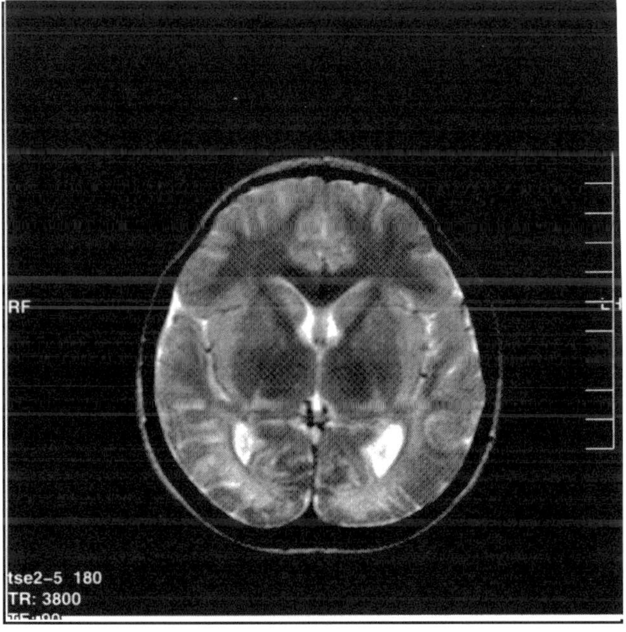

Figure 66a.

Figure 66 a-f. Longstanding hypoglisemic lesions. 4-year-old girl. T2W image reveals high signal in the occipital regions (a).

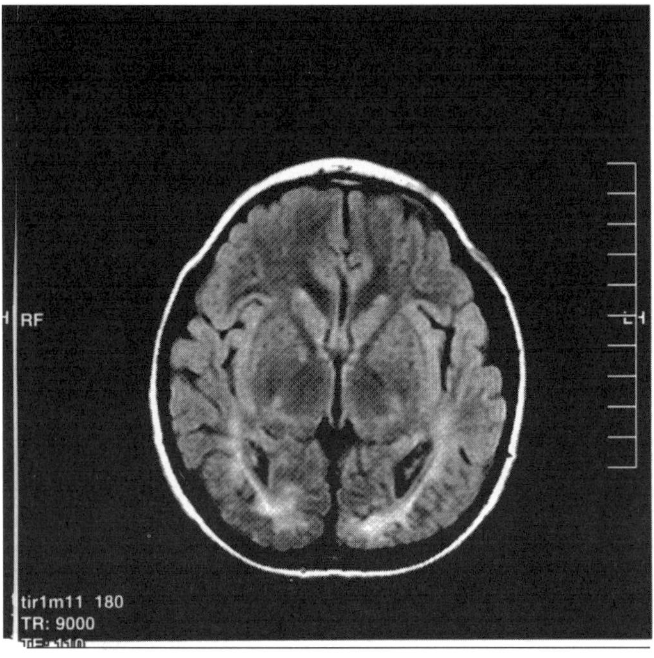

Figure 66b.

T1W image reveals thinning (destruction) in the posterior parts of the corpus callosum. Microcephaly is evident (c).

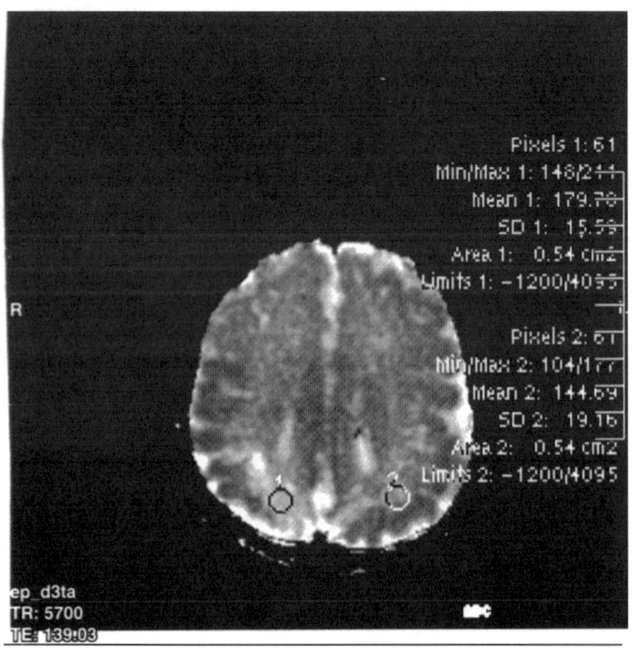

Figure 66d.

FLAIR image shows these as high signal changes, consistent with gliosis (b).

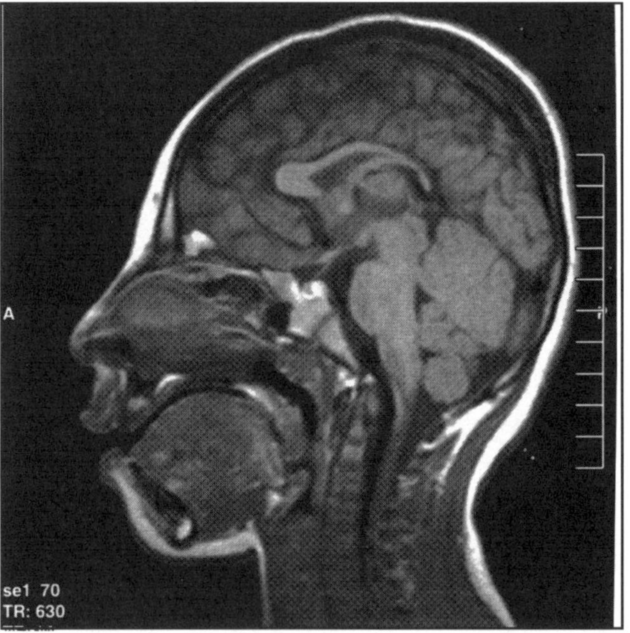

Figure 66c.

ADC map reveals high values (increased molecular motion) in these longstanding gliotic lesions: 1.79, and 1.44 X10^{-3} mm^2/sec (d).

ADC map again reveals a value of 1.87 $\times 10^{-3}$ mm^2/sec in the gliotic area. A higher than normal value is noted in the right frontal white matter: 1.18 $\times 10^{-3}$ mm^2/sec, secondary to retarded myelination (e). An ADC value of 1.89 $\times 10^{-3}$ mm^2/sec is shown in the gliotic area. The corpus callosum has similar high signal, hence high ADC value (arrow). Normal ADC value is shown from the right thalamus: 0.96 $\times 10^{-3}$ mm^2/sec (f).

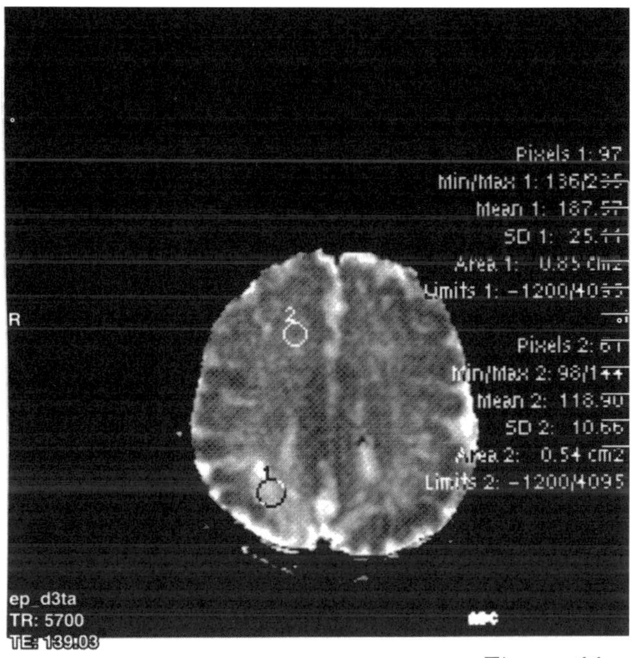

Figure 66e.

Reference
1   *Barkovich AJ. Pediatric neuroimaging
    Philadelphia, Lippincott Williams & Wilkins,
    2000*

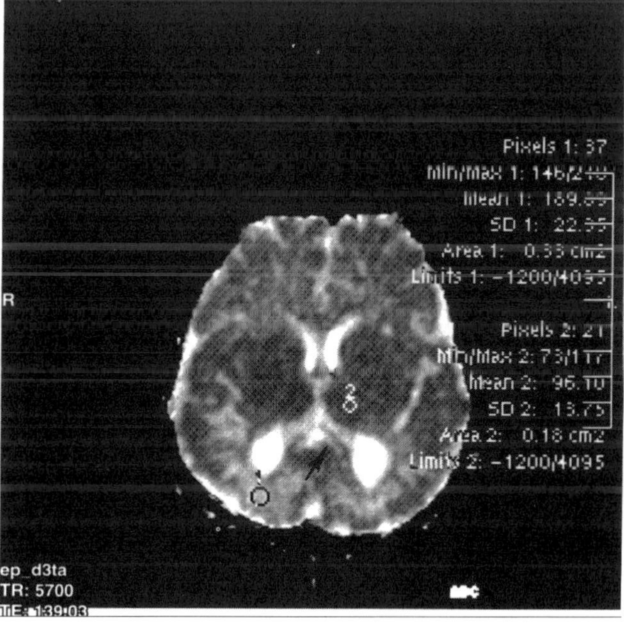

Figure 66f.

Figure 67 a-c. **Bilateral occipital porencephalic cavities.** 11-year-old girl. *a, b) SE T1W, and c) SE PDW MR images.* The caudal part of the corpus callosum (splenium) has been destroyed, and therefore it has an abnormal shape (arrow) (a). Axial images show bilateral porencephalic cavities (b, c). Note gliotic changes surrounding the cavities (arrows) (c).

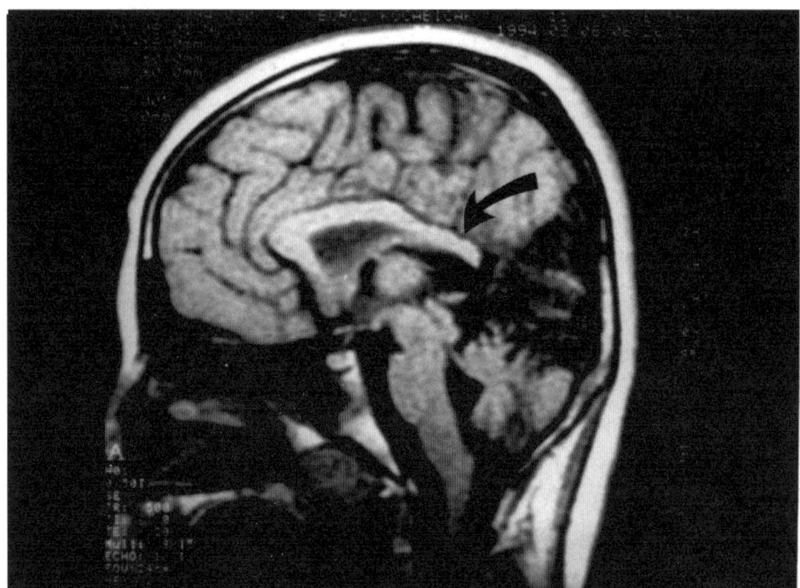

Figure 67a.

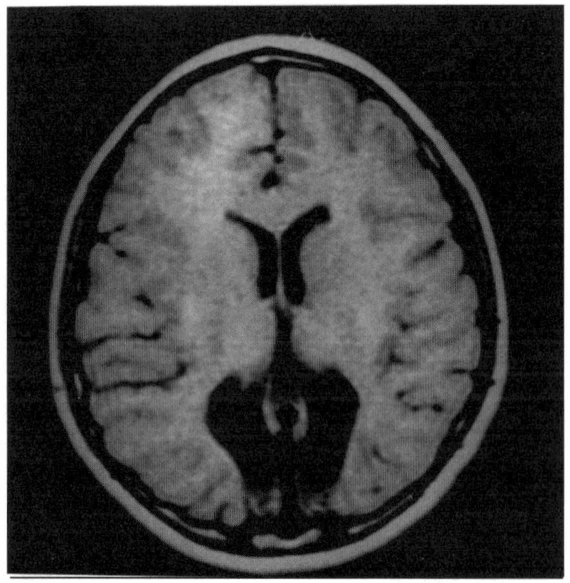

Figure 67b.

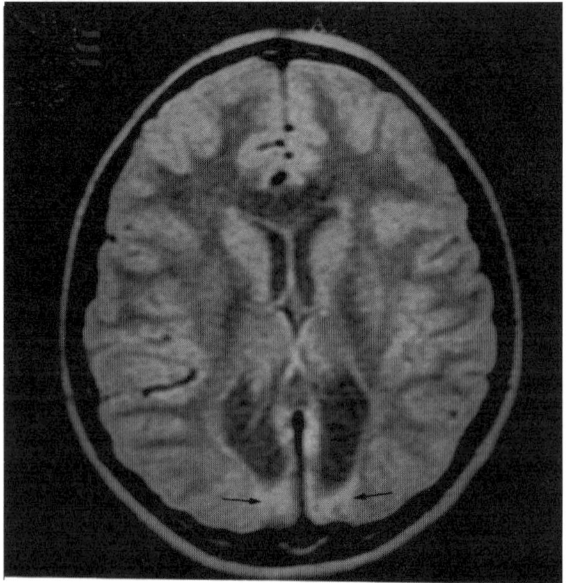

Figure 67c.

References

1.   *Truwit CL, Barkovich AJ, Koch TK, et al. Cerebral palsy: MR findings in 40 patients. AJNR 1992;13:67*
2.   *Osborn AG. Diagnostic neuroradiology. St. Louis, Mosby, 1994;54*
3.   *Barkovich AJ. Pediatric neuroimaging. New York, Raven Press, 1995;107*

Figure 68 a-c. **Occipital porencephalic cavity.** 8-year-old girl. *a, b) SE T1W, and c) SE T2W MR images.* The isthmus and the proximal part of the splenium show destruction. There is a large porencephalic cavity extending from the ventricle to the meninges (P). Also note the colpocephalic change (cc) of the left lateral ventricle (b, c).

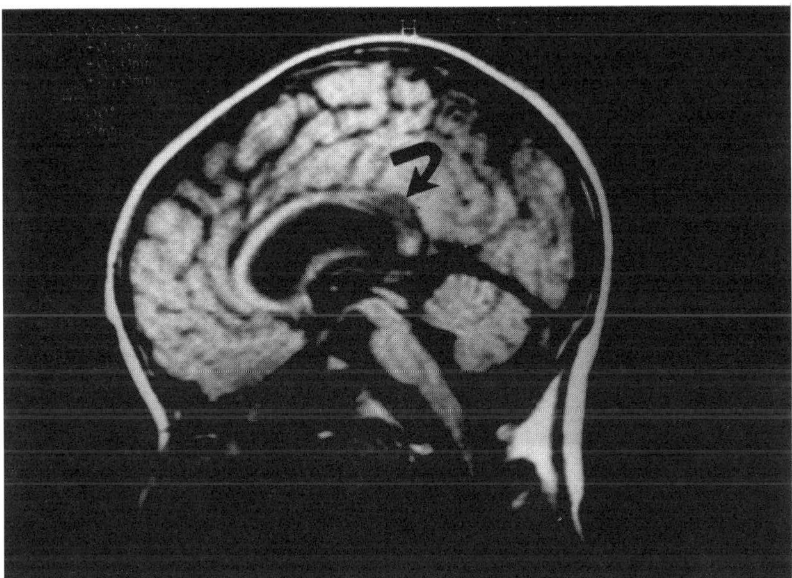

Figure 68a.

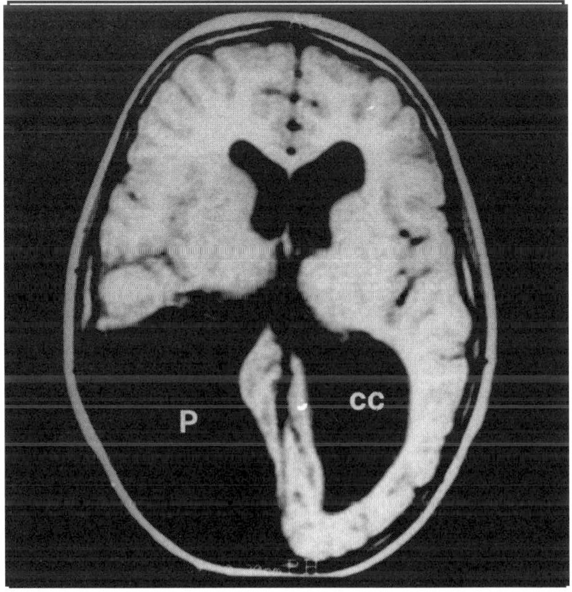

Figure 68b.

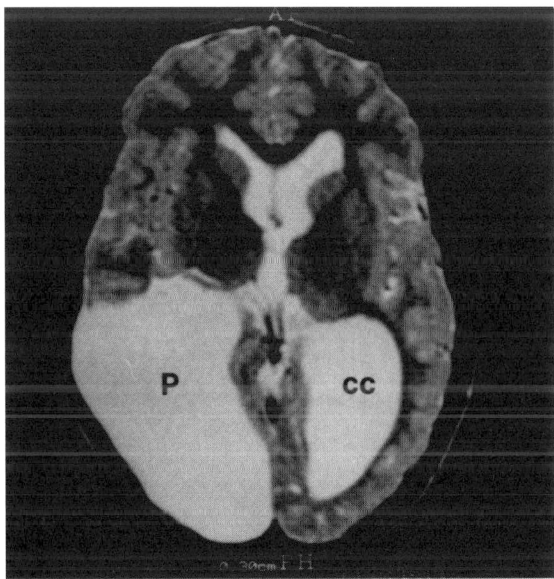

Figure 68c.

References
1. *Truwit CL, Barkovich AJ, Koch TK, et al. Cerebral palsy: MR findings in 40 patients. AJNR 1992;13:67*
2. *Osborn AG. Diagnostic neuroradiology. St. Louis, Mosby, 1994;54*
3. *Barkovich AJ. Pediatric neuroimaging. New York, Raven Press, 1995;107*

Lesions directly involving the corpus callosum

Figure 69 a-d. **Frontal porencephalic cavity.** 11-year-old girl. *a, b) SE T1W, c) SE PDW, and d) SE T2W MR images.* The body of the corpus callosum is very thin (arrow) (a). The condition is associated with a large frontal porencephalic cavity (P) (c, d, e). Note the surrounding gliosis manifesting as an hyperintense change (c, d).

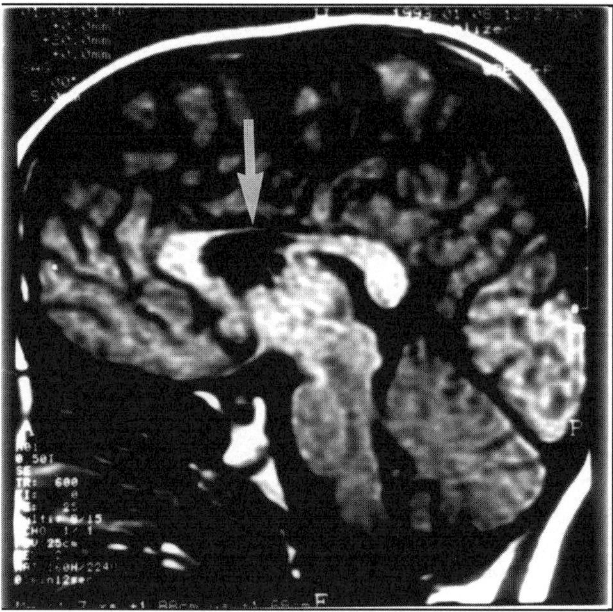

Figure 69a.

References
1. Truwit CL, Barkovich AJ, Koch TK, et al. Cerebral palsy: MR findings in 40 patients. AJNR 1992;13:67
2. Osborn AG. Diagnostic neuro-radiology. St. Louis, Mosby, 1994;54
3. Barkovich AJ. Pediatric neuro-imaging. New York, Raven Press, 1995;107

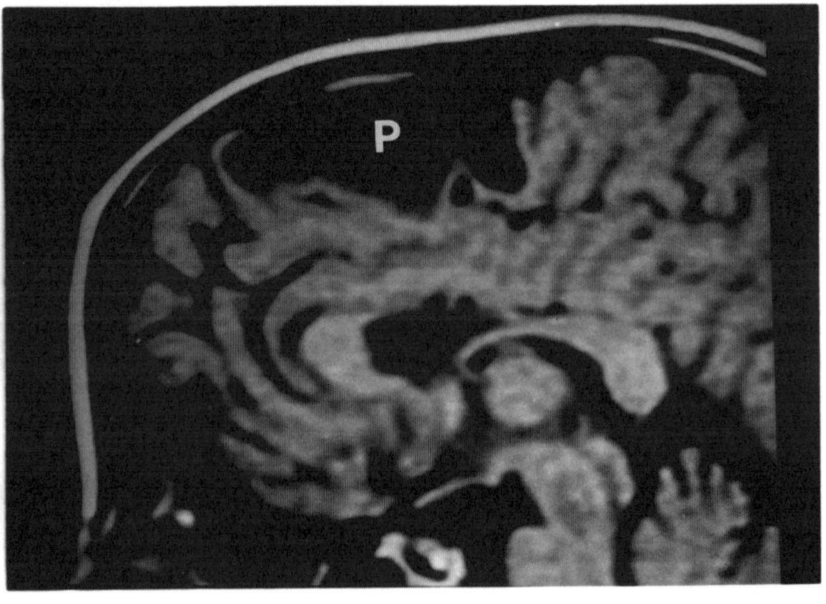

Figure 69b.

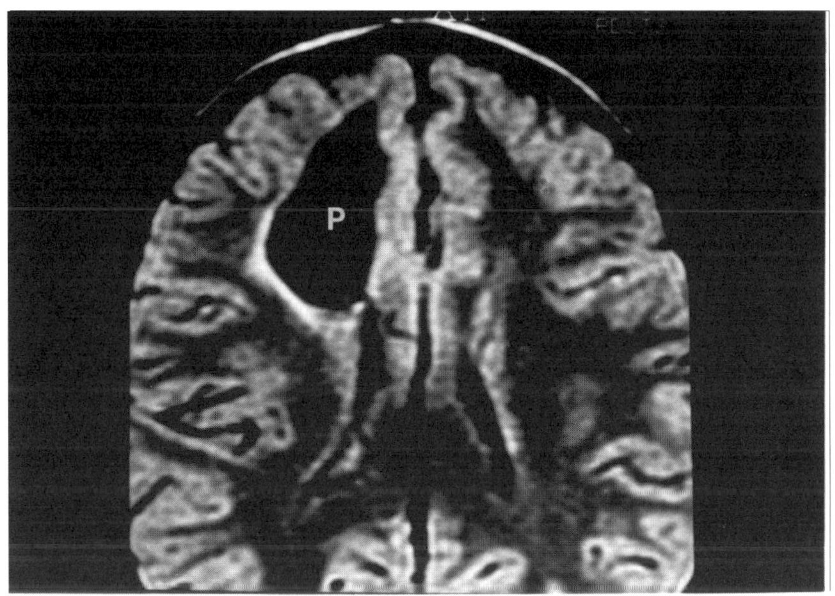

Figure 69c.

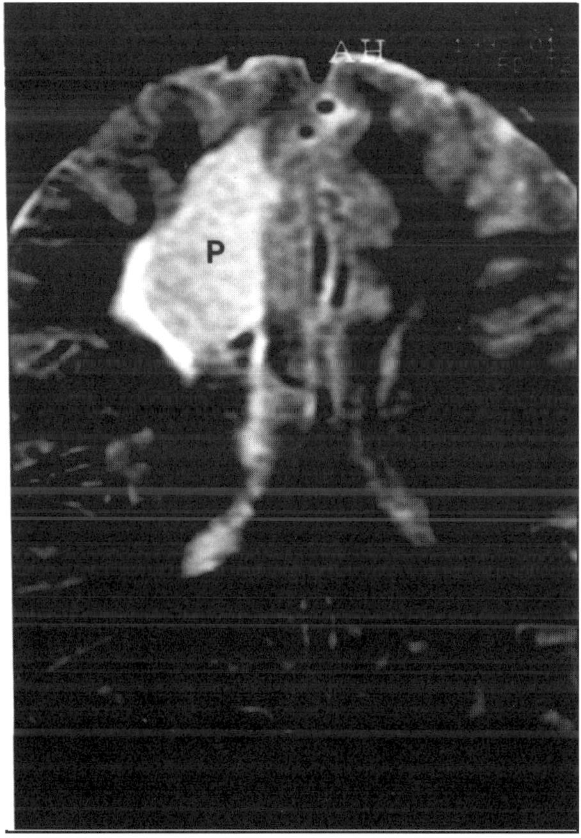

Figure 69d.

Figure 70 a-c. **Cerebral hemiatrophy.** 9-year-old boy. T1W image reveals destruction of the left hemisphere associated with passive dilatation of the lateral ventricle (a). FLAIR image reveals gliosis with apparent high signal (b). PSIF image (anisotropic diffusion sequence) shows high signal in the left hemisphere compared to the normal contralateral side. The left part of the corpus callosum is very thin (arrow) due to destruction from the perinatal ischemic condition causing cerebral hemiatrophy (c).

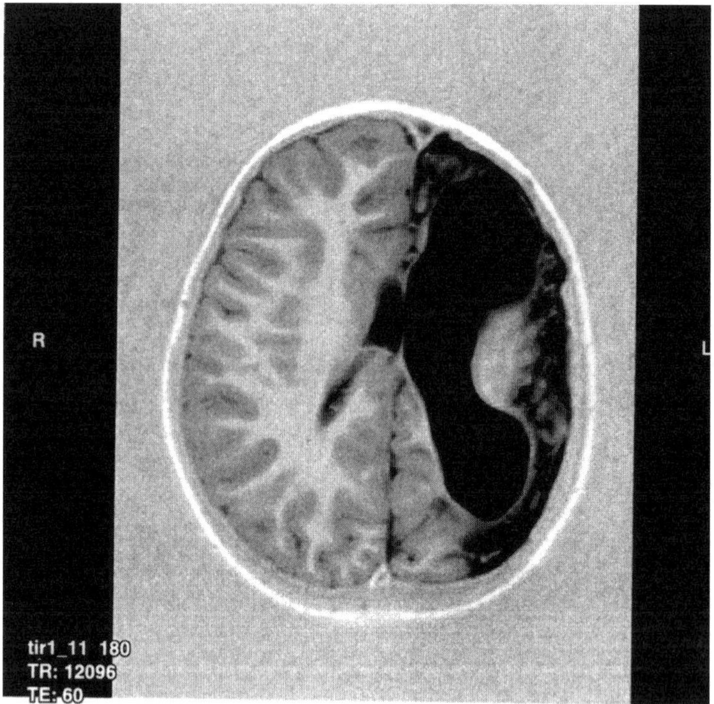

Figure 70a.

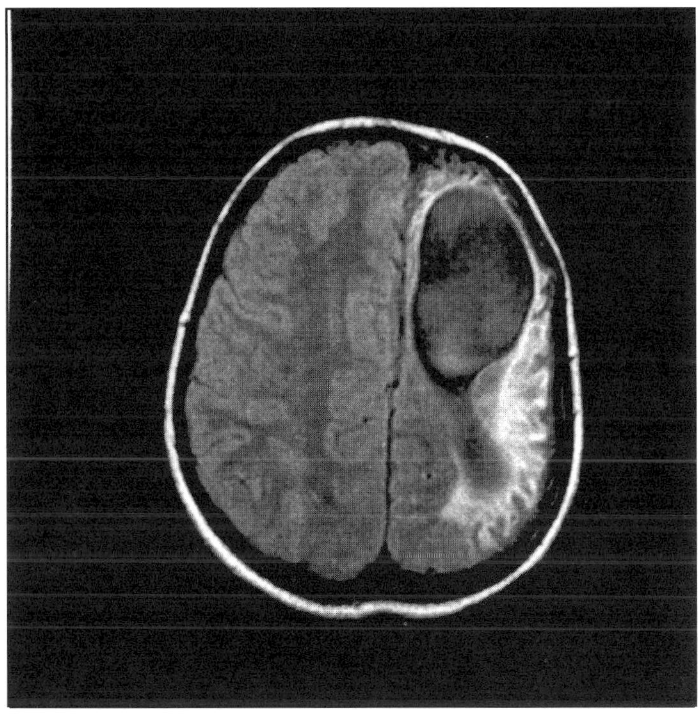

Figure 70b.

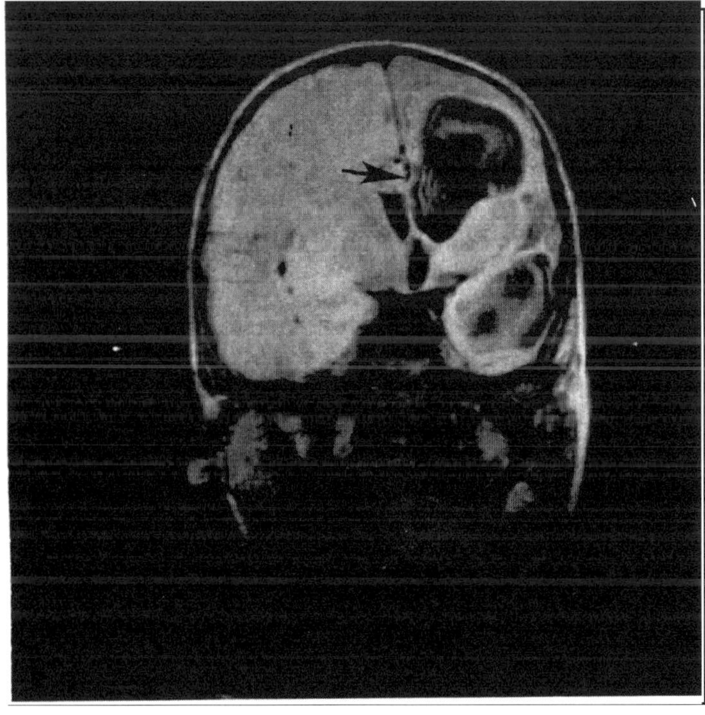

Figure 70c.

Figure 71 a, b. **Hydranencephaly (a partial form).** 14-month-old boy with congenital CMV infection. *a) SE T1W, and b) SE PDW MR images.* The parietal, temporal, and most of the frontal poles are absent (a, b). The body of the corpus callosum is very thin compared with the genu and splenium (arrow) (a), suggesting a widespread intrauterine ischemic event after the corpus callosum has been fully developed. This condition represents a partial form of hydranencephaly. The classical form of hydranencephaly is a global encephaloclastic disorder in which most of the cerebral hemispheres have been destroyed and replaced by membraneous sacs (leptomeninges) filled with CSF. The condition is considered to develop in the third to sixth months of gestation.

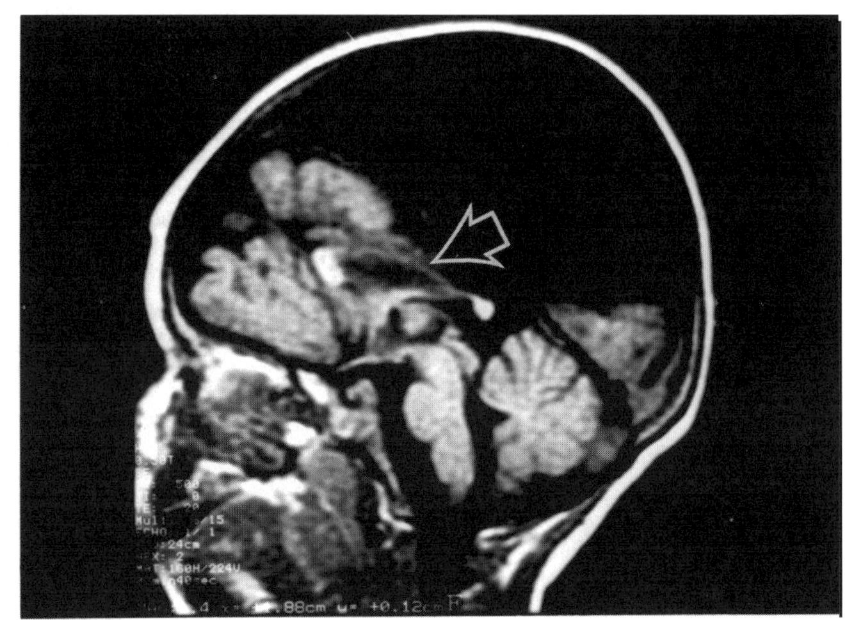

Figure 71a.

References
1. *Friede RL, Mikolasek J. Postencephalitic porencephaly, hydranencephaly or polymicrogyria. A review. Acta Neuropathol 1978;43:161*
2. *Barkovich AJ. Pediatric neuroimaging. New York, Raven, 1995;109*
3. *Halsey J, Allen N, Chamberlein HR. The morphogenesis of hydranencephaly. J Neurol Sci 1971;12:187*

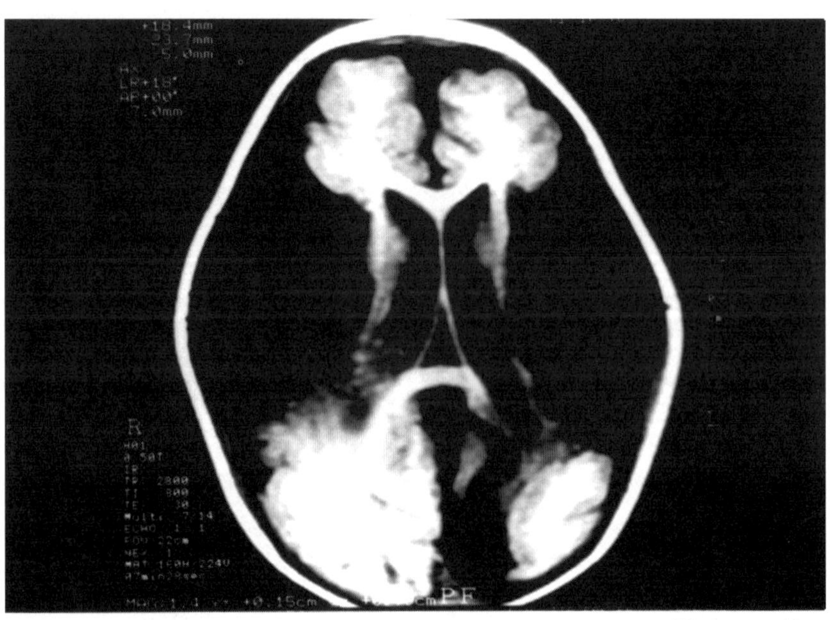

Figure 71b.

Figure 72 a, b. **Growing skull fracture.** 12-year-old girl. *a) and b) SE T1W MR images.* There is a porencephalic cavity (P) (a, b) and a growing skull fracture at the region of the anterior fontanelle (curved arrows) (b). Note that the corpus callosum has been extremely diminished in size and thickness (arrows) (a). The lateral ventricles are dilated. The condition occurred due to a birth trauma resulting in a dural tear, and a poren-cephalic cavity, leading to the growing skull fracture up to this age.

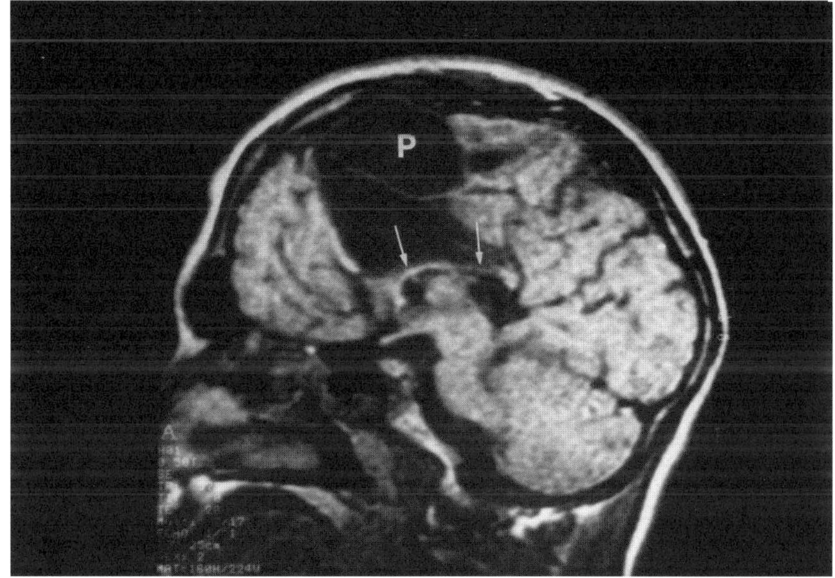

Figure 72a.

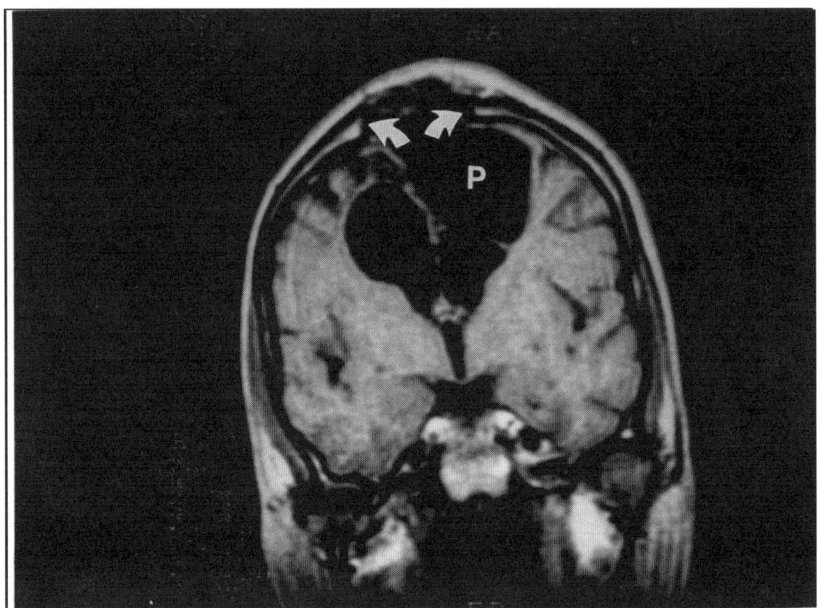

Figure 72b.

References
1. *Numerow LM, Krcek JP, Wallace CJ, et al. Growing skull fracture simulating a rounded lytic calvarial lesion. AJNR 1991;12:783*
2. *Kashiwagi S, Abiko S, Aoki H. Growing skull fracture in childhood. A recurrent case treated by shunt operation. Surg Neurol 1986;26:63*
3. *Tandon PN, Banerji AK, Bhatia R, et al. Cranio-cerebral erosion (growing fracture of the skull in children) Acta neurochir (Wien) 1987;88:1*

LESIONS DIRECTLY INVOLVING THE CORPUS CALLOSUM

INTRACALLOSAL LESIONS

Figure 73 a-f. **Intracallosal cyst.** 1-year-old boy. *a) SE T1W, b) SE PDW, and c) SE T2W MR images. Follow-up examination (two months later): d) SE T1W, e) SE PDW, and f) SE T2W MR images.* There is a cystic structure confined to the anterior part of the body of the corpus callosum, and its signal pattern follows that of cerebrospinal fluid (CSF) throughout the MR imaging sequences, suggesting that this is a true intracallosal cyst (arrows) (a-c). This cyst may be embryonic in origin or may be due to an acquired disorder such as traumatic laceration of the corpus callosum. On a follow-up MR imaging examination two months later, massive intracystic hemorrhage was detected, showing bright signal (arrow) (d). Note that the signal of the hemorrhagic products is also bright on the PDW (e) and T2W MR images (f) (circles), suggesting presence of extracellular methemoglobin, a subacute phase hemorrhagic product. This hemorrhagic condition was spontaneously resolved leaving behind an intracallosal cavity similar to that seen in the figures a, b and c (from reference 2). On the other hand, Marchiafava-Bignami disease, a demyelinating disorder which is believed to be caused by a toxin found in various alcoholic beverages, may show a similar intracallosal location, however, the signal pattern of the lesions in that disease does not follow that of CSF, and show a high-signal on SE proton density-weighted, and on T2W MR images, consistent with a demyelinating lesion.

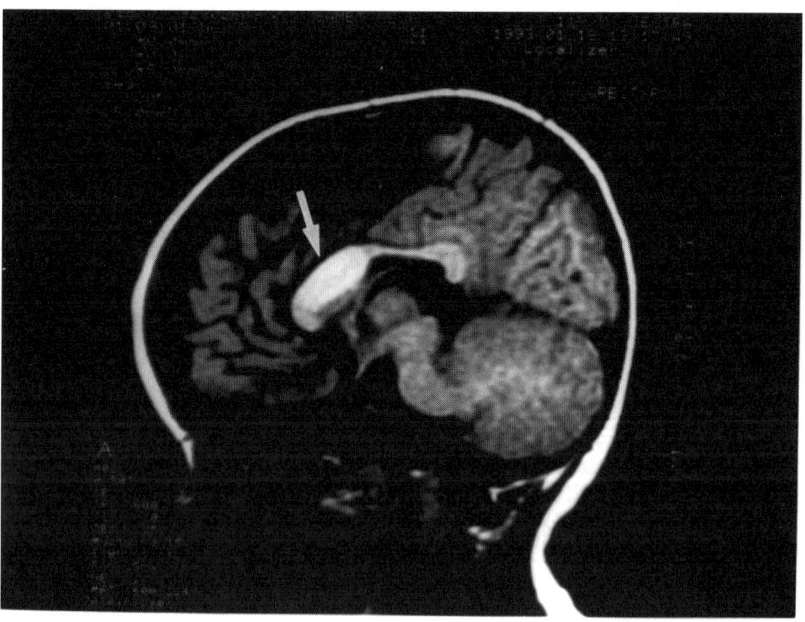

Figure 73a.

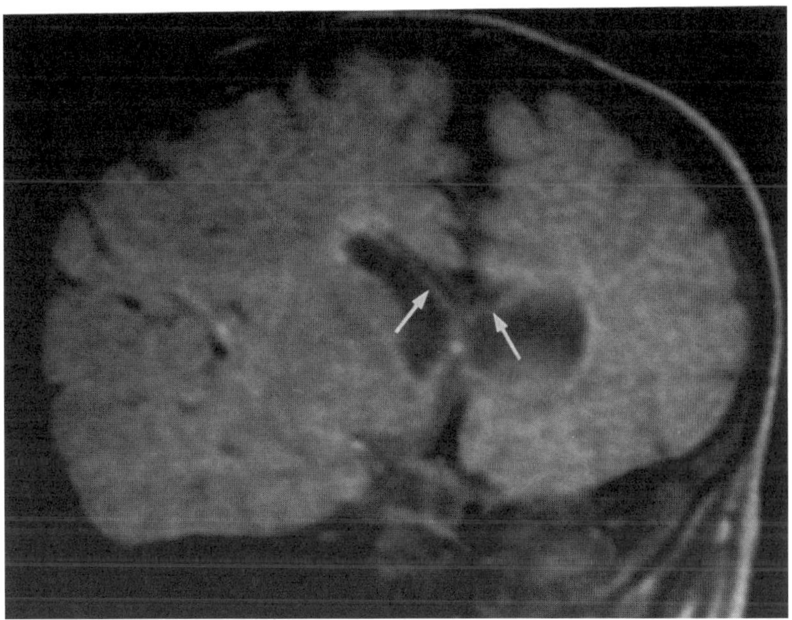

Figure 73b.

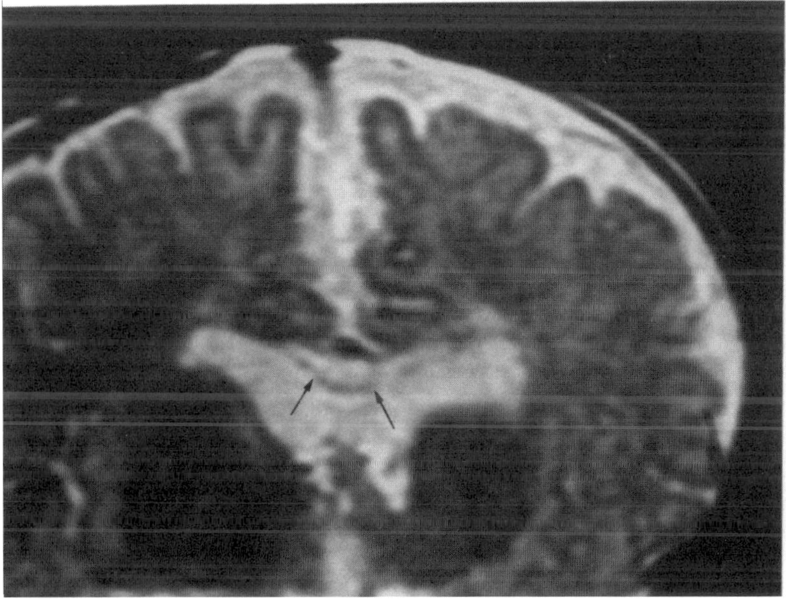

Figure 73c.

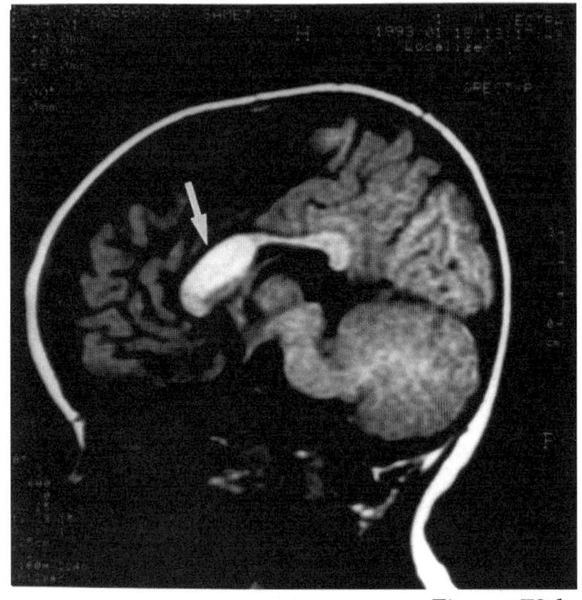

Figure 73d.

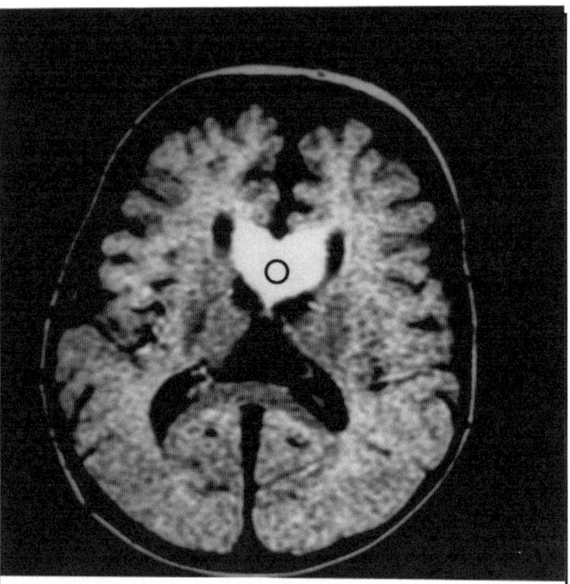

Figure 73e.

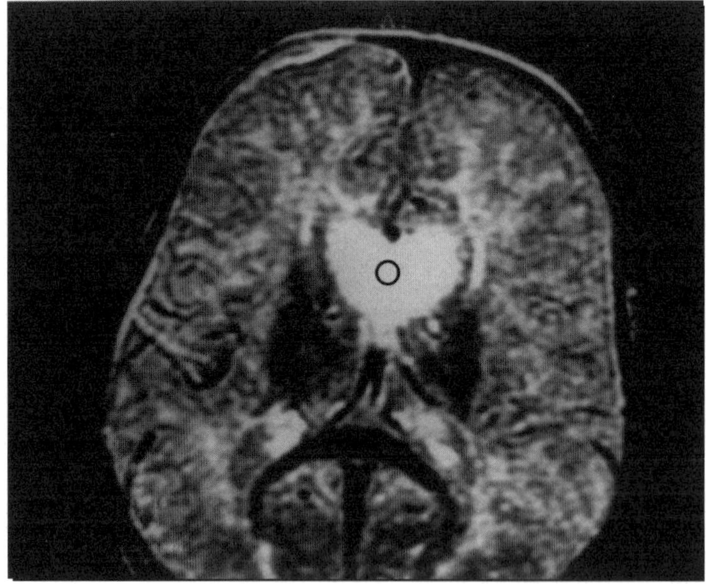

Figure 73f.

References
1. Besenski N, Jadro-Santel D, Grcevic N. Patterns of lesions of corpus callosum in inner cerebral trauma visualized by computed tomography. Neuroradiology 1992;34:126
2. Sener RN. Intracallosal cyst: MR demonstration. AJR 1994; 163:228
3. Osborn AG. Diagnostic neuroradiology. St. Louis, Mosby, 1994;763

Figure 74. **Posttraumatic callosal lacuna.** 15-year-old boy. *SE T1W MR image.* There is a lacuna located at the isthmus of the corpus callosum (arrow). The condition was a part of the lesions due to a posttraumatic shearing injury of the brain.

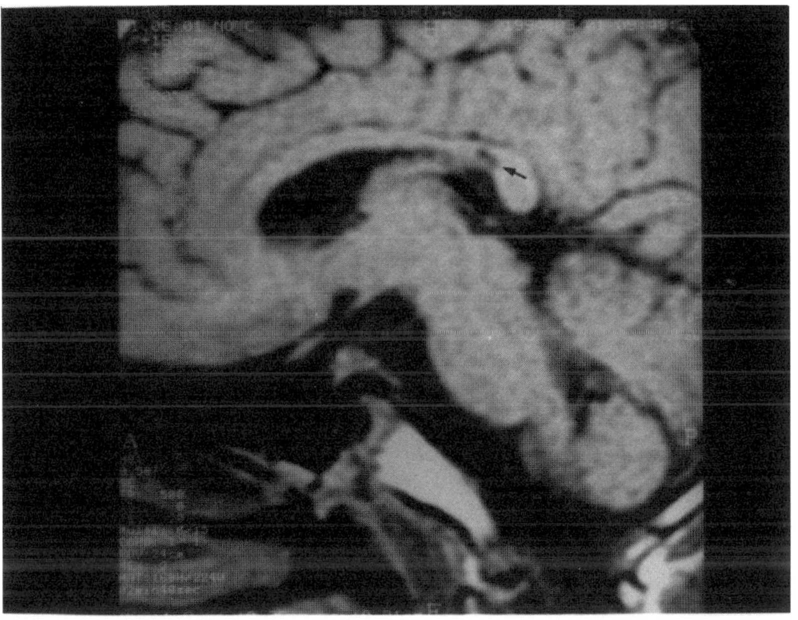

Figure 74.

Reference
1. Besenski N, Jadro-Santel D, Grcevic N. Patterns of lesions of corpus callosum in inner cerebral trauma visualized by computed tomography. Neuroradiology 1992;34:126

Figure 75 a,b. **Posttraumatic callosal destruction.** 3-year-old boy. CT scan reveals hemorrhage and surrounding edema (a). T1W image reveals that most of the corpus callosum is involved and destroyed by the condition (b).

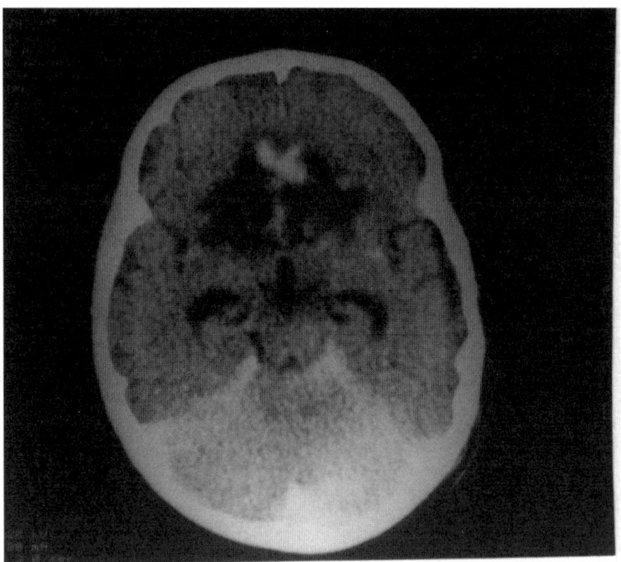

Figure 75a.

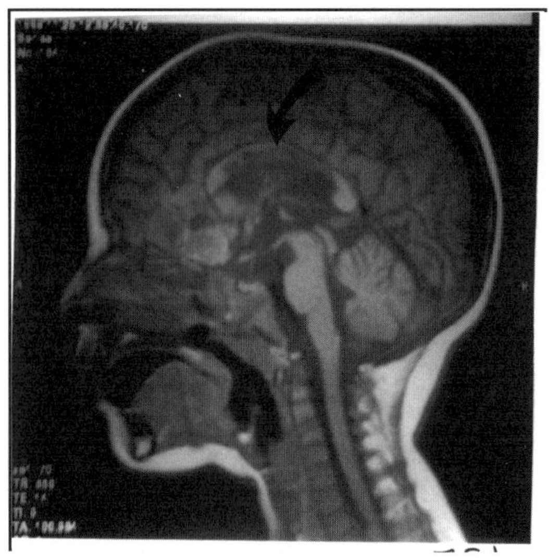

Figure 75b.

Figure 76 a-c. **Callosotomy for epilepsy.** 7-year-old girl. FLAIR image reveals presence of anatomic distortion and high signal in the left medial temporal region (arrow) (a).

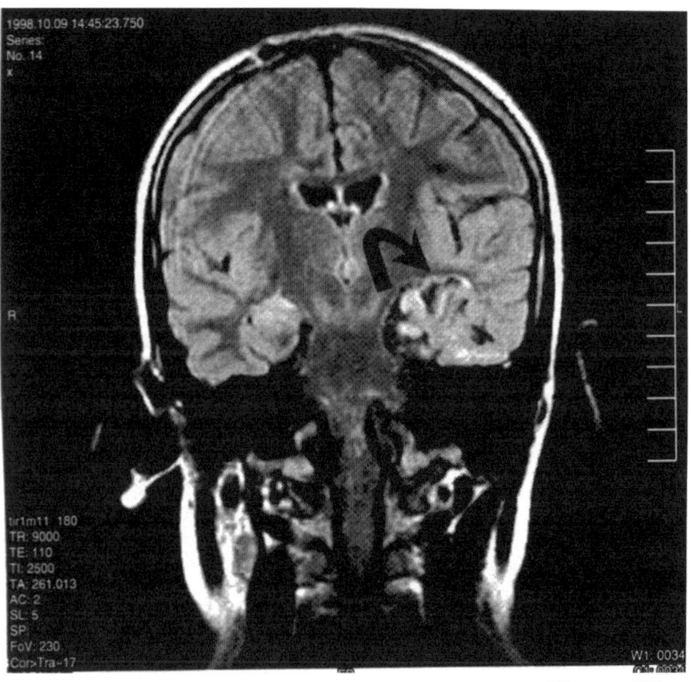

Figure 76a.

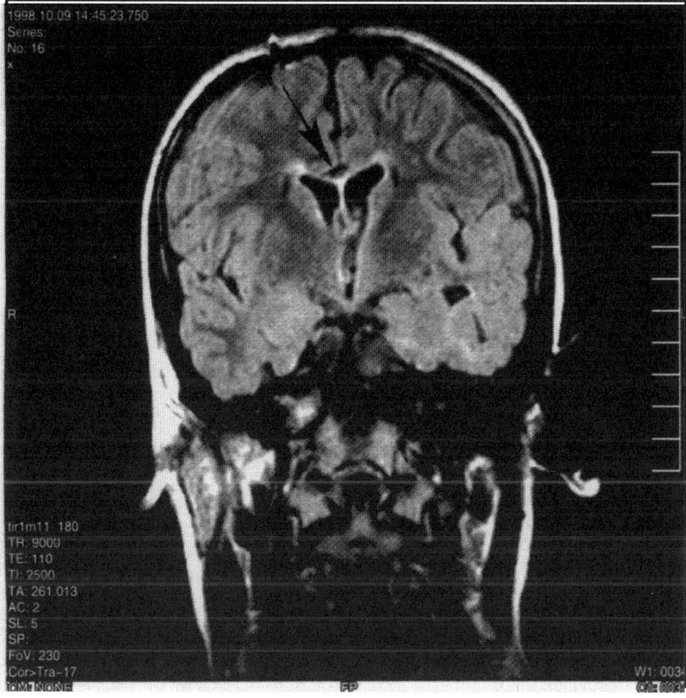

Figure 76b.

FLAIR image reveals a surgical defect in the corpus callosum (callosotomy) performed for intractable seizures (arrow) (b). Postsurgical defect is shown on T1W (turbo inversion recovery) image (arrow) (c).

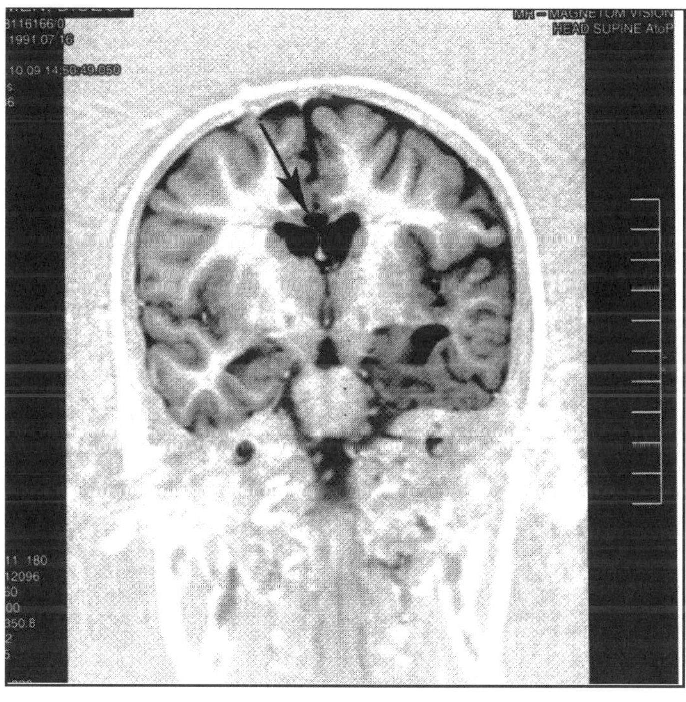

Figure 76c.

Figure 77 a, b. **Callosal irregularity** (associated with a longstanding intraventricular shunt tube for hydrocephalus). 12-year-old boy. *a) SE T1W, and b) IR T1W MR images.* The upper border of the corpus callosum shows widespread irregularity (arrows) (a). Axial image shows irregularity of the genu (small arrows), as well as the septum pellucidum (large arrow) (b). These changes were attributed to the effects of the longstanding shunt tube. Note thickening of the subcutaneous tissue at the occipital region, corresponding to the trace of the shunt tube.

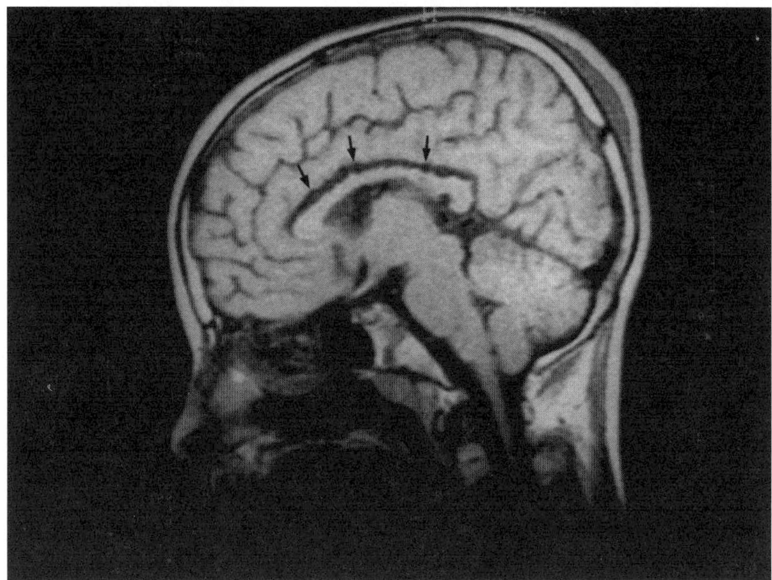

Figure 77a.

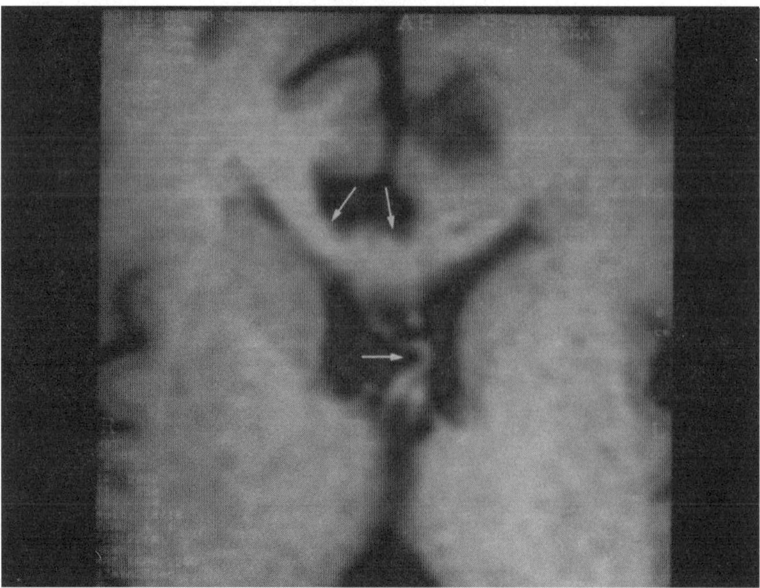

Figure 77b.

Figure 78 a, b. **Callosal irregularity** (associated with an arteriovenous malformation). 16-year-old girl. *a) SE T1W, and b) MR angiography (three dimensional time-of-flight) MR images.* Indentations at the upper border of the corpus callosum are noted (arrows) (a), created by the enlarged vessels of the extensive arteriovenous malformation (arrows) (b).

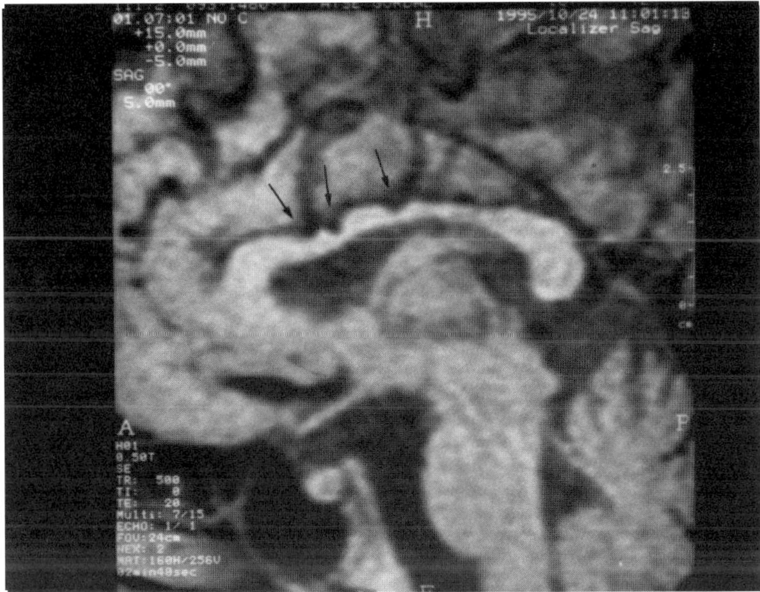

Figure 78a.

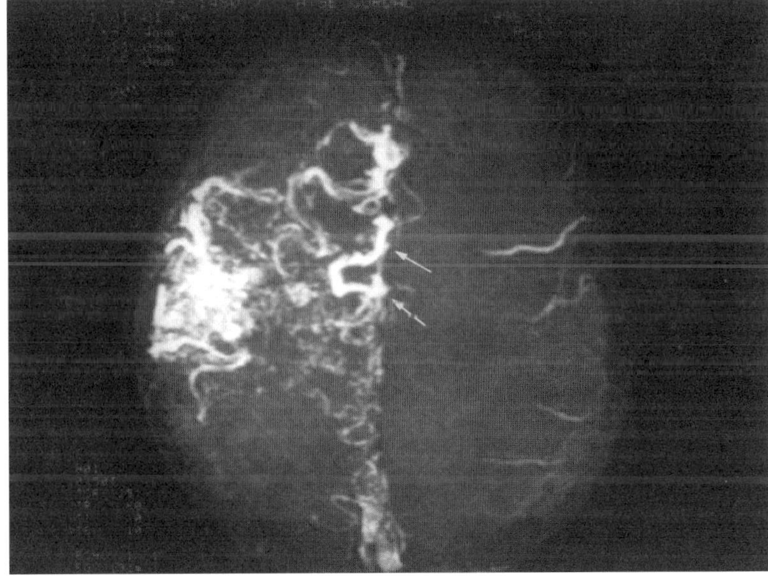

Figure 78b.

Figure 79 a-c. **Multiple sclerosis.** 28-year-old woman. *a, b and c) SE T2W MR images.* There are multiple demyelinating lesions in the cerebral parenchyma (a). Involvement of the corpus callosum is an expected feature in multiple sclerosis, manifesting as callosal lesions (arrows) (b), and callosal thinning (c). (case courtesy of Dr. M. Uygur, Izmir).

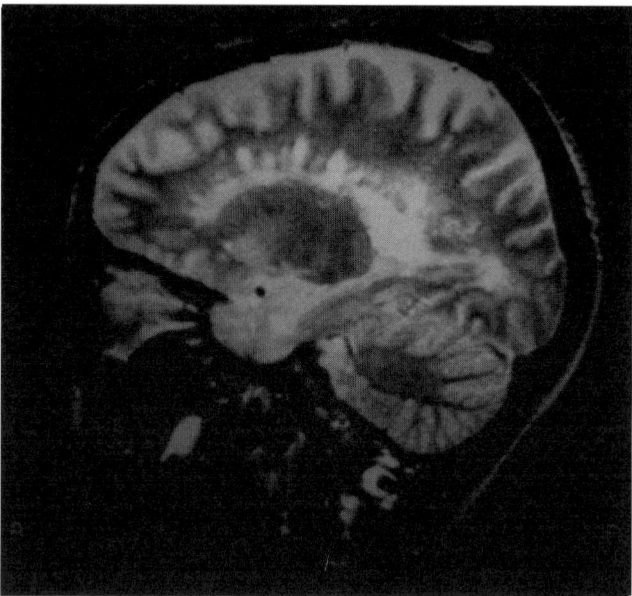

Figure 79a.

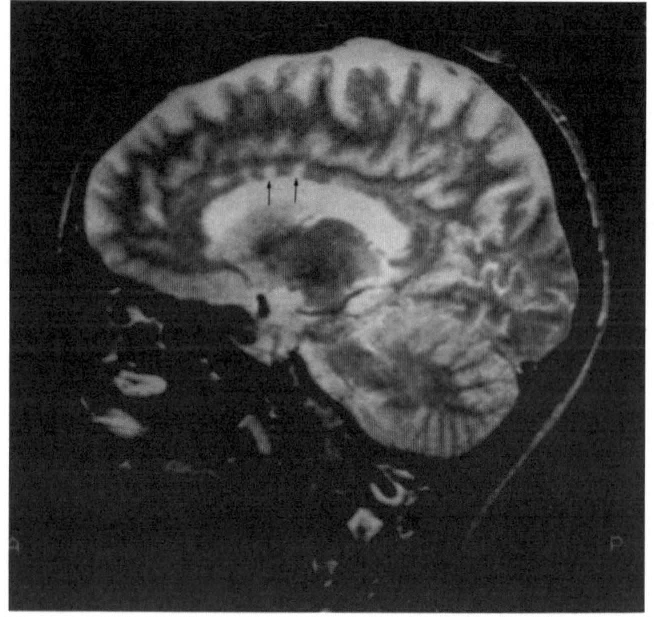

Figure 79b.

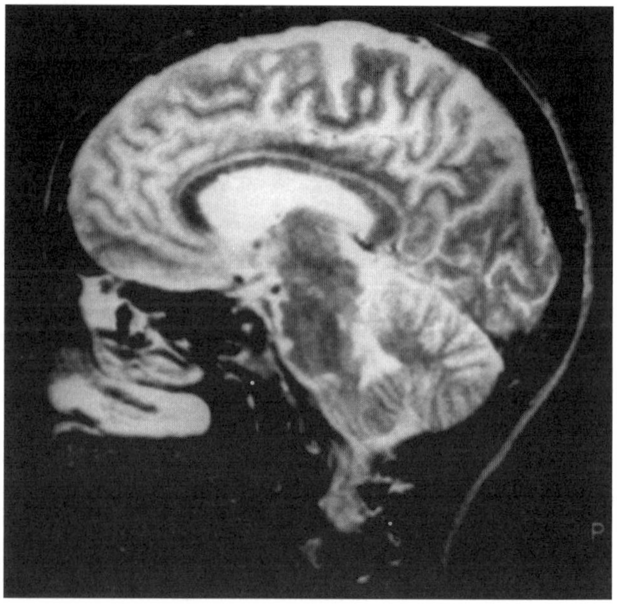

Figure 79c.

Reference
1.   *Osborn AG. Diagnostic neuroradiology. St. Louis, Mosby, 1994;755*

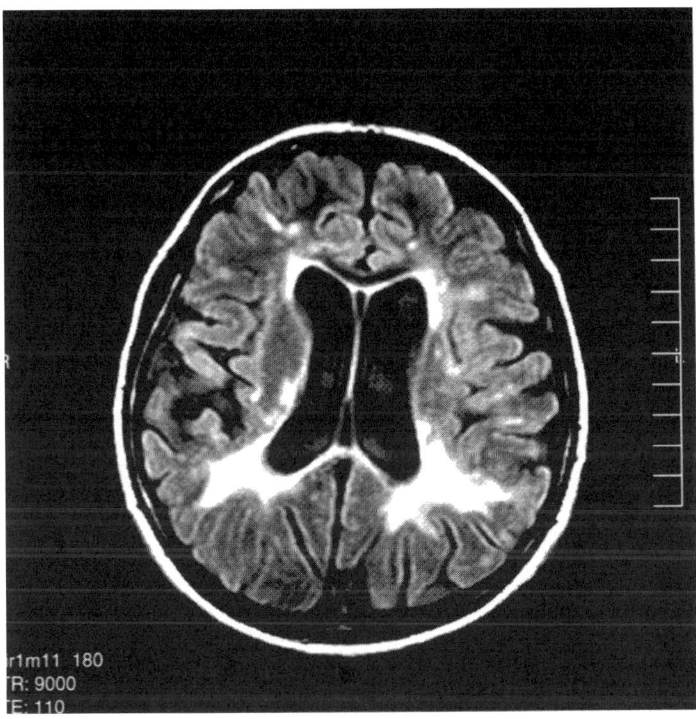

Figure 80a.

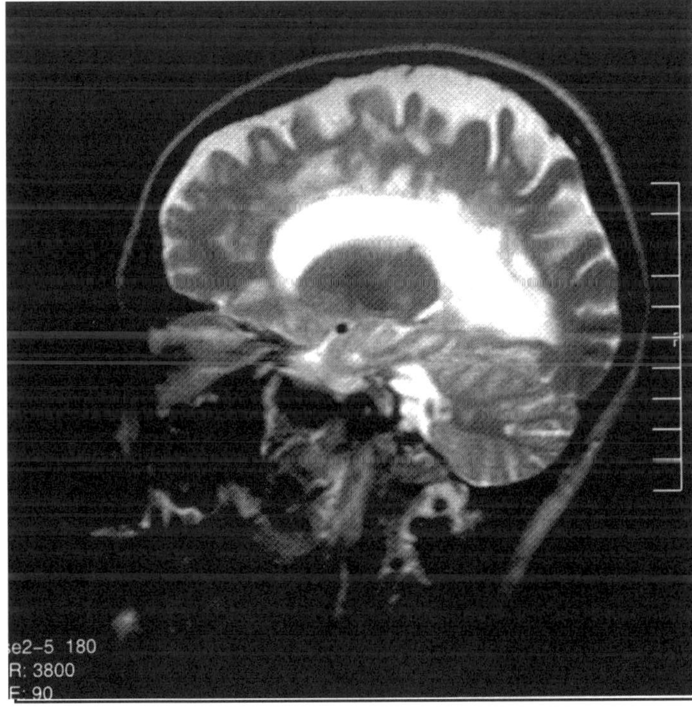

Figure 80b.

Figure 80 a-c. **Multiple sclerosis.** 31-year-old woman. FLAIR image reveals diffuse periventricular hyperintensities (a). Parasagittal T2W image reveals the plaques of MS (b). The corpus callosum is extremely thin due to diffuse, longstanding involvement with the condition (arrows) (c).

Figure 81 a-c. **Multiple sclerosis.** 43-year-old woman. FLAIR and T2 images show high-signal periventicular and intra-callosal high-signal changes (a,b). ADC map reveals a high ADC value in a plaque in the corpus callosum: 1.53 X 10^{-3} mm^2/sec. Values from other lesions are 1.45 and 1.51 X10^{-3} mm^2/sec. Normal ADC values are shown from the occipital regions for comparison: 0.78 and 0.84 X10^{-3} mm^2/sec (c). It should be noted that currently diffusion imaging (including ADC maps) can not differentiate between active and inactive MS lesions.

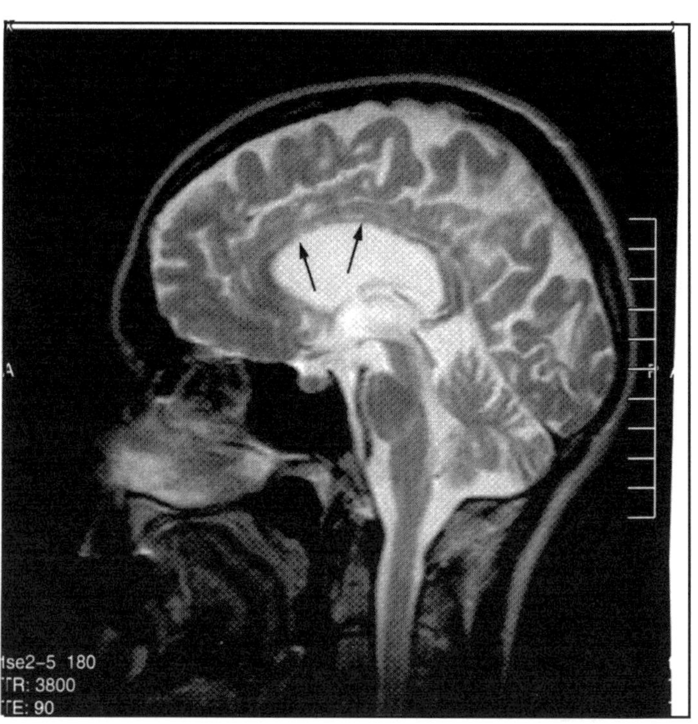

Figure 80c.

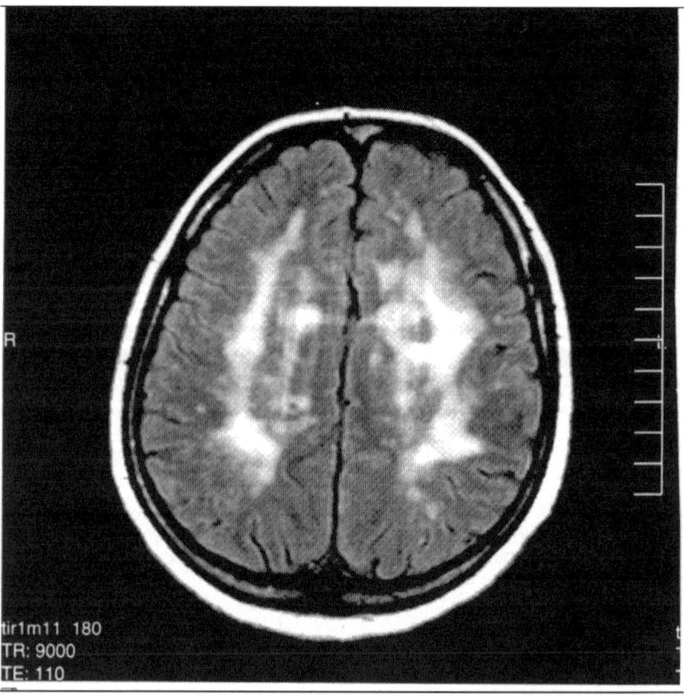

Figure 81a.

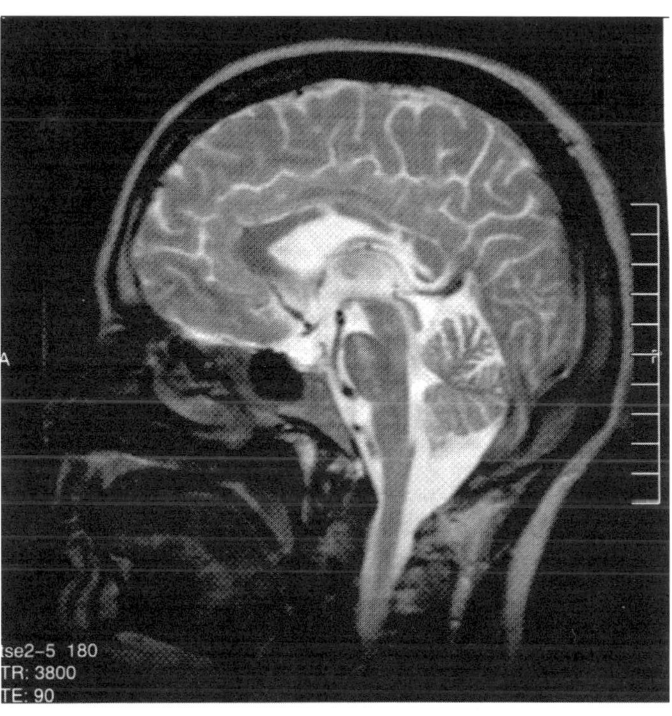

Figure 81b.

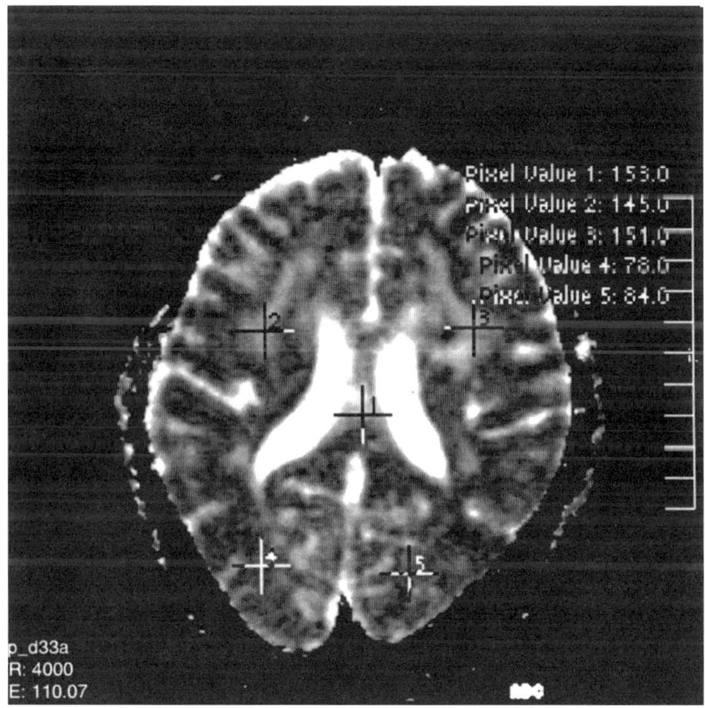

Figure 81c.

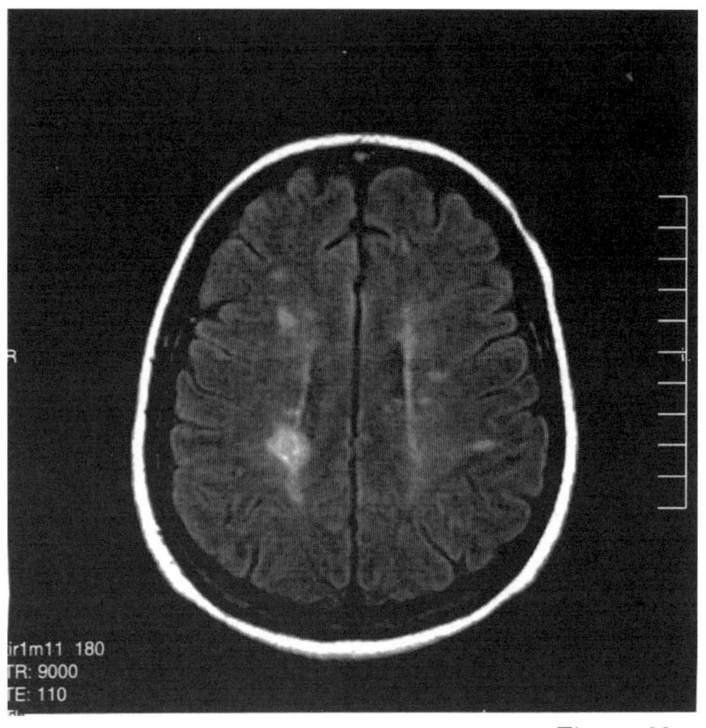

Figure 82a.

Figure 82 a-f. **Multiple sclerosis.** 58-year-old woman. FLAIR image reveals multiple ovale lesions of MS (a).

PSIF image (anisotropic diffusion sequence) by ROI (region of interest) evaluation reveals a high mean pixel value: 152 in a MS plaque, compared to a pixel value from the normal parenchyma: 82 (b).

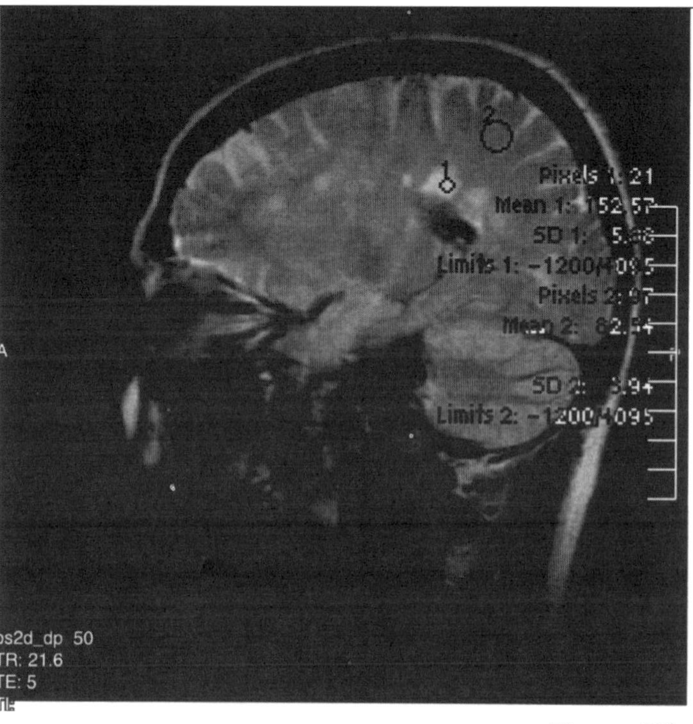

Figure 82b.

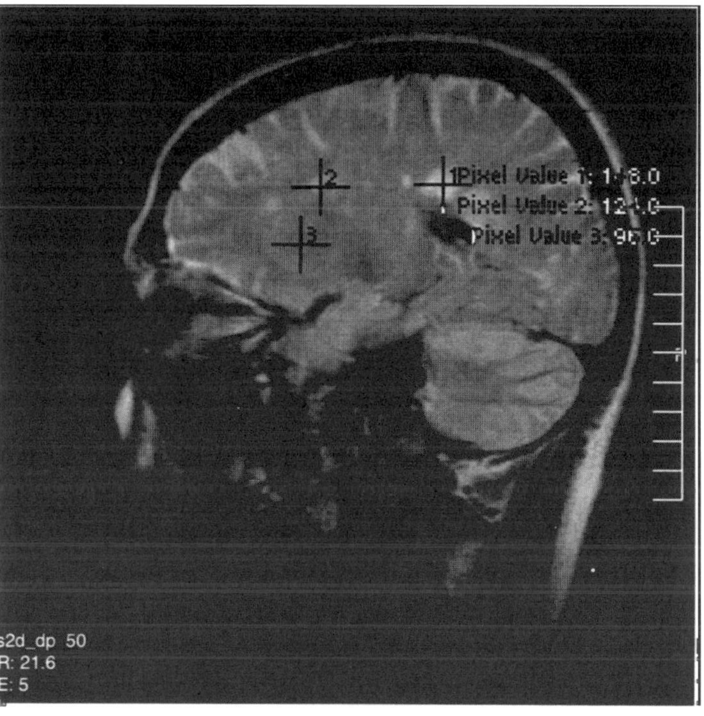

Figure 82c.

PSIF image, with pixel lens evaluation, reveals high pixel values from two MS lesions: 148 and 124. A normal value is: 96 (c). PSIF image reveals a high pixel value from an MS lesion in the corpus callosum: 126. Normal value from the corpus callosum is: 105, and from the parenchyma is: 91 (d).

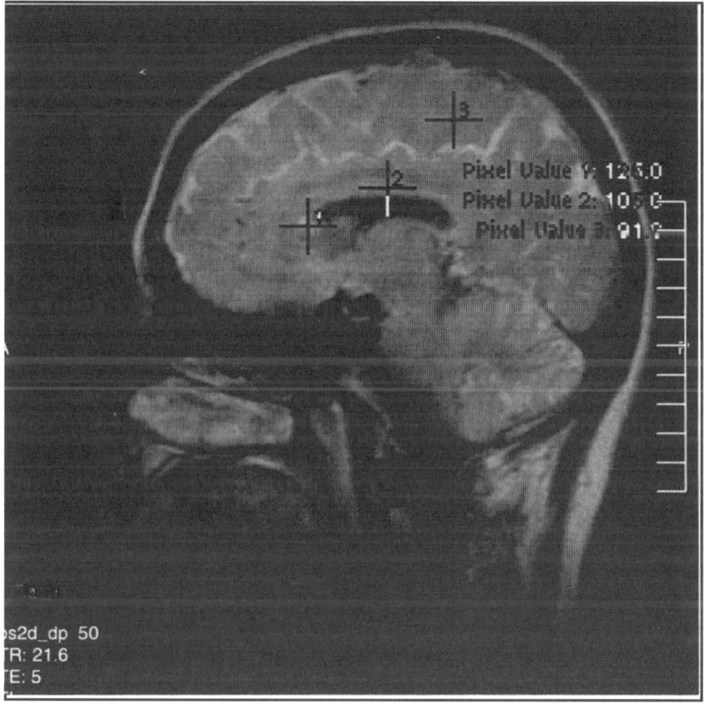

Figure 82d.

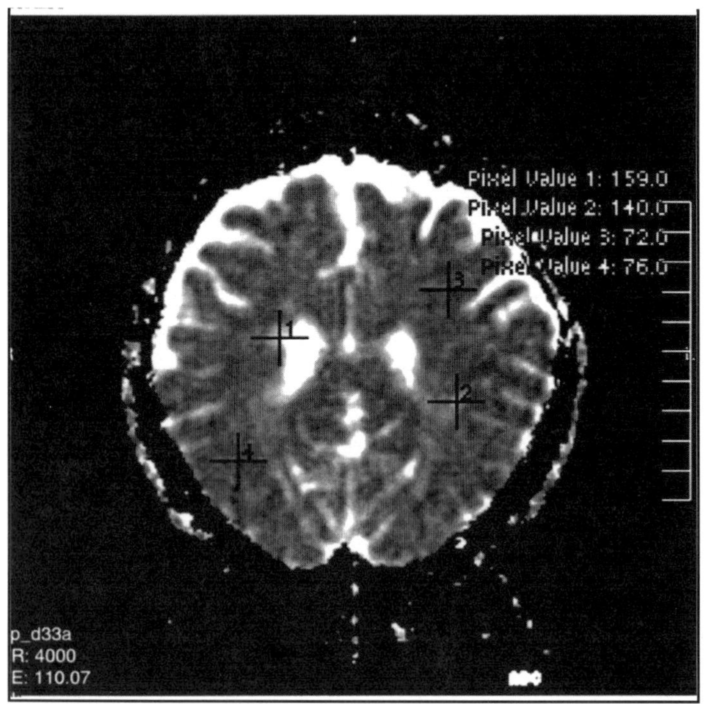

Figure 82e.

It should be noted that these pixel values obtained by PSIF (anisotropic diffusion) images can not be used for measurement of apparent diffusion coefficient (ADC) values. For calculation of ADC values echo-planar diffusion imaging should be used. In echo-planar diffusion imaging ADC values can directly be measured from ADC maps or by using the Stejskal-Tanner formula. ADC maps in this patient reveal high ADC values in the MS lesions: 1.59 and 1.40 $\times 10^{-3}$ mm^2/sec, compared to normal values from the parenchyma: 0.72, and 0.76 $\times 10^{-3}$ mm^2/sec (e). ADC map in a higher section reveals a high value: 2.00 $\times 10^{-3}$ mm^2/sec in a MS lesion. It is probable that the higher the ADC value in a MS lesion is, the higher the tissue disintegration. Normal parenchymal value is shown for comparison: 0.84 $\times 10^{-3}$ mm^2/sec (f).

References

1. *Sener RN. Diffusion MRI: apparent diffusion coefficient (ADC) values in the normal brain, and a classification of brain disorders based on ADC values. Comput Med Imaging Graph 2001; 25:299..*
2. *Barkovich AJ. Pediatric neuroimaging. Philadelphia, Lippincott Williams & Wilkins, 2000*
3. *Osborn AG. Diagnostic neuroradiology, St.Louis, Mosby, 1994*

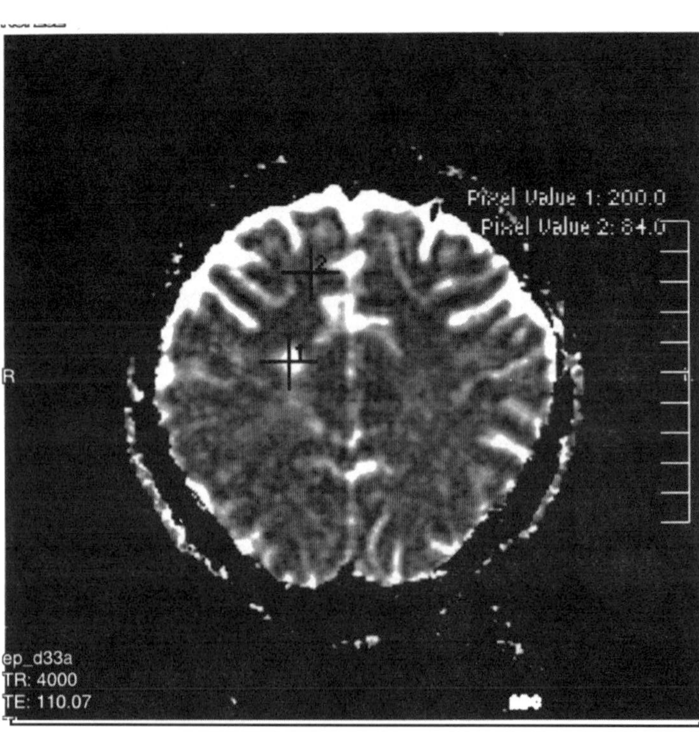

Figure 82f.

Figure 83 a, b. **Viral encephalitis.** 13-year-old boy. *a) SE T1W, and b) SE T2W MR images.* The genu of the corpus callosum has been thickened by a focal lesion (arrows) (a, b). Also note several hyperintense, hemispheral lesions (b). The condition was secondary to a longstanding viral encephalitis.

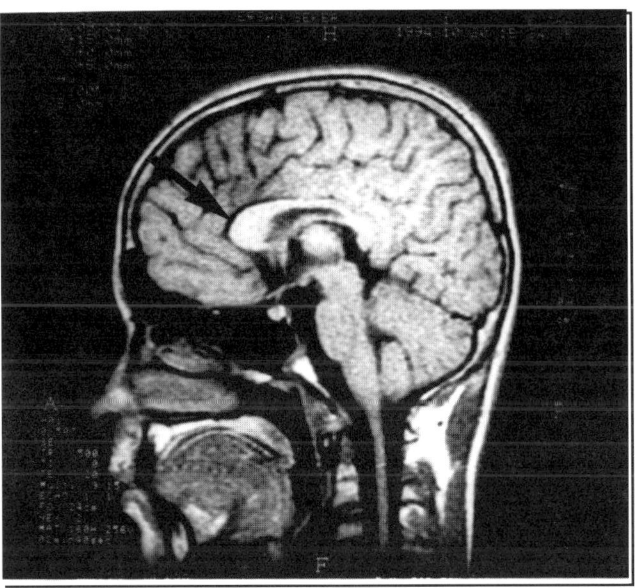

Figure 83a.

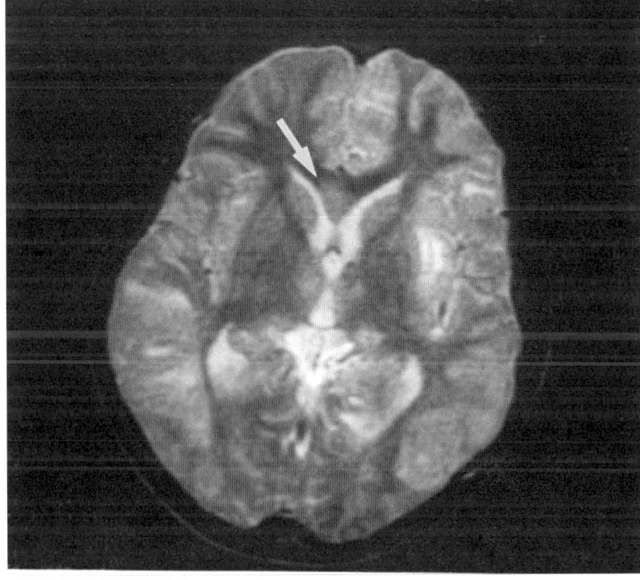

Figure 83b.

Reference
1.   Osborn AG. Diagnostic neuroradiology. St. Louis, Mosby, 1994;694

Figure 84 a-c. **Viral encephalitis.** 7-year-old boy. *a and b) SE T2W MR images at age 4 years, c) follow-up, SE T1W MR image at age 7 years.* There is an almost spherical, hyperintense lesion at the region of the isthmus of the corpus callosum (arrows) (a, b). Also note several hyperintense, hemispheral lesions. Follow-up MR image 3 years later shows an apparent thinning of the isthmus (arrow) associated with an isthmal-splenial kinking (c).

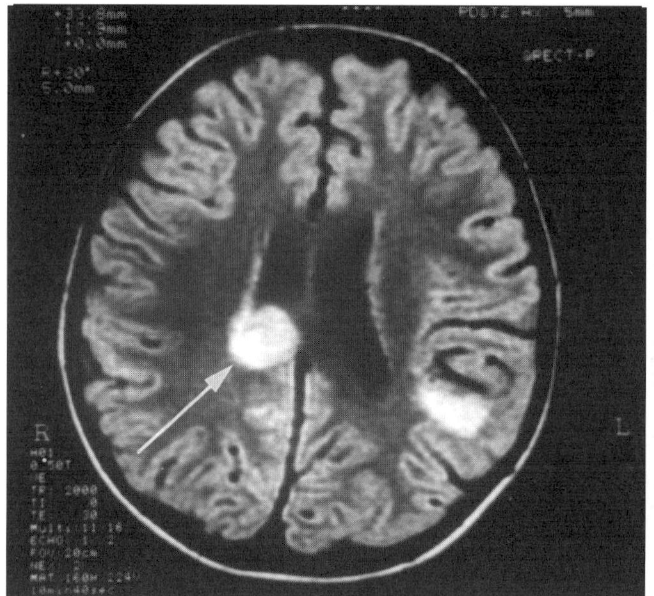

Figure 84a.

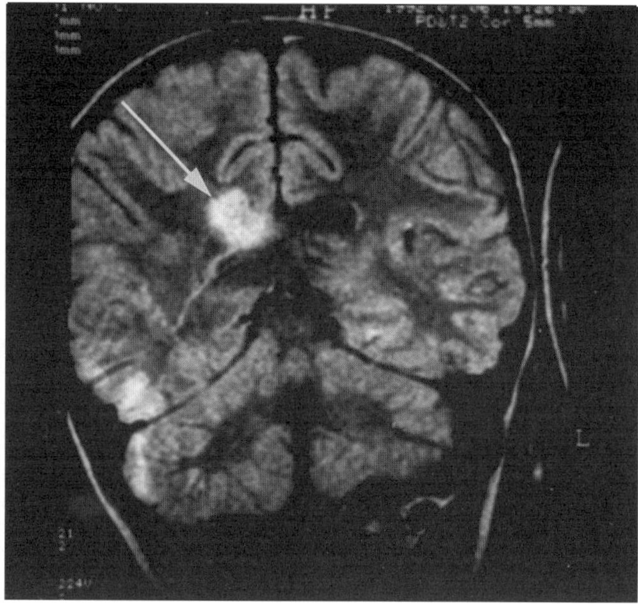

Figure 84b.

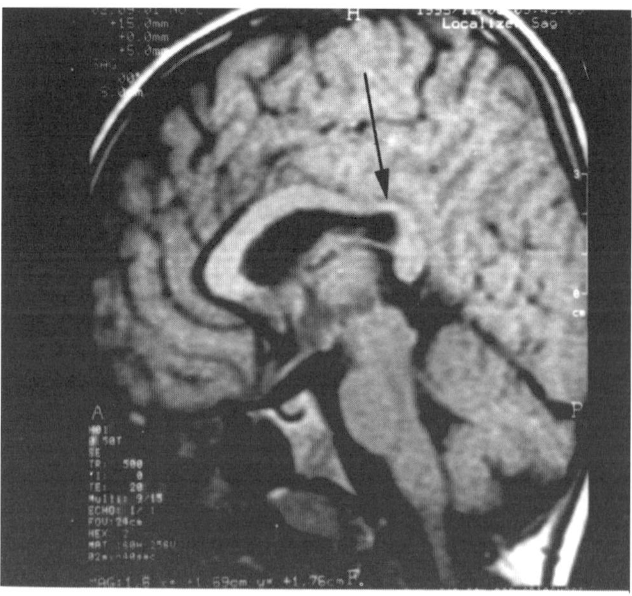

Figure 84c.

Reference
1.   Osborn AG. Diagnostic neuroradiology. St. Louis, Mosby, 1994;694

Figure 85 a-d. **Viral encephalitis.** 5-year-old boy. *a, b) SE T1W MR image, c) SE T2W MR image, and d) SE T1W MR image after administration of contrast medium.* There are two hypointense, focal lesions in the genu of the corpus callosum (arrows) (a, b, d), which became hyperintense on proton density and T2W images (arrow) (c), suggesting a demyelination disorder. No enhancement of the lesions was noted (d). No other lesion in the brain parenchyma was evident. Laboratory work-up disclosed an infectious condition due to varicella zoster. (case courtesy of Dr. R. Savas, Heidelberg).

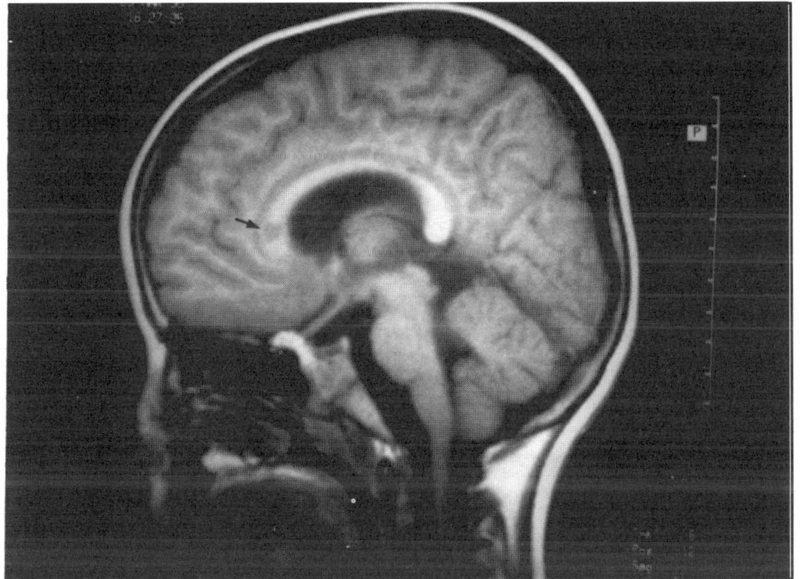

Figure 85a.

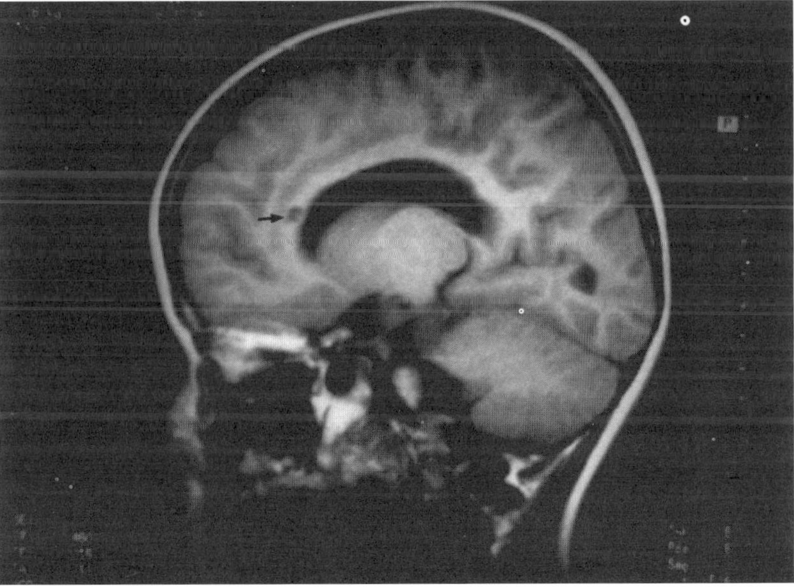

Figure 85b.

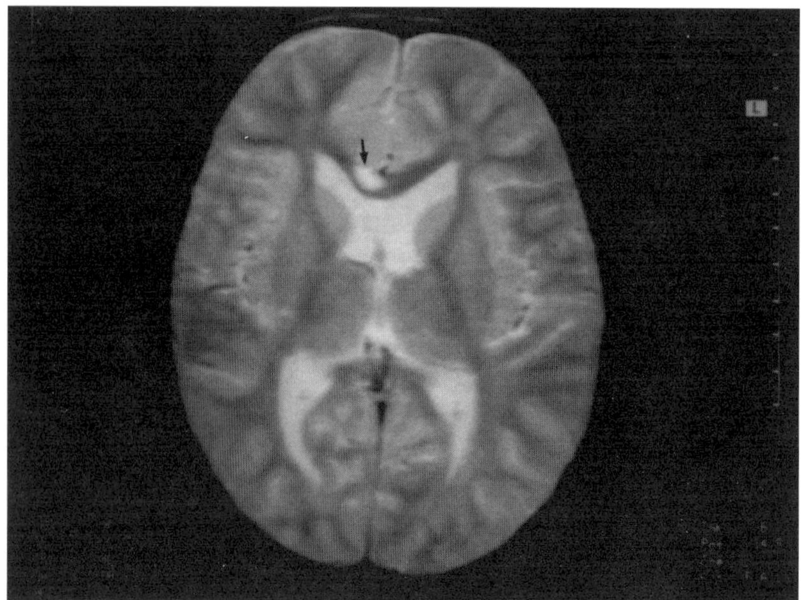

Figure 85c.

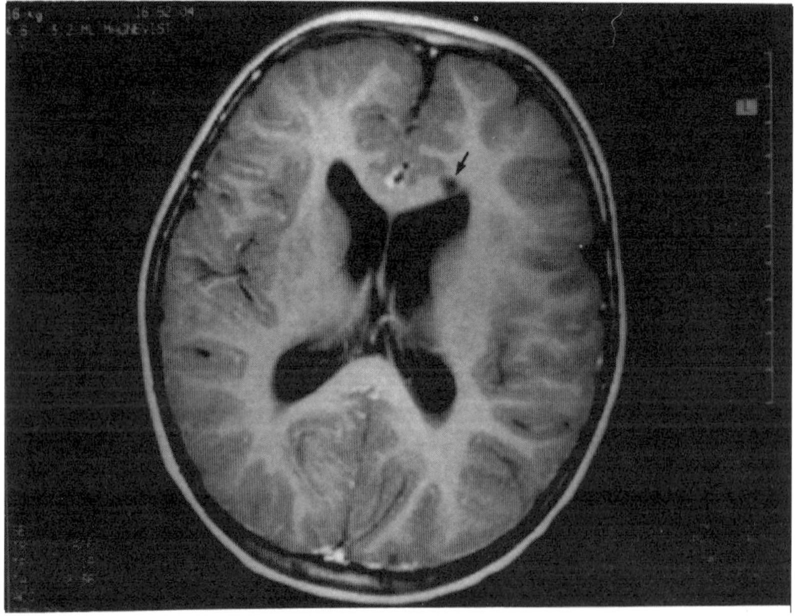

Figure 85d.

Reference
1.   Osborn AG. Diagnostic neuroradiology. St. Louis, Mosby, 1994;694

Figure 86 a-d. **Longstanding herpesvi-
rus infection.** 2-year-old girl. FLAIR
image reveals hyperintense changes in
the left temporal and frontal lobes (a).
Extension of the lesion to the left side
of the corpus callosum (arrow) is demonstrated by FLAIR images (b,c). ADC
map reveals high ADC values at the
lesion sites: 1.35 and 1.45 X10^{-3} mm^2/
sec, compared to normal value of the
contralateral frontal lobe: 0.82 X10^{-3}
mm^2/sec (d).

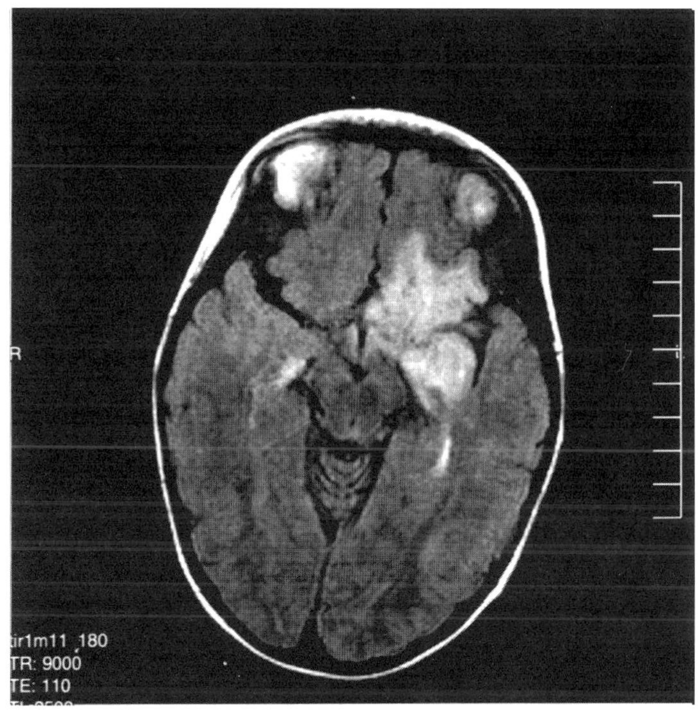

Figure 86a.

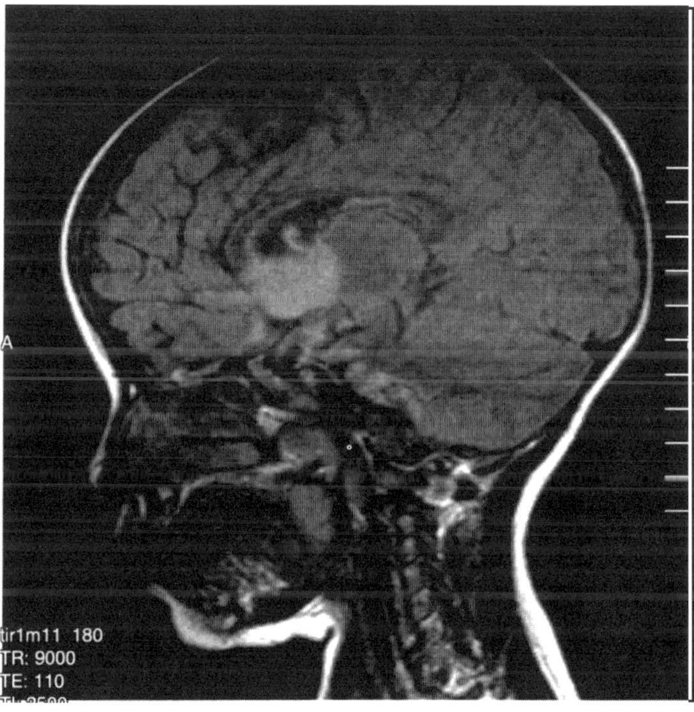

Figure 86b.

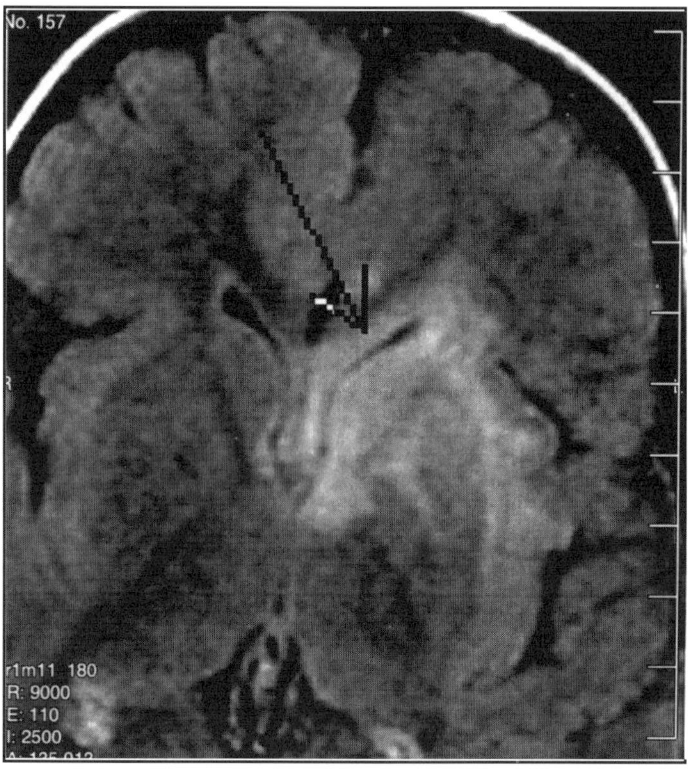

Figure 86c.

References
1. *Barkovich AJ. Pediatric neuroimaging. Philadelphia, Lippincott Williams & Wilkins, 2000*
2. *Osborn AG. Diagnostic neuroradiology, St.Louis, Mosby, 1994*

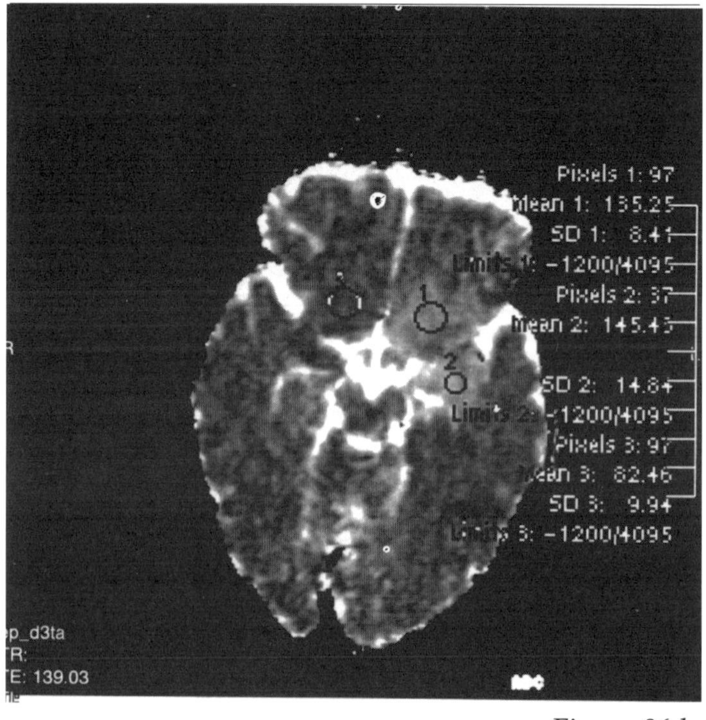

Figure 86d.

Figure 87 a-c. **Canavan's disease.** 2-year-old boy. *a) SE T1W, b) SE PDW, and c) SE T2W MR images.* The genu of the corpus ·callosum has apparently been thickened (arrow) (a), while the caudal parts are relatively normal. Axial images show diffuse white matter involvement including the subcortical arcuate fibers, and cortical thinning due to Canavan's disease. Note the thickened genu (circles) (b, c). This lesion in the callosal genu appears to be an unusual finding in Canavan's disease. On the other hand, in adrenoleukodystrophy involvement of the splenium is commonly seen.

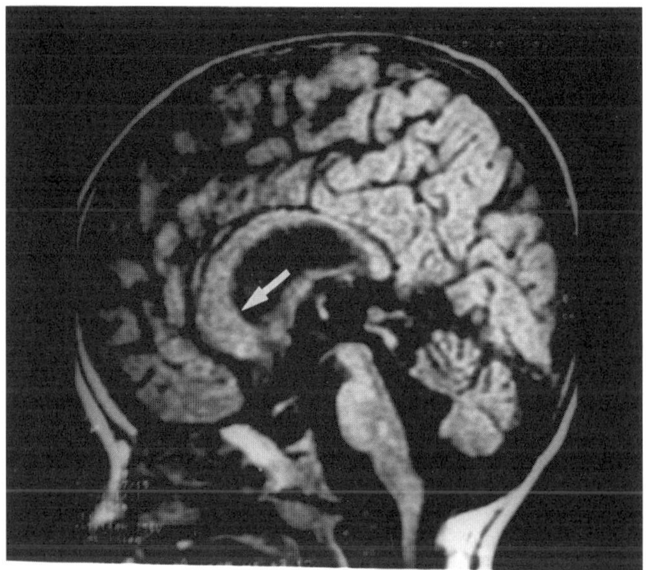

Figure 87a.

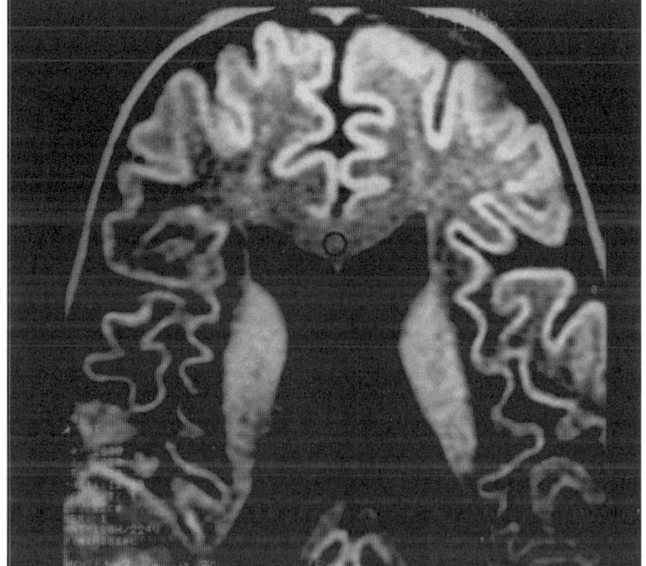

Figure 87b.

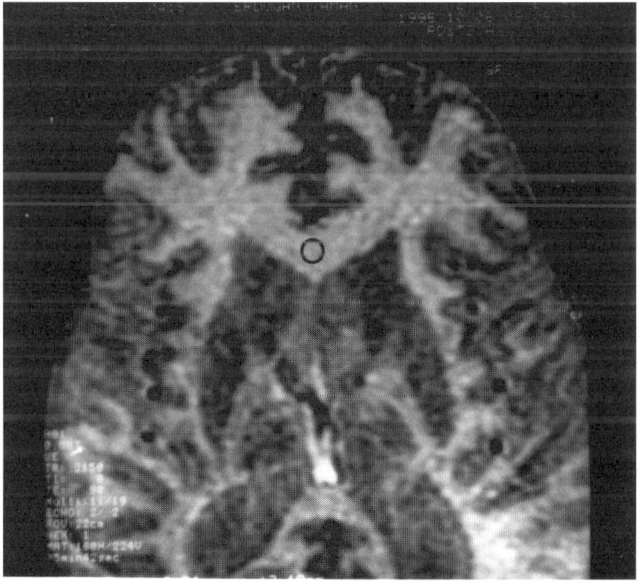

Figure 87c.

Reference

1. *Osborn AG. Diagnostic neuroradiology. St. Louis, Mosby, 1994;732*

Figure 88 a-h. **Adrenoleukodystrophy.** 11-year-old boy. FLAIR image reveals prominent hyperintensity in the frontal lobes (a). This type of involvement is unusual for adrenoleukodystrophy. *In adrenoleukodystrophy, usually the occipital lobes and the posterior parts of the corpus callosum are involved, and frontal lobe involvement is usually seen in Alexander's disease.* Sagittal, T1W images reveal hypointense appearances in the genu of the corpus callosum (arrows) (b,c). ADC map clearly shows the hyperintense changes. ADC measurements with ROI evaluations reveal high ADC values in the affected frontal lobe: 1.48 and 1.48 $X10^{-3}$ mm^2/sec. Normal parenchymal value is shown: 0.84 $X10^{-3}$ mm^2/sec (d). ADC map in a lower section reveals a higher ADC value in the frontal white matter: 2.03 $X10^{-3}$ mm^2/sec, compared

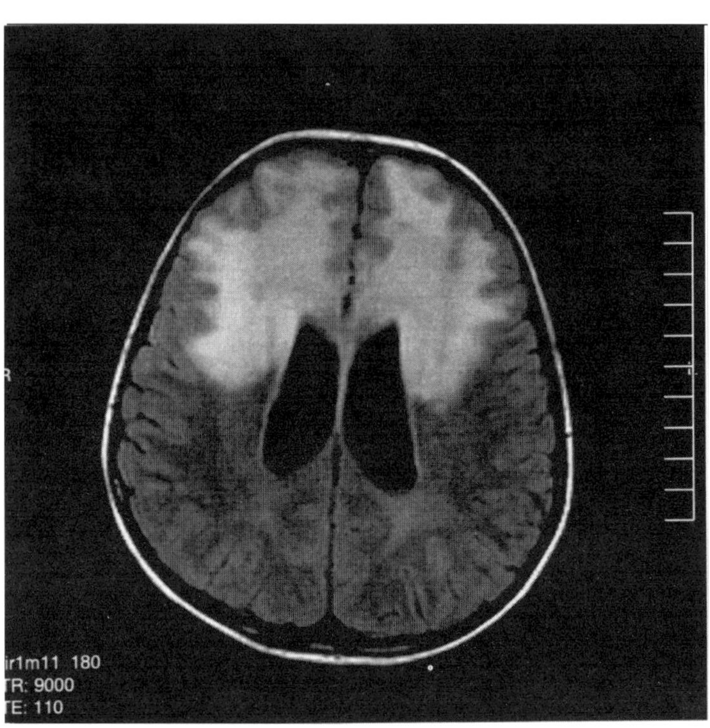

Figure 88a.

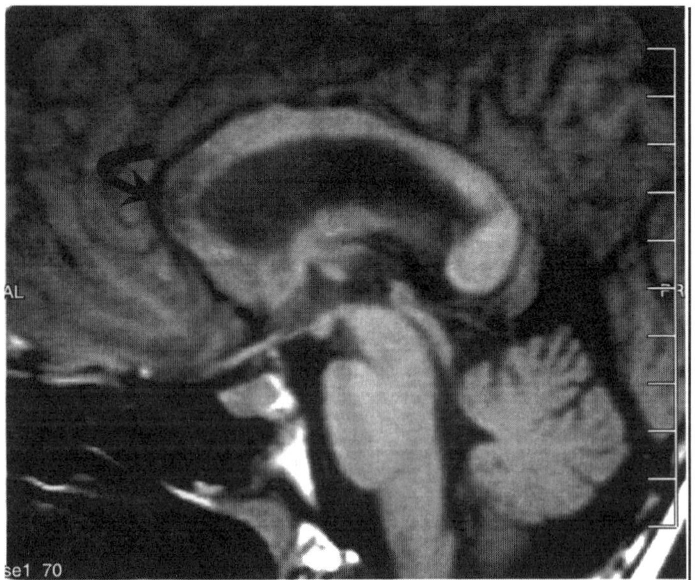

Figure 88b.

to those of the normal occipitoparietal white matters: 0.68 and 0.83 $X10^{-3}$ mm^2/sec (e). Chemical-shift, proton MR spectroscopy (TR=1500 msec, TE=40 msec) reveals a decreased NAA (N-acetyl aspartate) peak, compared to the peaks of creatine, and choline, a common pattern in leukodystrophies (f). Spectroscopy (TR=1500 msec, TE=40 msec) in another voxel again reveals a decreased NAA peak, compared to that of choline. Also, noted are double peaks at 3.50, and 3.56 ppm belonging to glycine, and myoinositol, respectively. The height of the myoinositol peak is normal, however, that of glycine is probably high, representing presence of excitotoxic brain damage. Also noted are prominent double peaks at 1.1 and 1.3 ppm belonging

to macromolecules (g). Normal spectrum is shown for comparison from a normal region of the patient's brain (h).

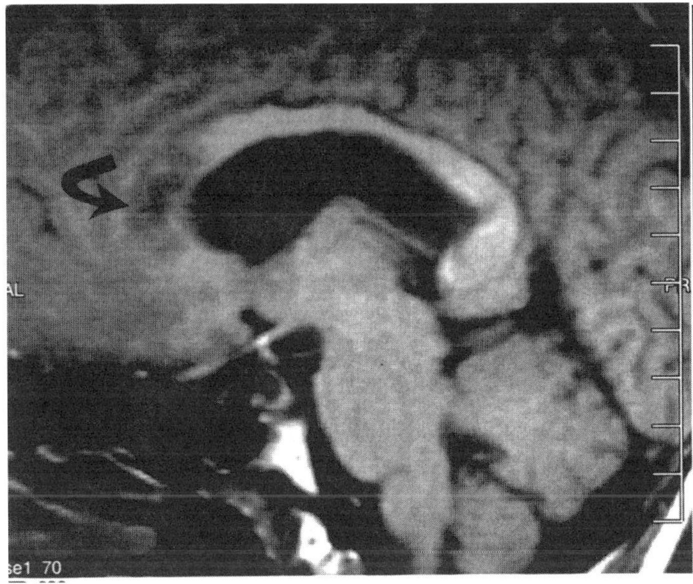

Figure 88c.

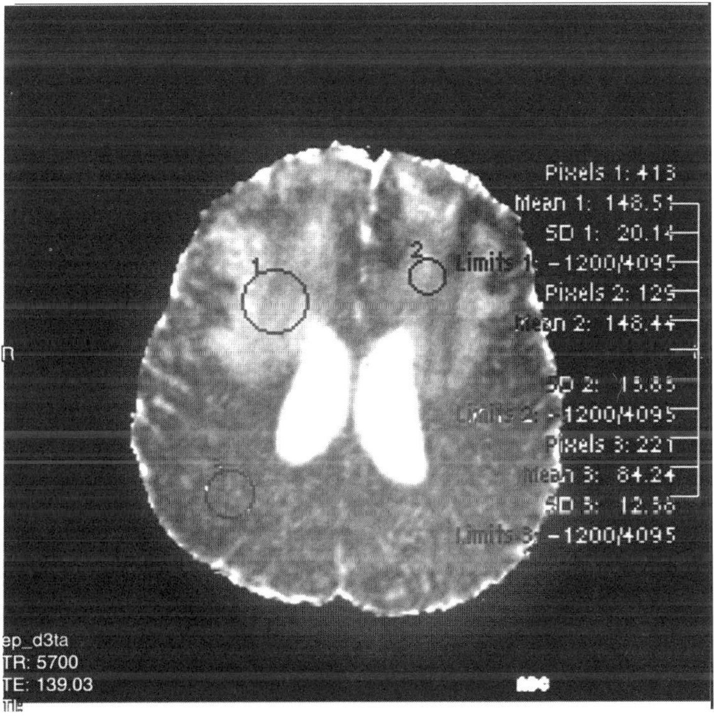

Figure 88d.

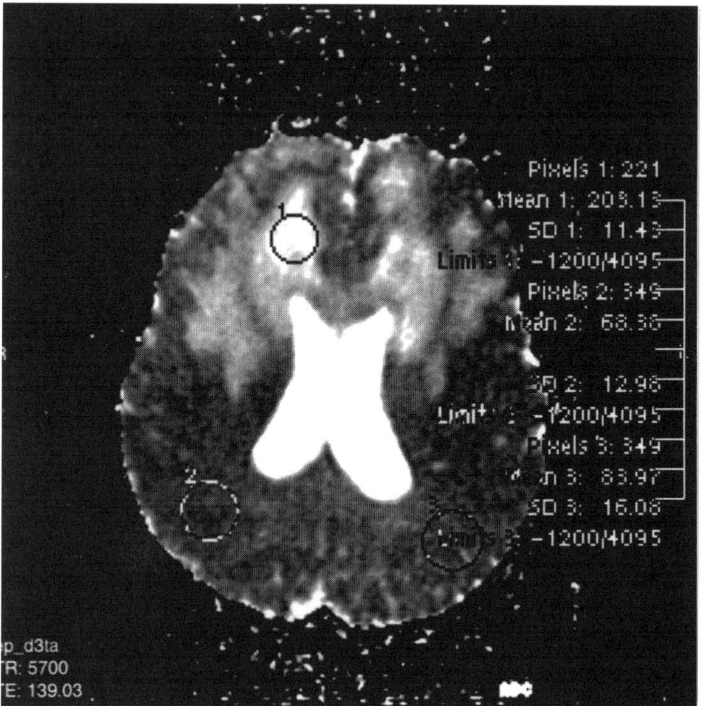

Figure 88e.

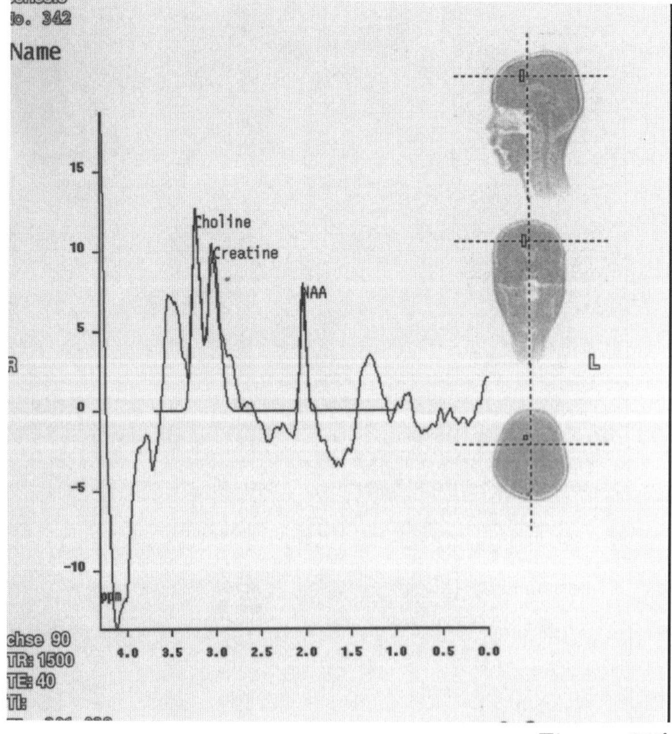

Figure 88f.

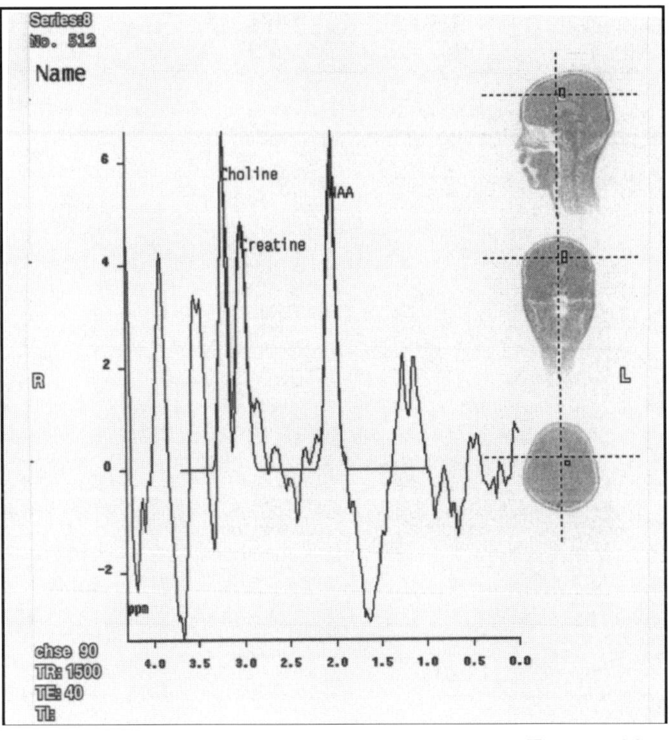

Figure 88g.

References
1. *Barkovich AJ. Pediatric neuroimaging. Philadelphia, Lippincott Williams & Wilkins, 2000*
2. *Osborn AG. Diagnostic neuroradiology, St.Louis, Mosby, 1994*

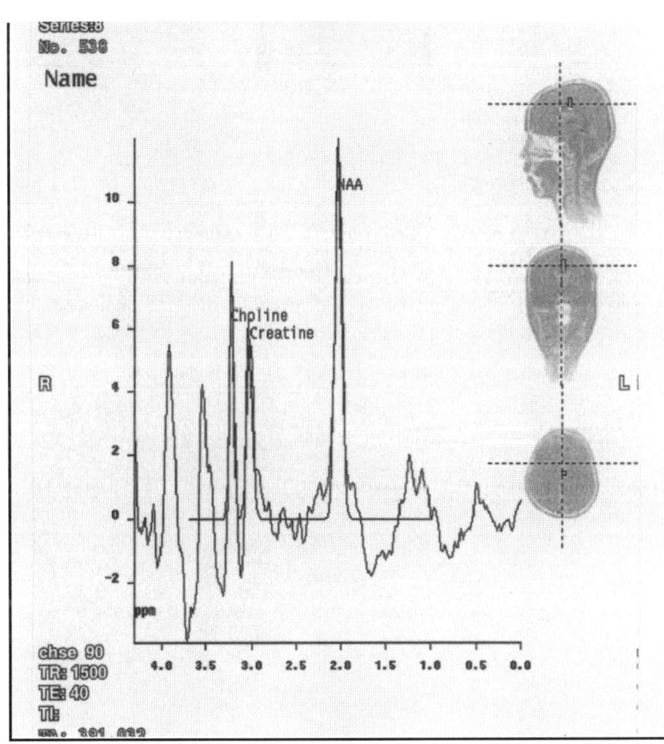

Figure 88h.

Figure 89 a-d. **Metachromatic leukodystro-phy.** 1.5-year-old boy. Diffusion images are shown: *b=0 image is actually a T2-weighted image; b=500S sec/mm² image contains partial T2 information referred to as T2-shine through; and b=1000S sec/mm² image is the true diffusion image (S is slice select gradient). ADC map is also shown.* b=0 image (T2-weighted) image reveals signal abnormality (high signal) involving the deep white matter, and peripheral white matter is spared, suggesting metachromatic leukodystrophy The corpus callosum is also involved, and thickened. (a). b=500S sec/mm² (with T2 info in part) image has similar appearance (b). b=1000S sec/mm² (true diffusion) image reveals an unusual high-signal in the deep white matter including the corpus callosum (arrow). This mimicks ischemia (cytotoxic edema), however, the condition was not associated with ischemia. Therefore, this abnormal signal probably reflects restriction of molecular movement of water in these regions with disordered myelination (c). ADC map reveals low ADC values in the abnormal deep white matter (indicated by pixels 1 and 4): 0.43 and 0.53 X10⁻³ mm²/sec, similar to that of ischemia. Otherwise, normal parenchymal ADC values are evident from different regions, including peripheral white matter and cortex: 0.80, 1.00, 0.94, and 0.88 X10⁻³ mm²/sec. There is a place in the peripheral white matter with a slightly higher ADC value: 1.09 X10⁻³ mm²/sec (d).

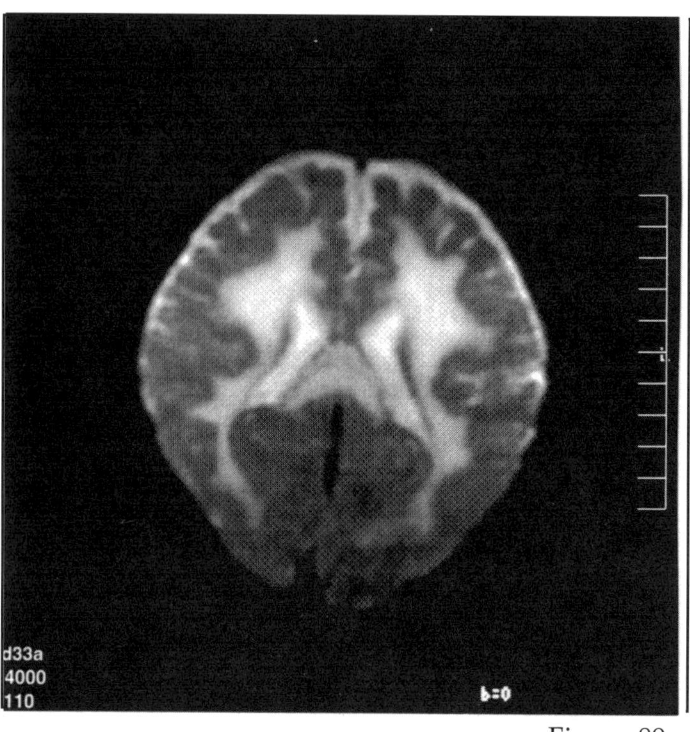

Figure 89a.

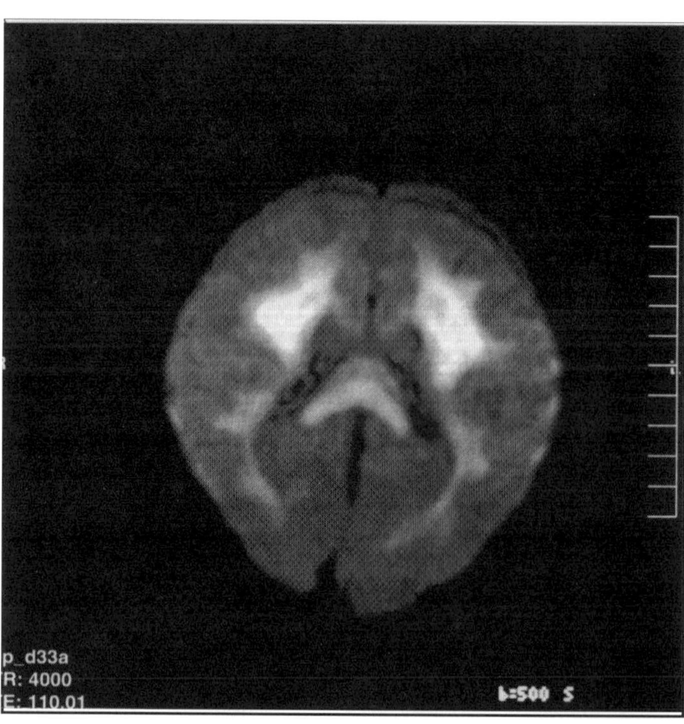

Figure 89b.

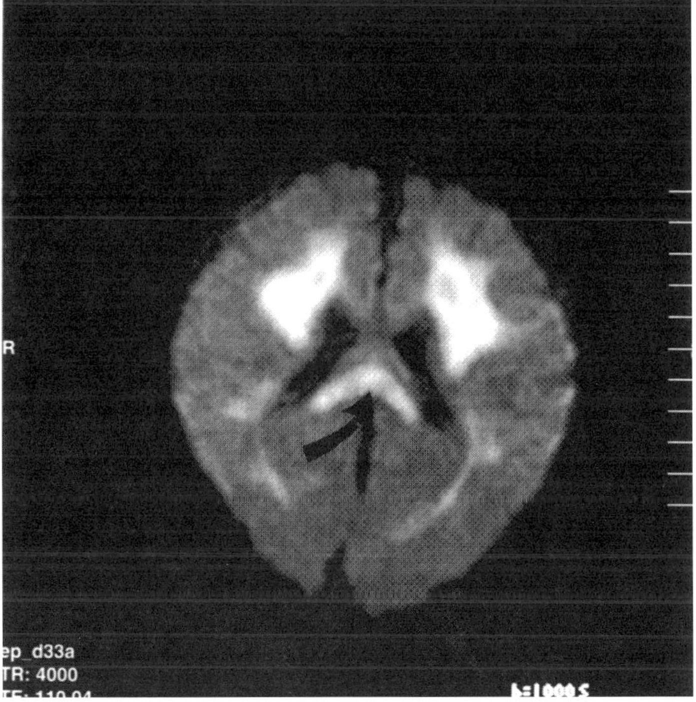

Figure 89c.

References
1. *Sener RN. Diffusion MRI: apparent diffusion coefficient (ADC) values in the normal brain, and a classification of brain disorders based on ADC values. Comput Med Imaging Graph 2001; 25:299.*
2. *Barkovich AJ. Pediatric neuroimaging. Philadelphia, Lippincott Williams & Wilkins, 2000*
3. *Osborn AG. Diagnostic neuroradiology, St.Louis, Mosby, 1994*

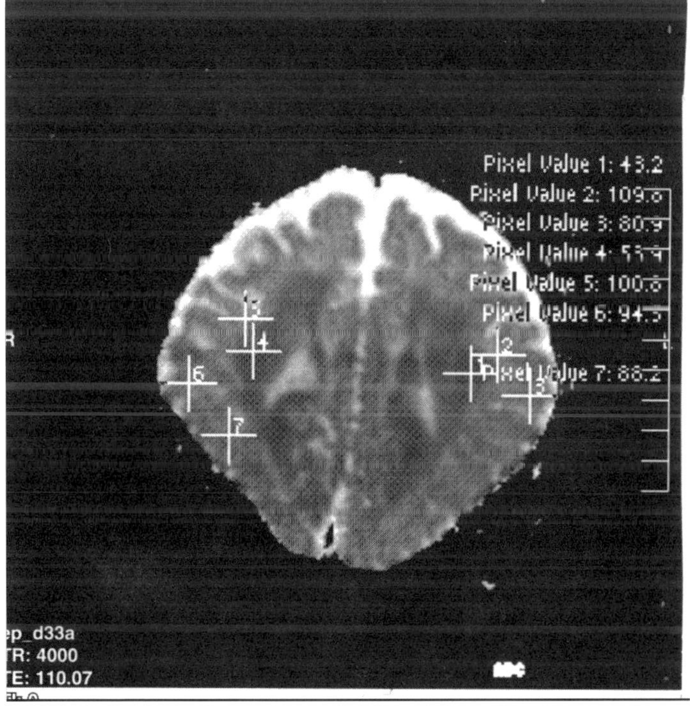

Figure 89d.

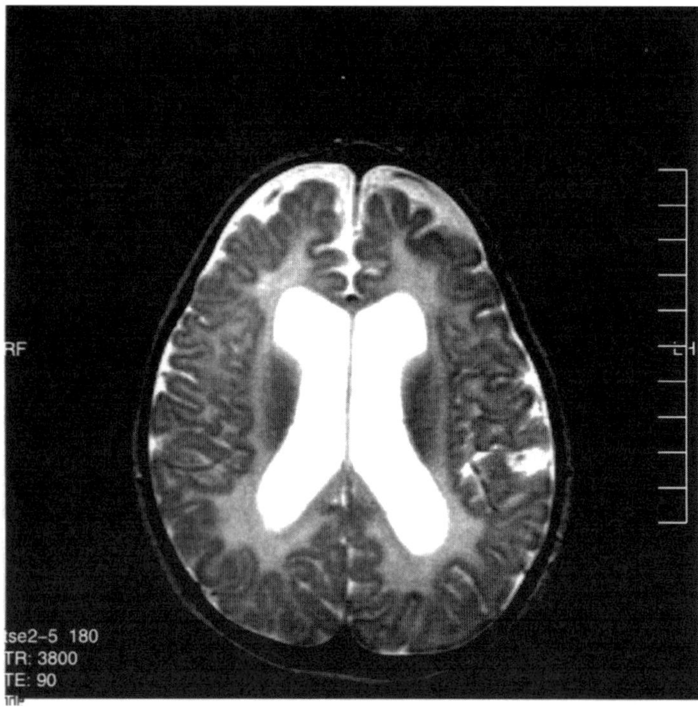

Figure 90a.

Figure 90 a-d. **Metachromatic leukodystrophy.** 1.5-year-old girl. T2W image reveals signal abnormality diffusely involving the deep white matter. Peripheral white matter is spared, suggesting metachromatic leukodystrophy (a). Diffuse callosal thinning is associated with the condition. Note hypoplasia of the inferior vermis (b). b=1000T sec/mm^2 (true diffusion) image reveals an unusual high signal in the deep white matter (mimicking ischemia). This high signal, however, represents some kind of a restriction of movement of water molecules among the axons in this disease with disorder of myelination (c). PSIF (anisotropic diffusion) image also reveals high signal, and a high pixel value: 172 in the affected white matter. Normal pixel value is shown from peripheral white matter: 100. Therefore, presence of high signal, and high pixel values in the PSIF sequence also represent restriction of motion of water molecules, however, true ADC value calculations can not be done by the PSIF sequence. For this echo-planar diffusion imaging is required (d).

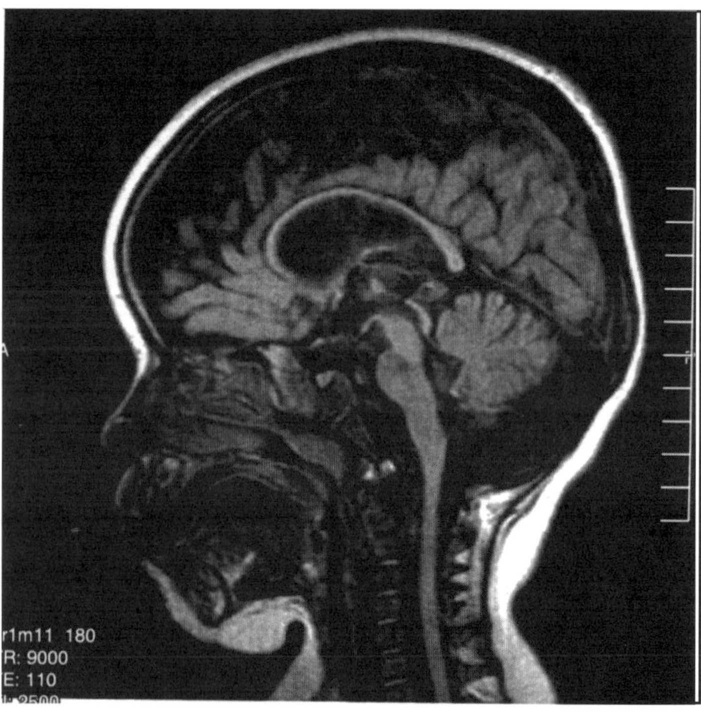

Figure 90b.

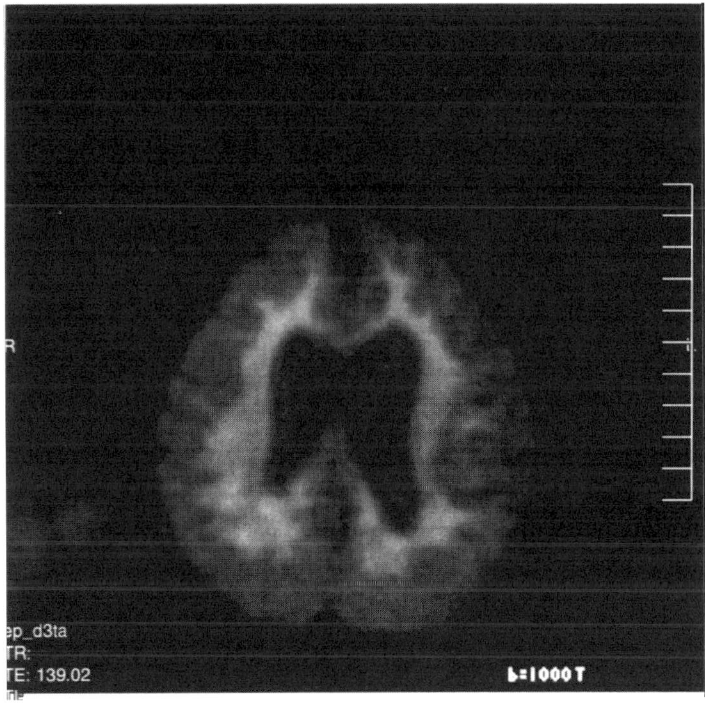

Figure 90c.

References

1. *Sener RN. Diffusion MRI: apparent diffusion coefficient (ADC) values in the normal brain, and a classitication ot brain disorders based on ADC values. Comput Med Imaging Graph 2001; 25:299*

2. Barkovich AJ. Pediatric neuroimaging. Philadelphia, Lippincott Williams & Wilkins, 2000

3. *Osborn AG. Diagnostic neuroradiology, St.Louis, Mosby, 1994*

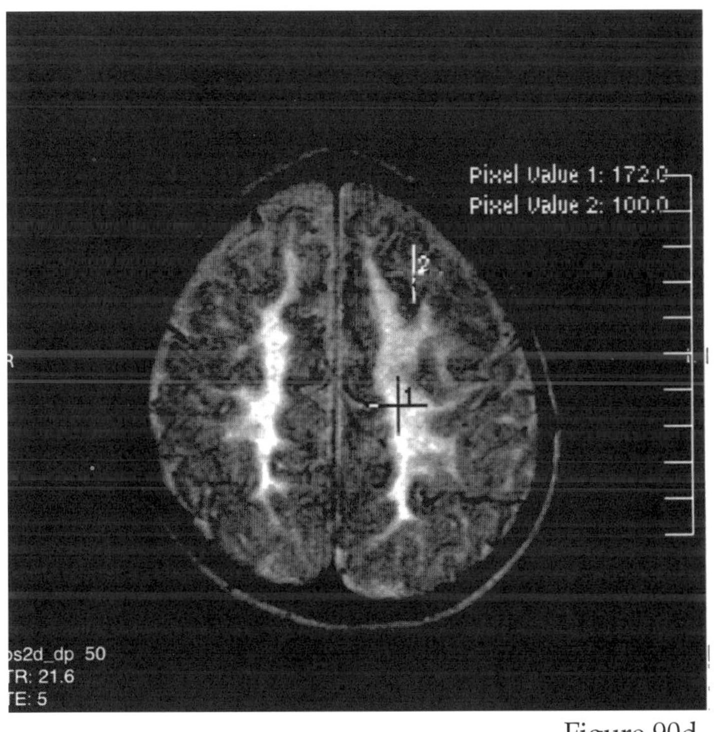

Figure 90d.

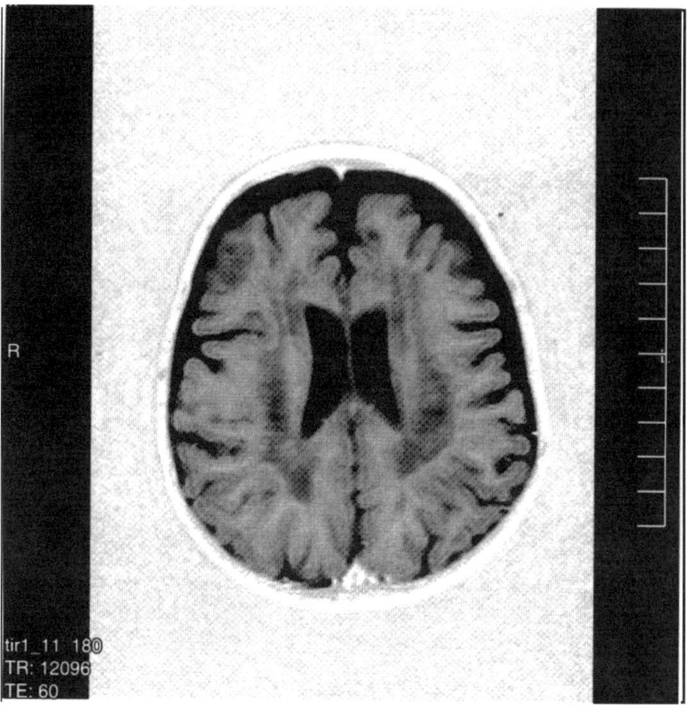

Figure 91a.

Figure 91 a-j. **Mucopolysaccharidosis (Sly's disease).** 11-month-old girl. T1W (turbo inversion recovery) image reveals periventricular low signal regions representing dilated Virchow-Robin spaces (a)

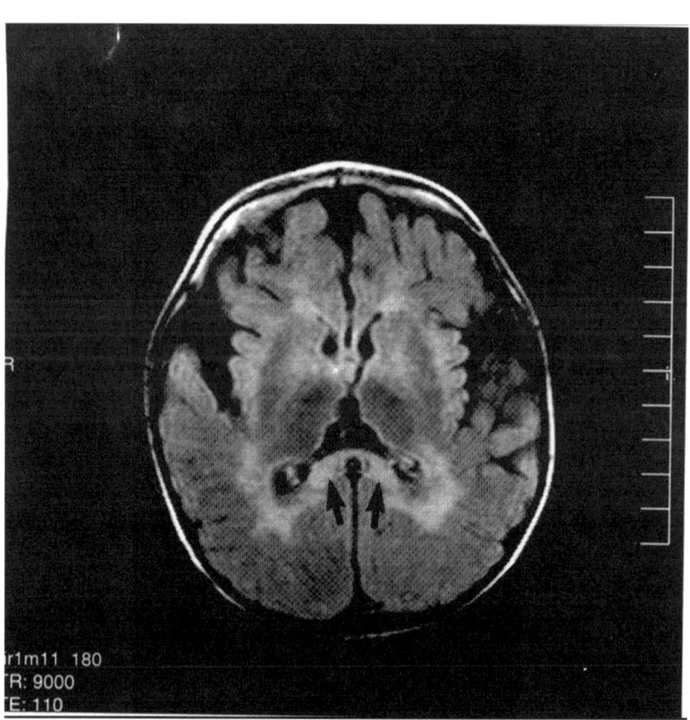

Figure 91b.

FLAIR image shows high-signal changes in deep white matter as well as in the corpus callosum (arrows) (b). Localizer images (T1W) from the periventricular regions partly including the corpus callosum are shown from a single-volume proton MR spectroscopy (c,d). Single-volume proton MR spectroscopy (TR=1500 msec, TE=135 msec) reveals a prominently decreased NAA peak, and increased choline peak. Such a pattern could be observed in a tumor. However, herein NAA decrease represents presence of insufficient amount of neurons and axons in the corresponding regions. The high choline peak represents insufficient myelination. Creatine peak appears normal, as it is a generally stable peak related with energy state of the tissue (e). Localizer is shown from a chemical-shift (multivolume) spectroscopic imaging (f). Chemical-shift proton MR spectroscopy

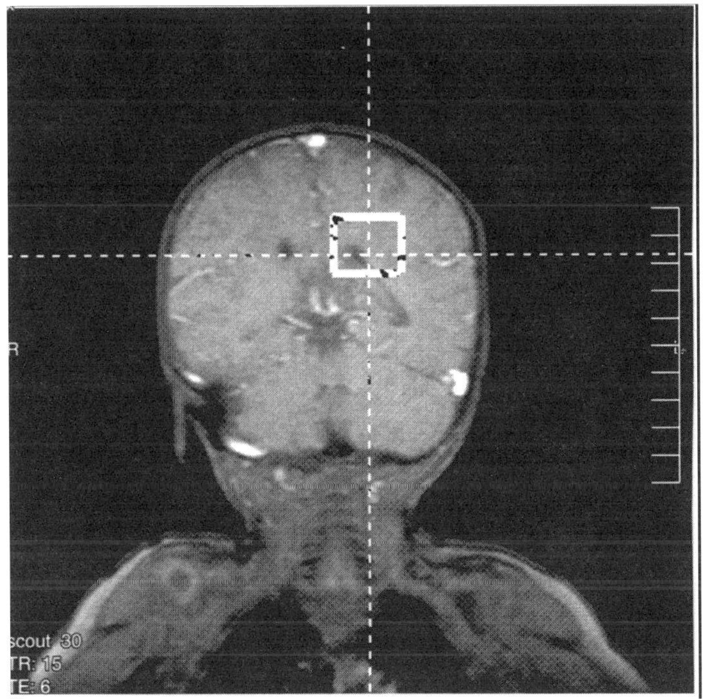

Figure 91c.

(TR=1500 msec, TE=40 msec) from a voxel lateral to that shown on the single-volume spectroscopy, again reveals a high choline peak, and a low NAA peak. However, at this region the amplitudes and integral values of these peaks were closer to normal, compared to the former spectroscopy (g). Transverse *peak information map* from each voxel on the chemical-shift spectroscopy reveals abnormal spectra close to the periventricular regions including the corpus callosum at the row on the right hand side (arrow), compared to relatively normal ones located laterally (h). Coronal *peak information map* again reveals abnormal spectra close to the periventricular regions (arrow), compared to those located laterally (i). Map showing integral values of NAA in each voxel on the chemical-shift spectroscopy reveals lower values close to the periventricular regions (arrow) (j).

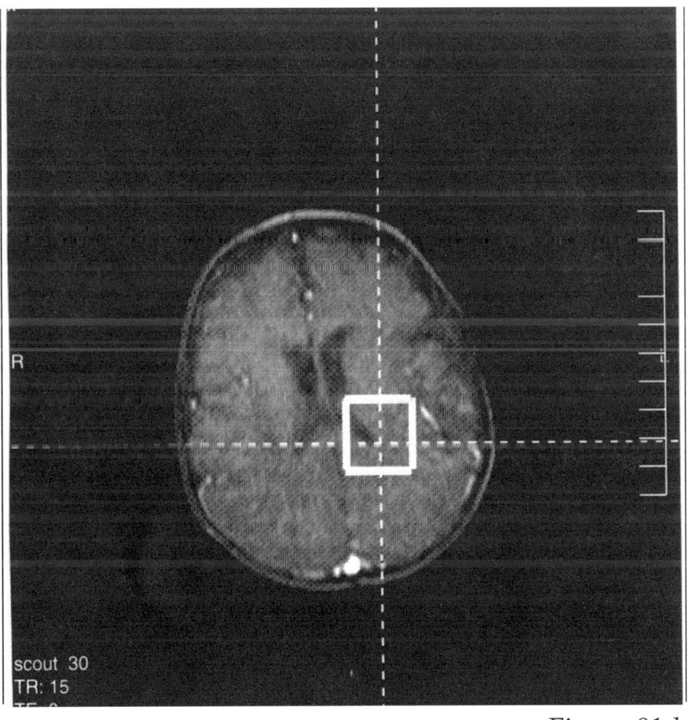

Figure 91d.

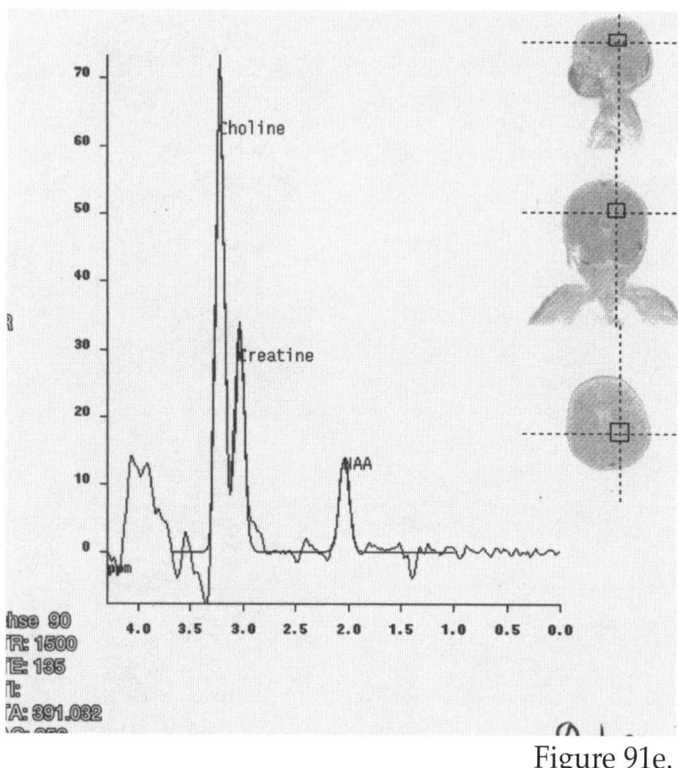

Figure 91e.

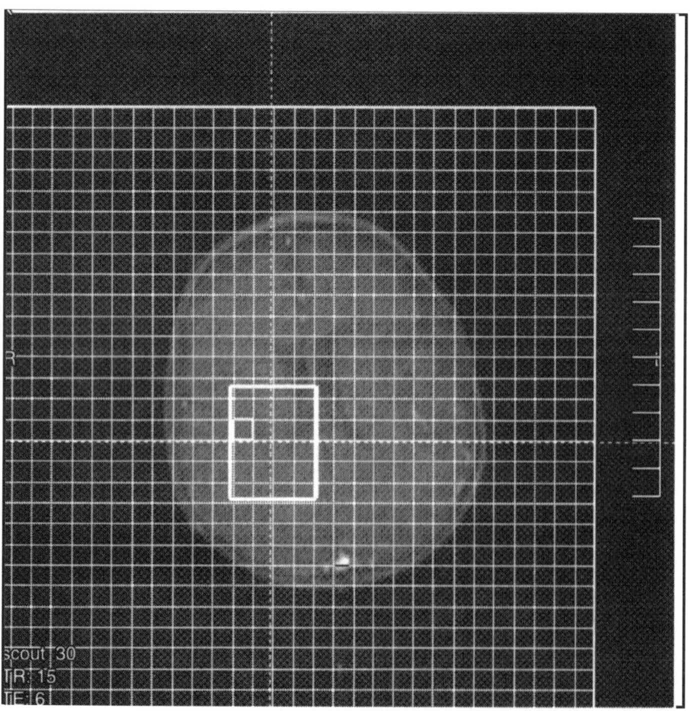

Figure 91f.

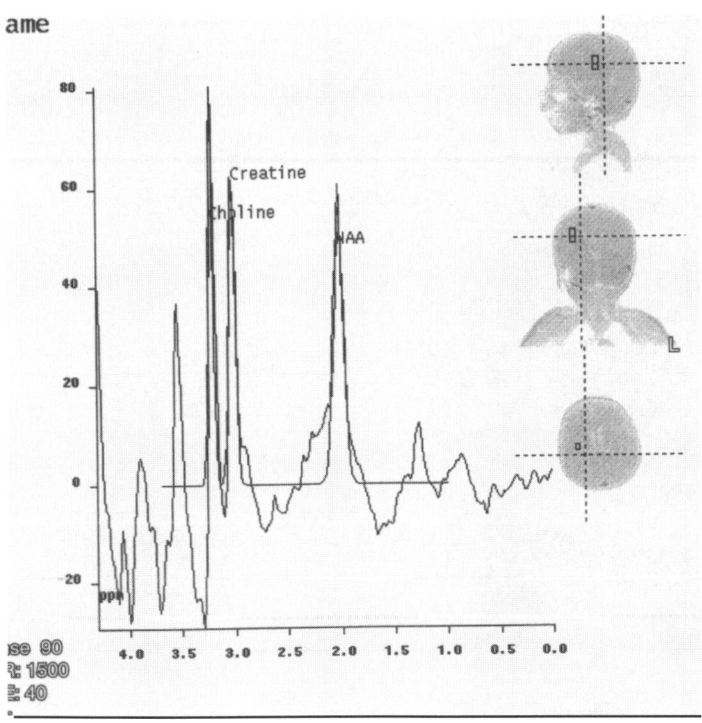

Figure 91g.

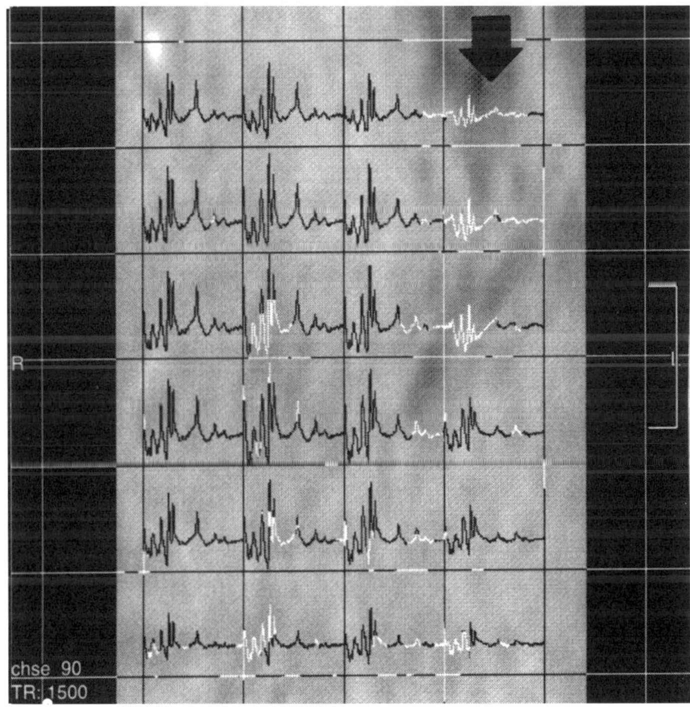

Figure 91h.

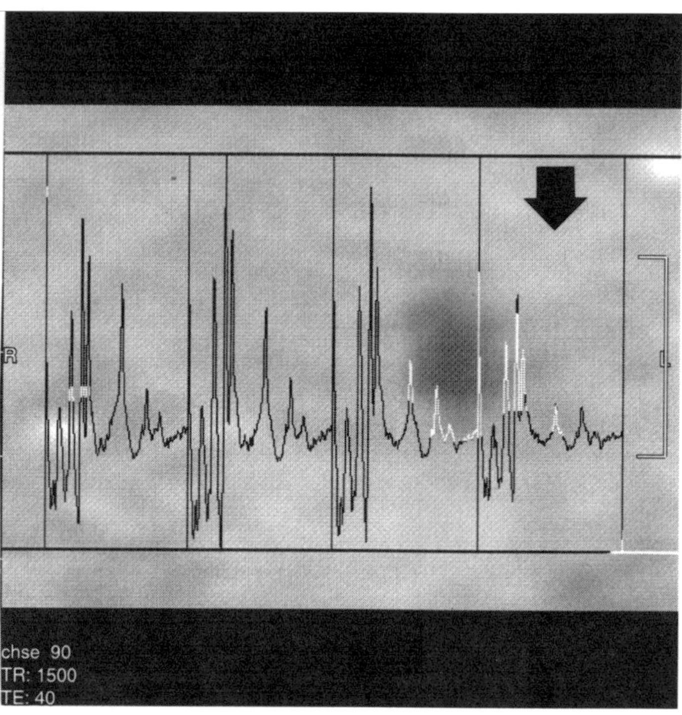

Figure 91i.

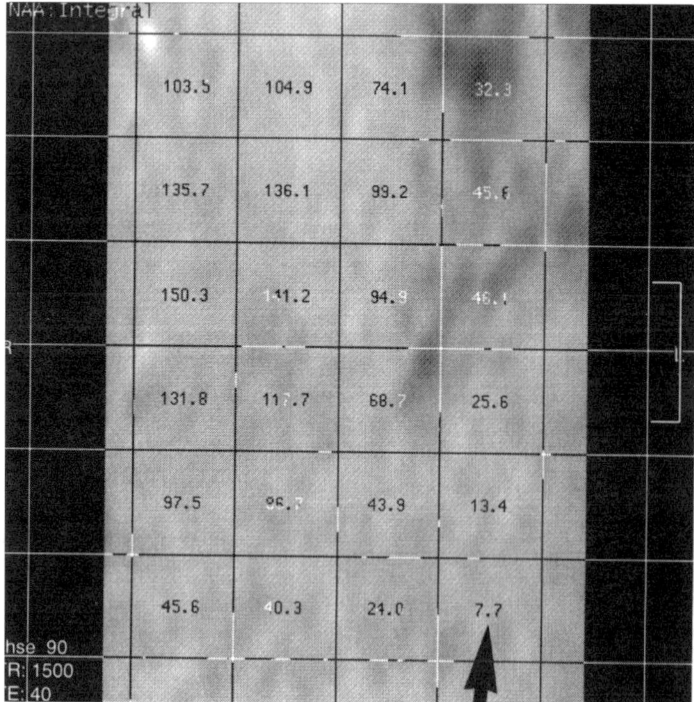

Figure 91j.

Figure 92 a-f. **Mucopolysaccharidosis (Scheie's disease).** 2-year-old girl. T2W images reveal high signal due to dilated Virchow-Robin spaces (a-c). The corpus callosum is diffusely thinned (d). ADC maps reveal high values in the periventricular areas, as well as in the corpus callosum: 1.43, 1.12, 1.26, 1.20, 1.19, 1.19, 1.10, and 1.27 X10^{-3} mm^2/sec (e,f).

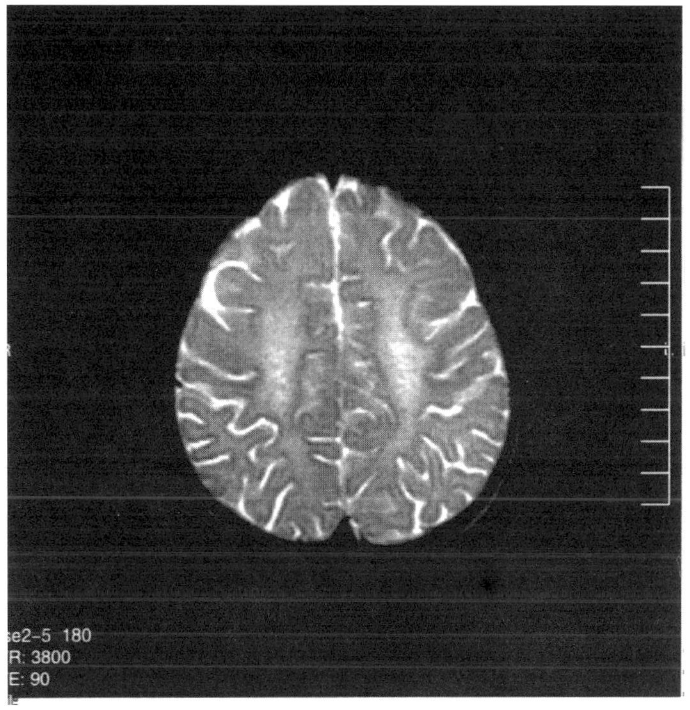

Figure 92a.

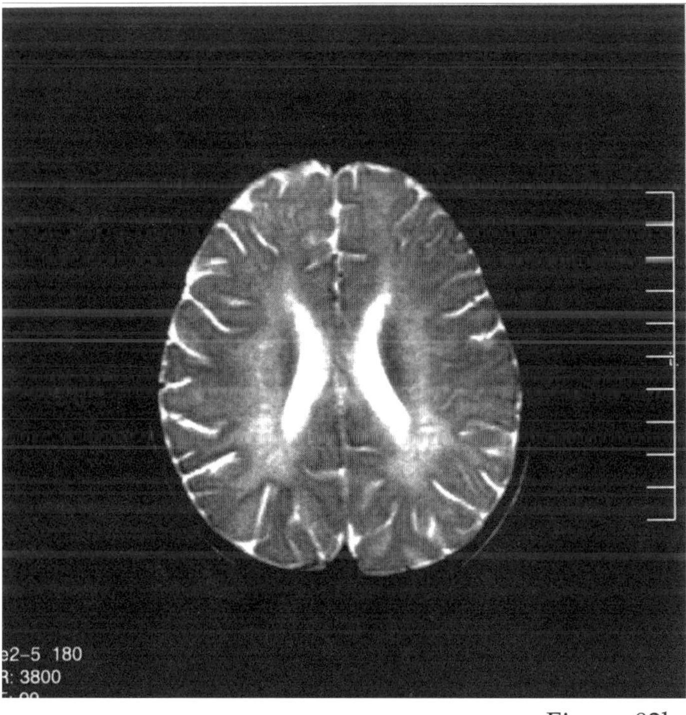

Figure 92b.

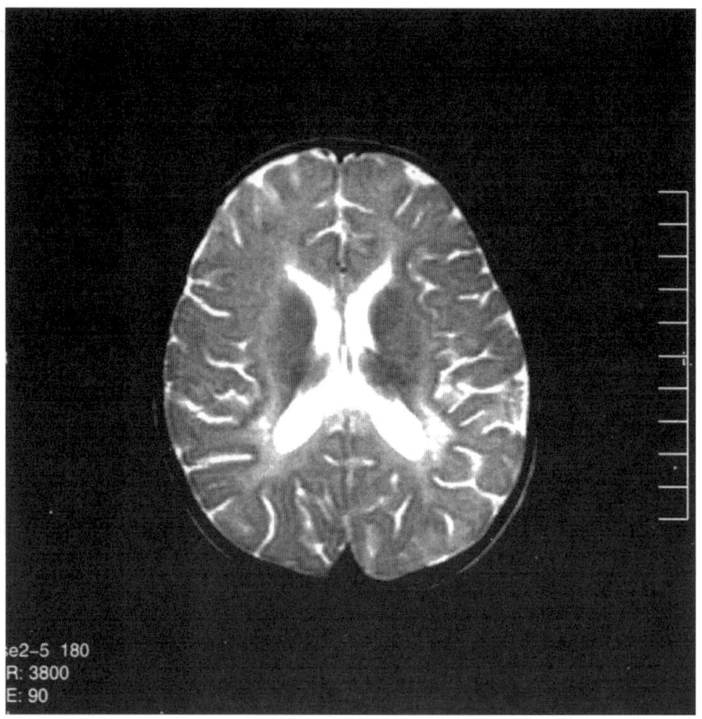

Figure 92c.

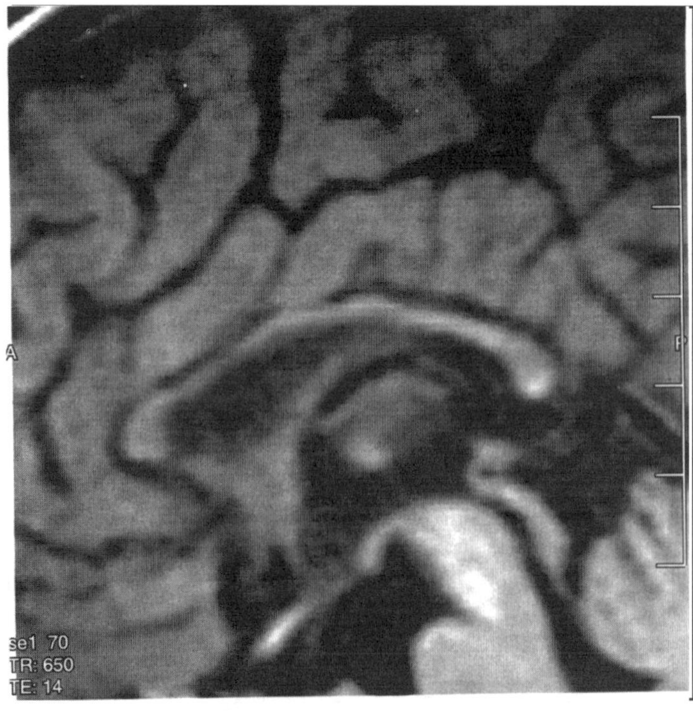

Figure 92d.

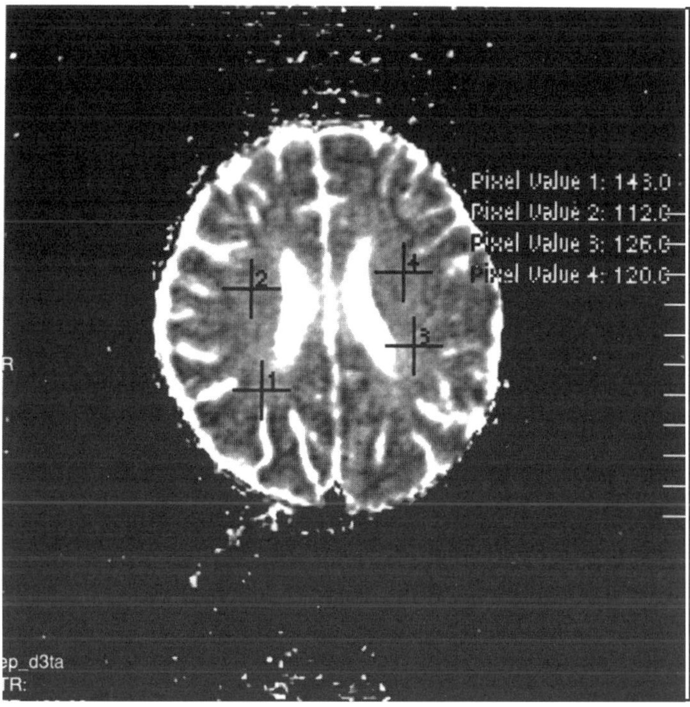

Figure 92e.

References
1. *Sener RN. Diffusion MRI: apparent diffusion coefficient (ADC) values in the normal brain, and a classification of brain disorders based on ADC values. Comput Med Imaging Graph 2001; 25:299*
2. Barkovich AJ. Pediatric neuroimaging. Philadelphia, Lippincott Williams & Wilkins, 2000
3. *Osborn AG. Diagnostic neuroradiology, St.Louis, Mosby, 1994*

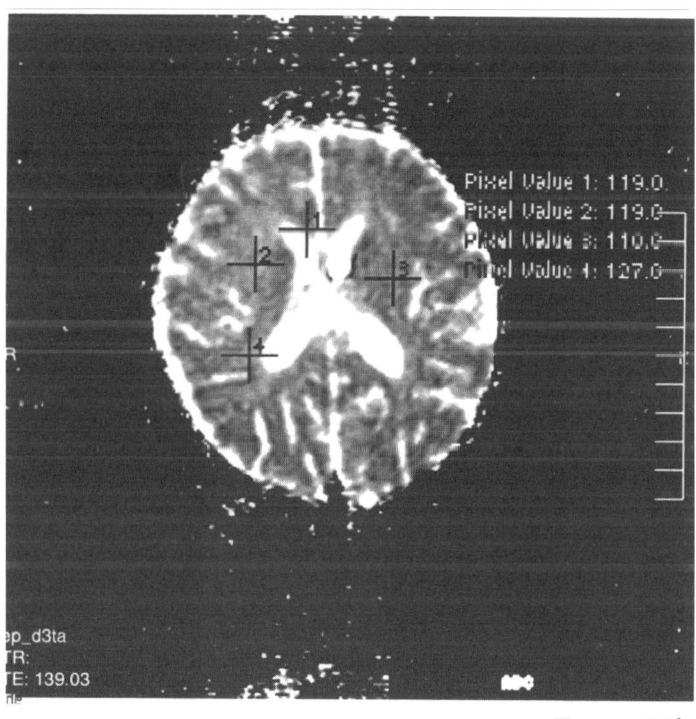

Figure 92f.

Figure 93 a-g. **van der Knaap syndrome** *(diffuse leukoencephalopathy associated with cystic degeneration of the white matter).* 4-year-old girl. Sagittal T1W images reveal a diffusely thinned corpus callosum in this diffuse type of leukoencephalopathy. The hypophysis gland is extremely thin (a,b).

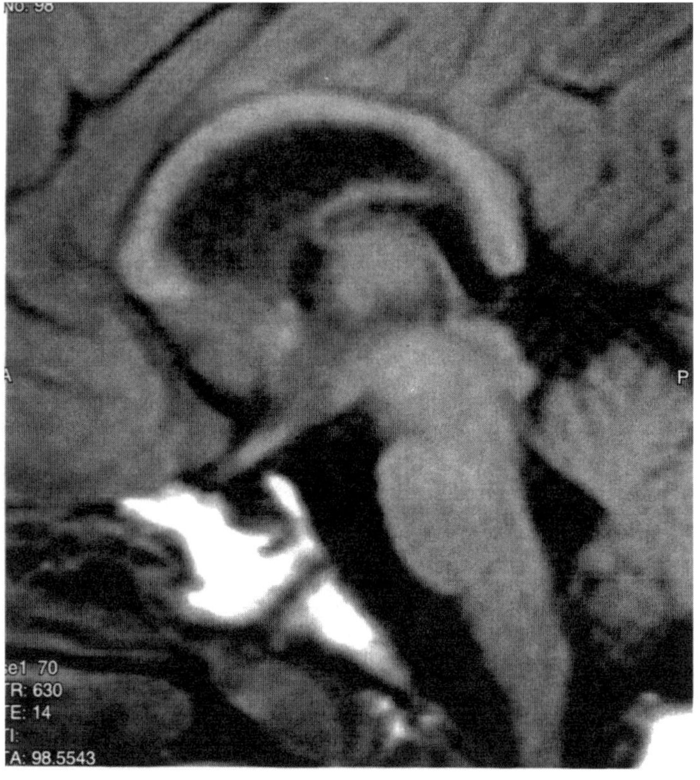

Figure 93a.

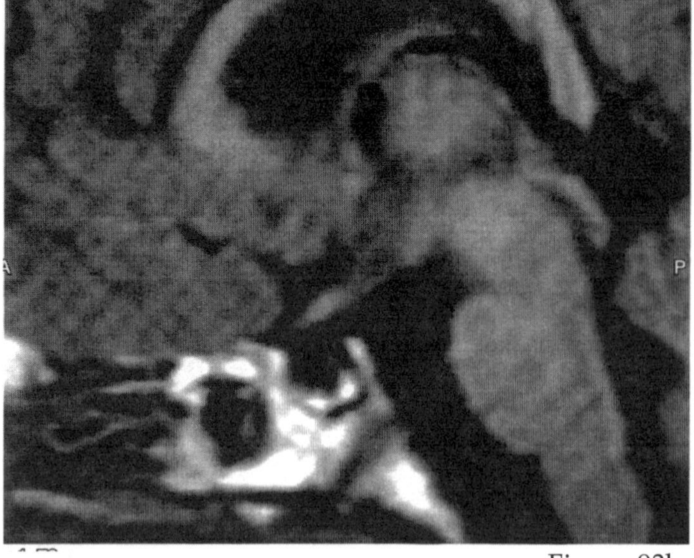

Figure 93b.

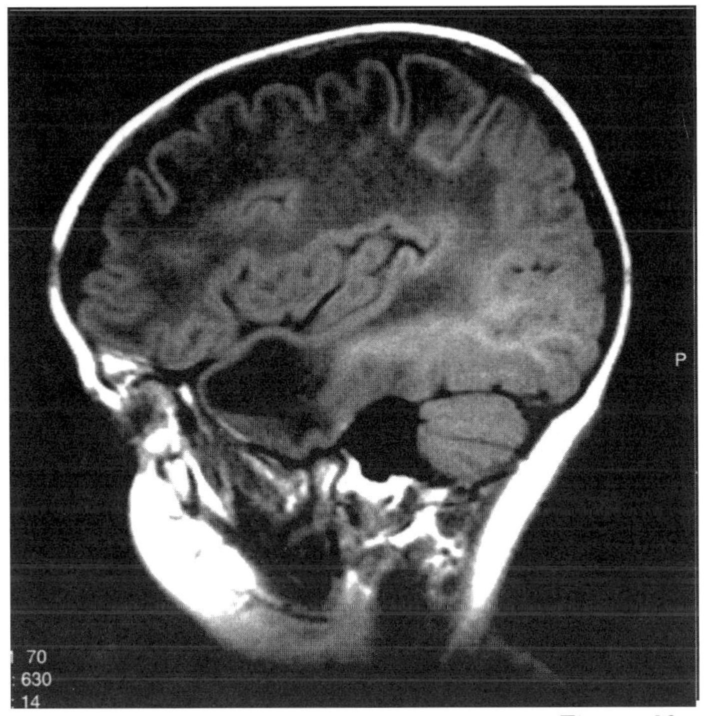

Figure 93c.

Sagittal T1W image reveals typical cystic degeneration at the tip of the temporal lobe, hypointense white matter, and thinned cortices (c). FLAIR image reveals diffuse signal abnormality in the white matter. Characteristic temporal cysts (cystic degeneration of white matter) are evident (d).

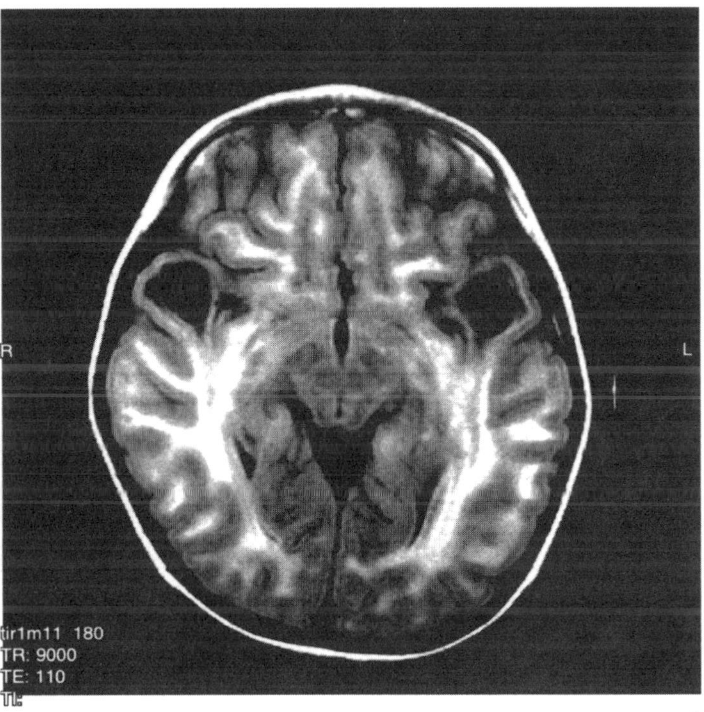

Figure 93d.

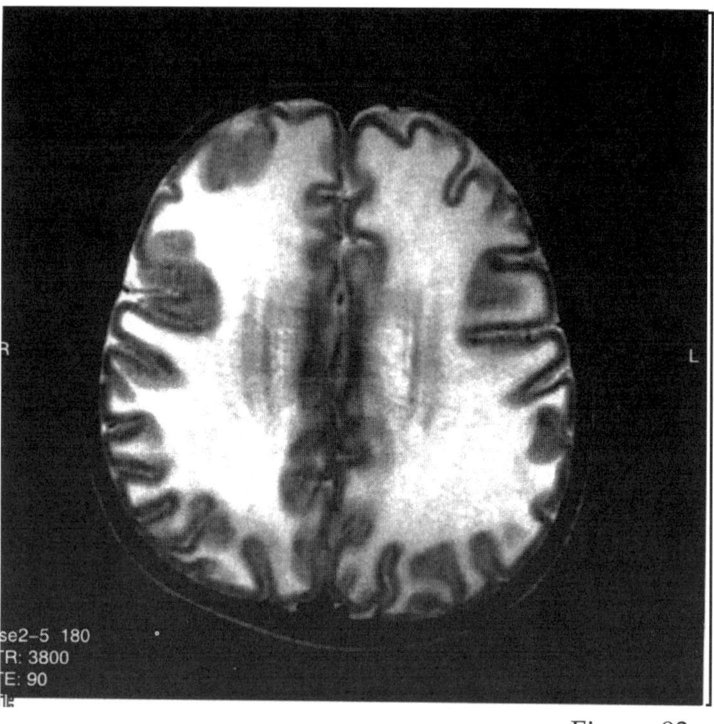

Figure 93e.

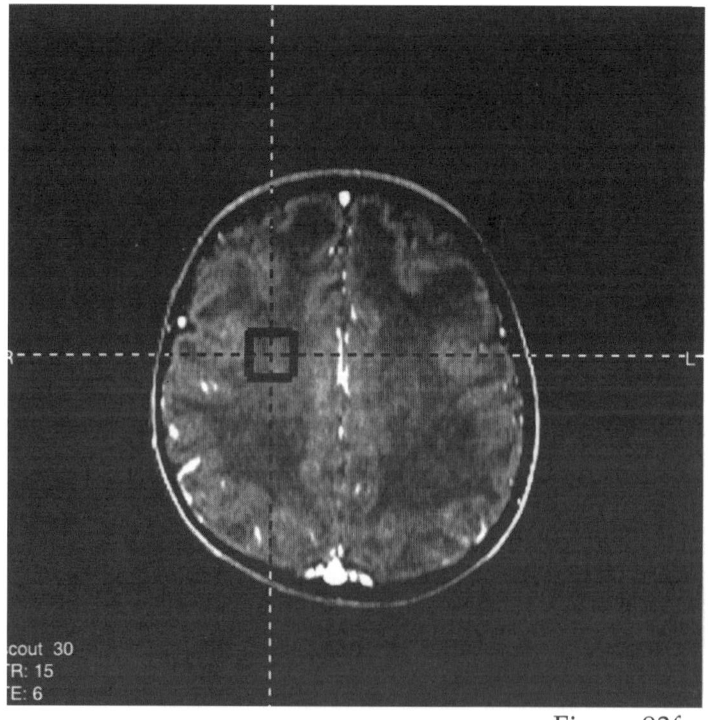

Figure 93f.

T2W image reveals diffuse high signal of the white matter and thin cortices (e). Localizer (T1W) of single-volume spectroscopy is shown (f).

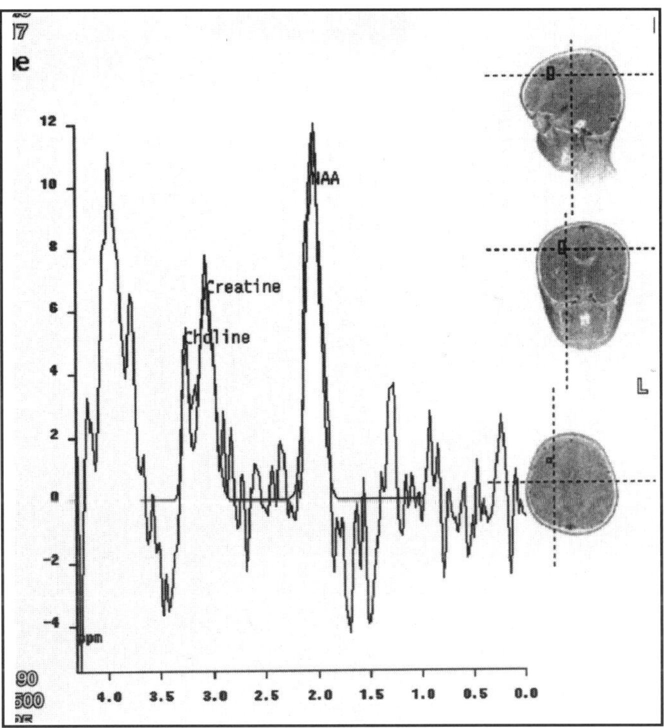

Figure 93g.

Proton MR spectroscopy (TR=1500 msec, TE=135 msec) reveals normal relationships of the major metabolites, NAA, creatine, and choline (g). The clinical findings in this disease are slowly progressive, and spectroscopy from the parenchyma remains normal or near normal until late stages of the disease.

References

1.　*van der Knaap MS, Barth PG, Stroink H, et al. Leukoencephalopathy with swelling and a discrepantly mild clinical course in eight children. Ann Neurol 1995;37:324*
2.　*van der Knaap MS, Wevers RA, Kure S, et al. Increased cerebrospinal fluid glycine: a biochemical marker for a leukoencephalopathy with vanishing white matter. J Child Neurol. 1999;14:728.*
3.　*Sener RN. van der Knapp syndrome: MR imaging findings including FLAIR, diffusion imaging, and proton MR spectroscopy. Eur Radiol 2000;10:1452*

Figure 94 a-d. **Infiltrating glioma (gliomatosis cerebri).** 32-year-old man. FLAIR image reveals a hyperintense lesion in the right frontal lobe extending to the corpus callosum, and passing to the contralateral hemisphere. Note the ground glass appearance of the lesion (a). Post-contrast T1W image reveals no enhancement (b).

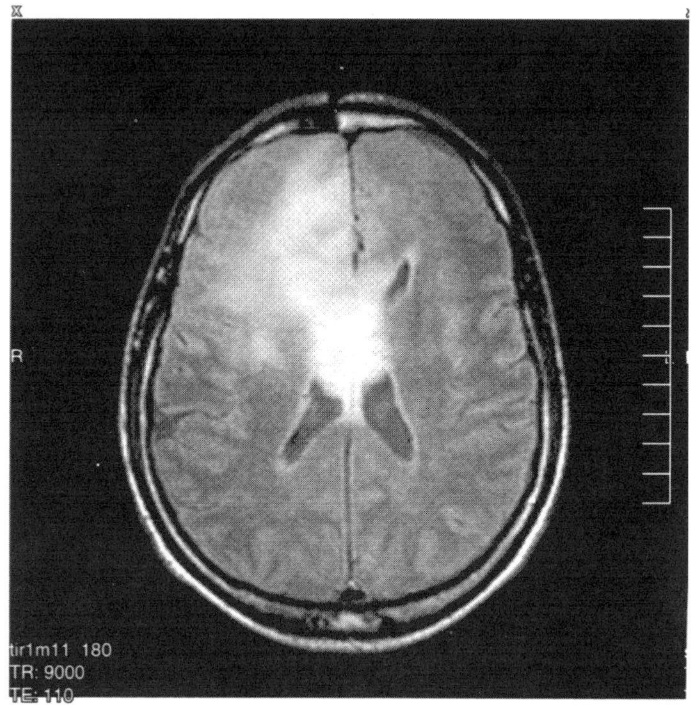

Figure 94a.

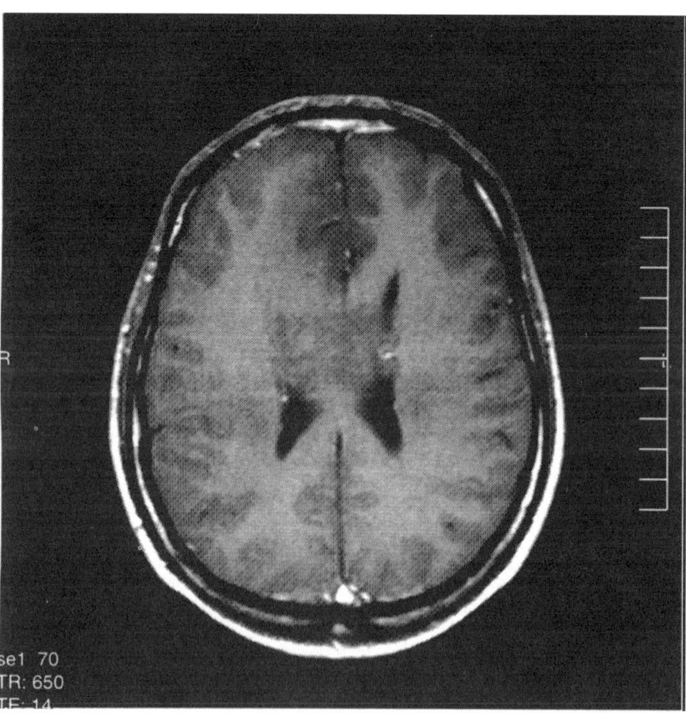

Figure 94b.

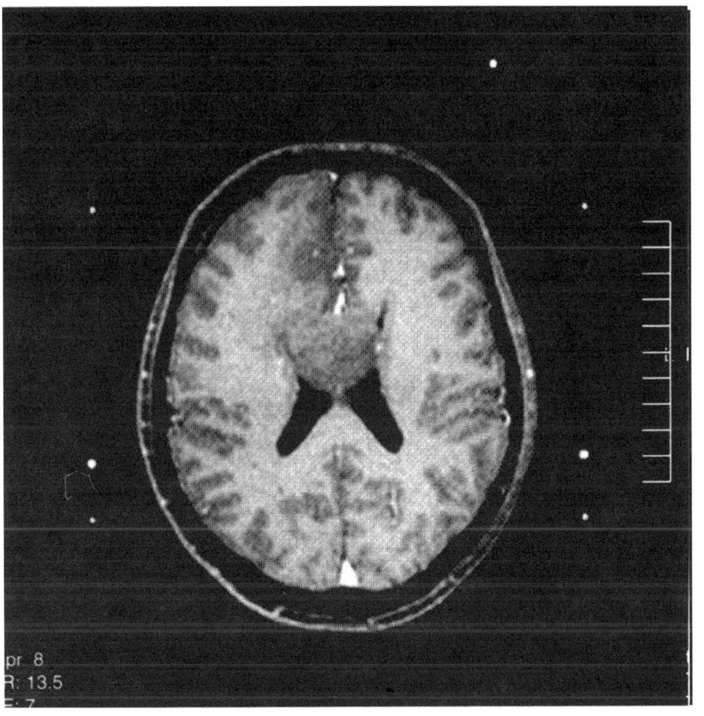

Figure 94c.

MPR image (T1W) obtained during stereotaxic biopsy is shown (c). Single-volume proton MR spectroscopy (TR=1500 msec, TE=135 msec) reveals a decreased NAA peak and increased choline peak. NAA decrease represents destruction of neurons and axons. Choline increase reflects increased membrane turnover (i.e. increased cell membrane destruction, and increased production of neoplastic cells and their membranes). The integral value of NAA is: 35.90, and that of choline is 52.94. Creatine has an integral value of 30.89. Therefore, NAA/Choline ratio is: 0.67; NAA/Creatine ratio is: 1.16; and Choline/Creatine ratio is: 1.71 (d). Generally, changes in these ratios become more prominent correlating with malignant features in a tumor. Also, in malignant tumors lactic acid, lipids and other macromolecules, myoinositol, and glycine peaks tend to increase.

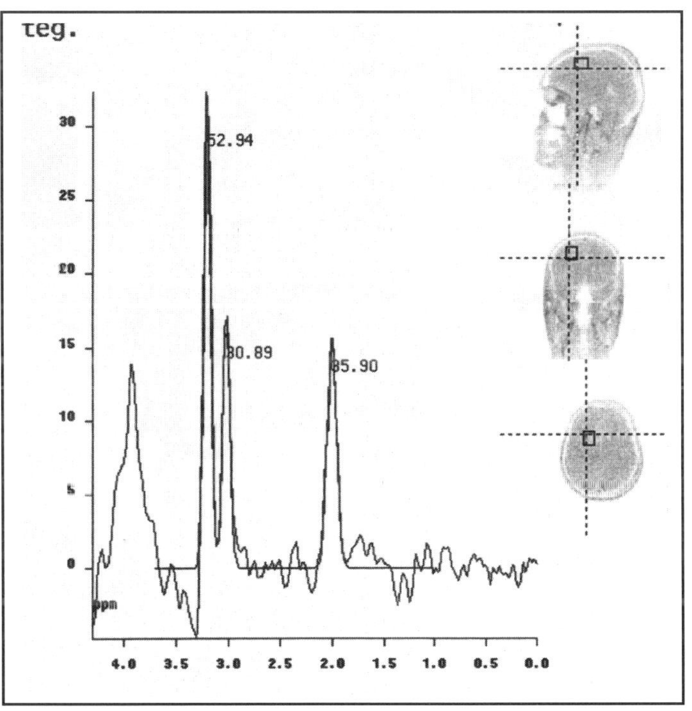

Figure 94d.

Figure 95 a-c. **Gliomatosis cerebri.** 82-year-old man. *a) SE TlW MR image, b) SE T1W MR image after administration of contrast medium, and c) SE PDW MR image.* The splenium of the corpus callosum has apparently been thickened showing a round configuration (circle) (a). Axial images show thickening of the genu (circles) (b, c) and an abnormal signal (hyperintensity) (c), representing an infiltrating tumor crossing the splenium and spreading to both hemispheres, gliomatosis cerebri. Note absence of contrast enhancement (b).

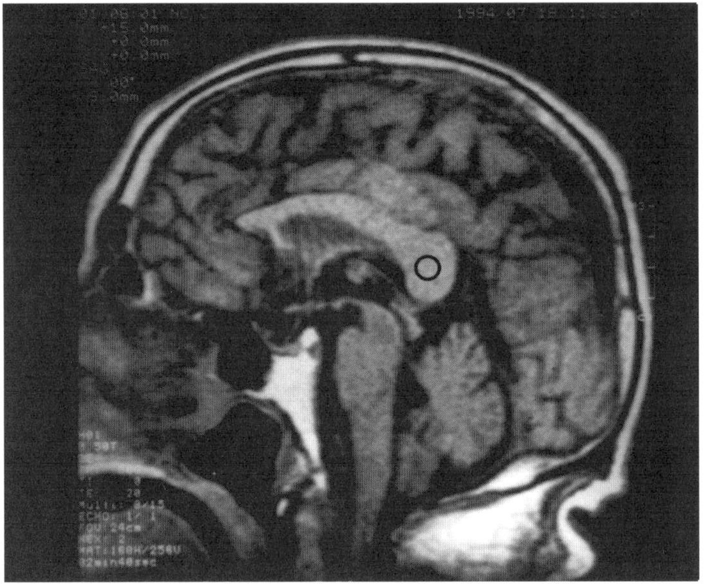

Figure 95a.

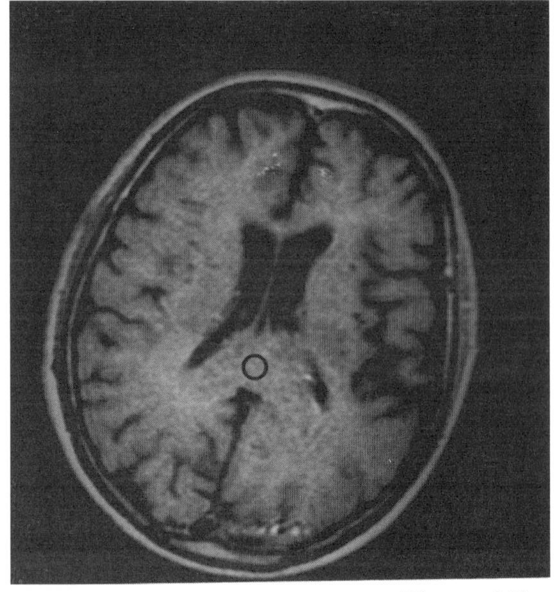

Figure 95b.

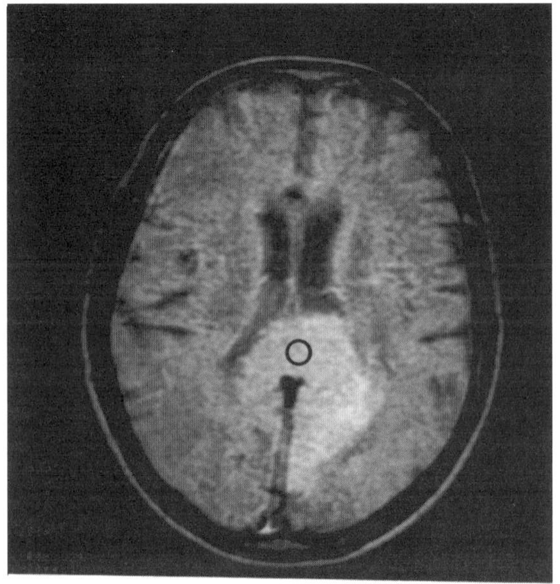

Figure 95c.

Reference
1.   *Osborn AG. Diagnostic neuroradiology. St. Louis, Mosby, 1994;550*

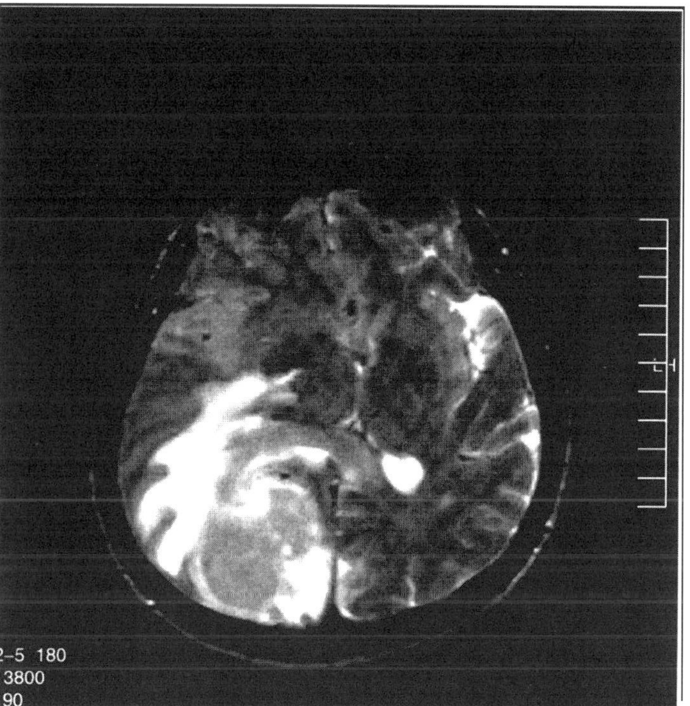

Figure 96a.

Figure 96 a-g. **Non-Hodgkin lymphoma (B-cell).** 46-year-old man. T2W image reveals a relatively low-signal tumor with surrounding edema in the right occipital lobe with extension to the corpus callosum (a). b=1000S sec/mm^2 (true diffusion) image reveals high signal of the tumor and in its callosal extension. High signal on true diffusion image represents hypercellularity of this metastatic tumor (b).

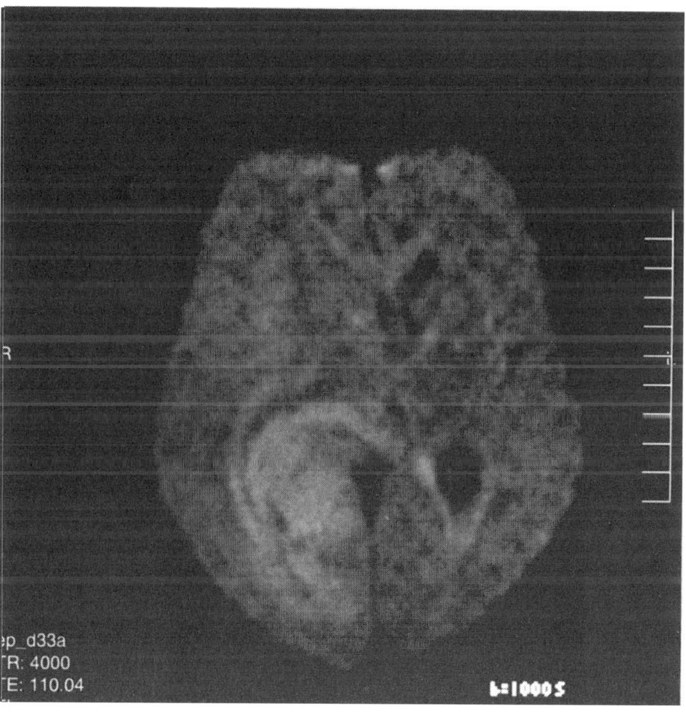

Figure 96b.

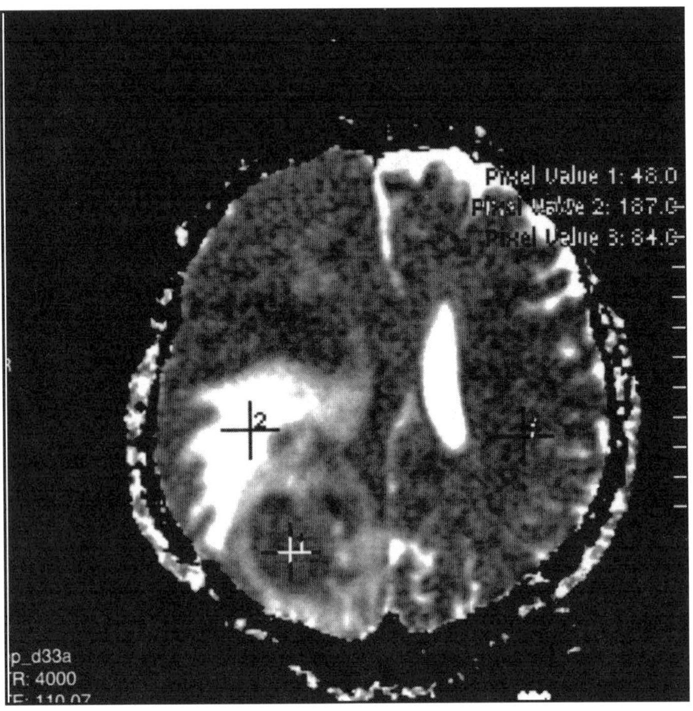

Figure 96c.

ADC map reveals a low ADC value: 0.48 $\times 10^{-3}$ mm²/sec in the tumor. Surrounding vasogenic edema has a high value: 1.87 $\times 10^{-3}$ mm²/sec. Normal parenchymal value is shown: 0.84 $\times 10^{-3}$ mm²/sec (c). Low ADC values from the bulk of the tumor: 0.46 and 0.57 $\times 10^{-3}$ mm²/sec, normal parenchymal values: 0.69 and 0.69 $\times 10^{-3}$ mm²/sec, and a high value of surrounding vasogenic edema: 1.94 $\times 10^{-3}$ mm²/sec are shown (d).

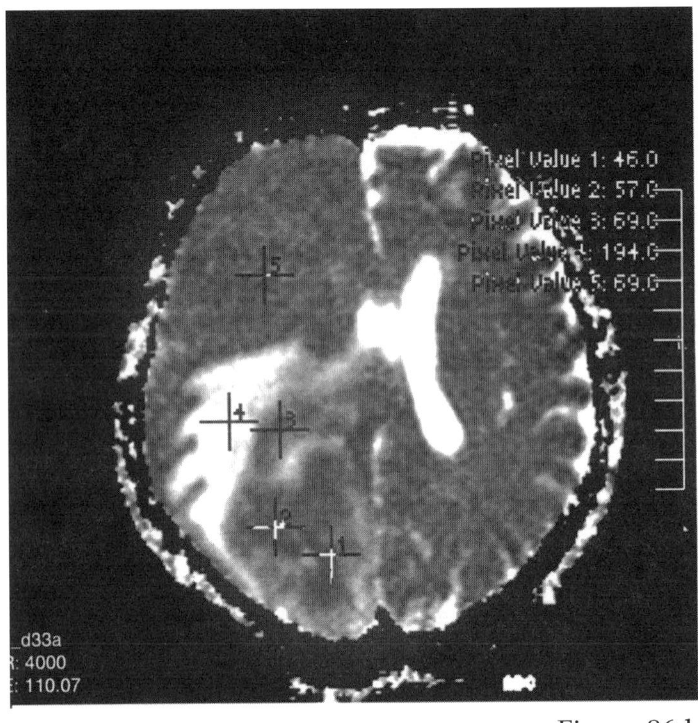

Figure 96d.

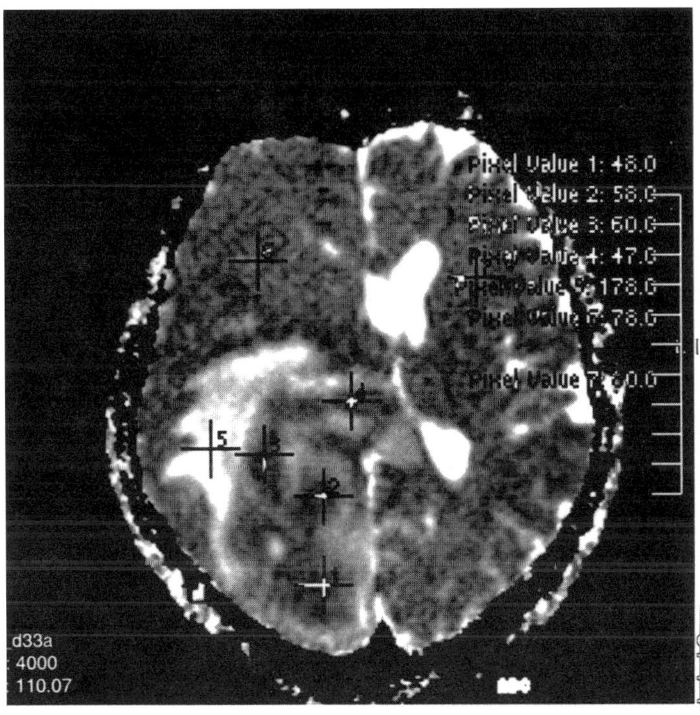

Figure 96e.

The tumor and its callosal extension reveal low ADC values: 0.48, 0.58, 0.60, and 0.47 X 10^{-3} mm^2/sec. Vasogenic edema has a high value: 1.78 X10^{-3} mm^2/sec. Two normal ADC values from the parenchyma are shown: 0.78 and 0.80 X10^{-3} mm^2/sec (e).

Spectra from a chemical-shift imaging (TR=1500 msec, TE=135 msec) in two different voxels (f,g) reveal apparently low NAA, and high choline peaks. Low NAA represents neuroaxonal destruction, and high choline represents increased membrane turnover. Creatine appears to be prominently decreased in one of the spectra (f). Low creatine indicates high metabolic status of the tumor. There is a prominent lactic acid peak at 1.33 ppm (below the baseline). High lactate corresponds to carbonhydrate catabolism. Prominent peaks from 1.30 to 0.80 ppm represents lipids and other macromolecules. Presence of high lipid peaks represent accumulation of membrane lipids in the tissue.

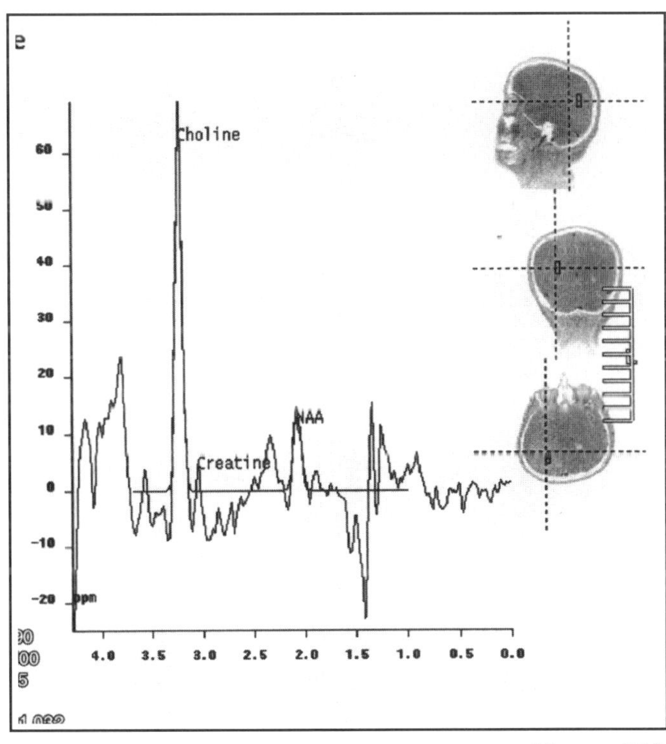

Figure 96f.

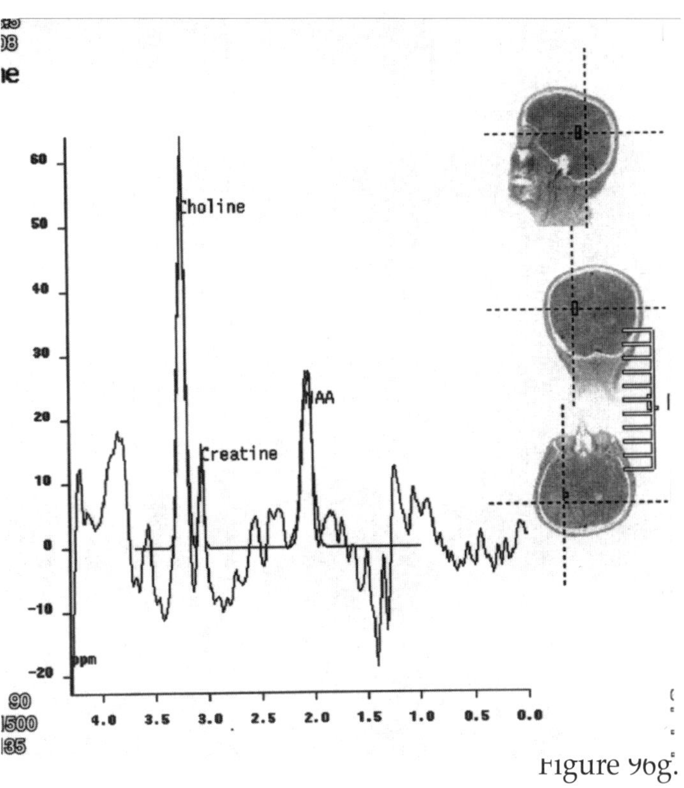

Figure 96g.

Reference

1.   *Kuroda I, Kawasaki T, Haraoka S, et al. autopsy report of primary cns b-cell lymphoma indistinguishable from multiple sclerosis - diagnosis with the immunoglobulin gene rearrangements analysis. J Neurol Sci 1992;111: 173*

Figure 97 a-c. **Polycystic brain.** 9-year-old girl. *a, b) SE T1W and c) SE T2W MR images.* There are numerous intraparenchymal cysts (a-c) which also involve the corpus callosum (arrows) (a, b). The cysts represented extremely dilated Virchow-Robin spaces. The patient also had changes consistent with ectodermal dysplasia. There was no apparent clinical correspondence with respect to such widespread cysts, and the patient only had learning difficulties. The condition was not associated with any form of mocopolysaccharidoses (from reference 1).

References

1. Sener RN. Polycystic brain (cerebrum polycystica vera) associated with ectodermal dysplasia: a new neurocutaneous syndrome. Pediatr Radiol 1994;24:116
2. Bacheschi LA, Magalhaes ACA, Mathias SC. Multiple cystic lesions in white matter without clinical manifestations (unidentified black holes). Neuroradiology (suppl) 1995;37:246
3. Lynch SA, Hall K, Precious S, et al. Two further cases of Sener syndrome: frontonasal dysplasia and dilated Virchow-Robin spaces. J Med Genet 2000;37:466

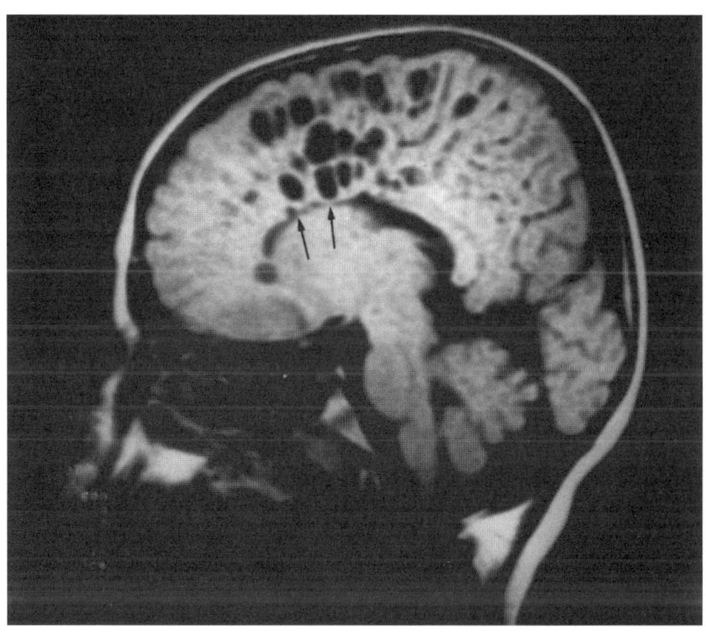

Figure 97a.

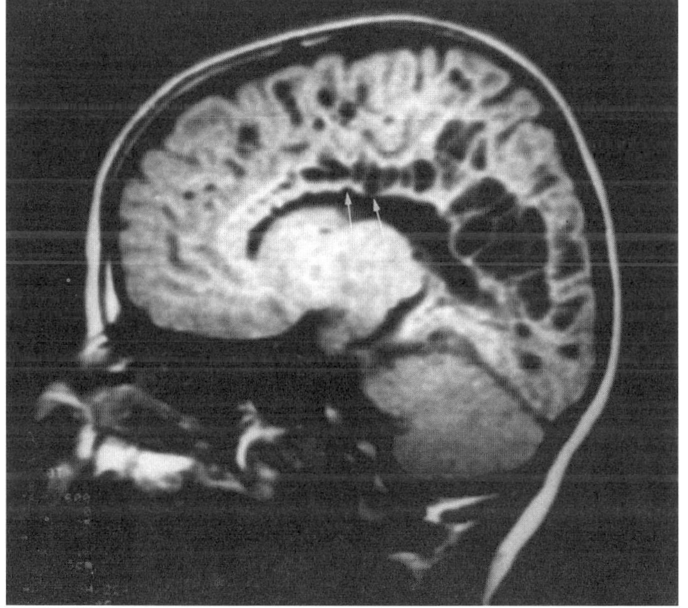

Figure 97b.

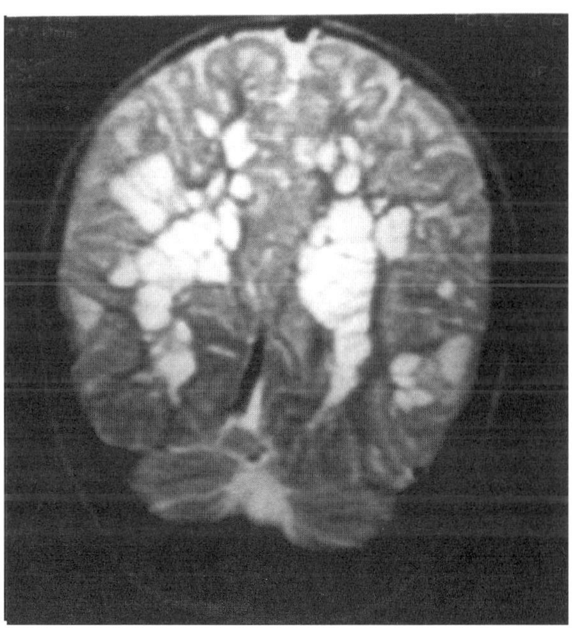

Figure 97c.

Figure 98 a-c. **Infarct.** 65-year-old man. *a, b) SE T1W and c) SE PDW MR images.* There is a lesion consistent with a subacute phase infarct at the territory of the left anterior cerebral artery which involves the body of the corpus callosum (circles) (a, b, c). Also note several zones of chronic infarcts and periventricular chronic ischemic changes (b, c)

Reference
1. Osborn AG. Diagnostic neuroradiology. St.Louis, Mosby, 1994;343

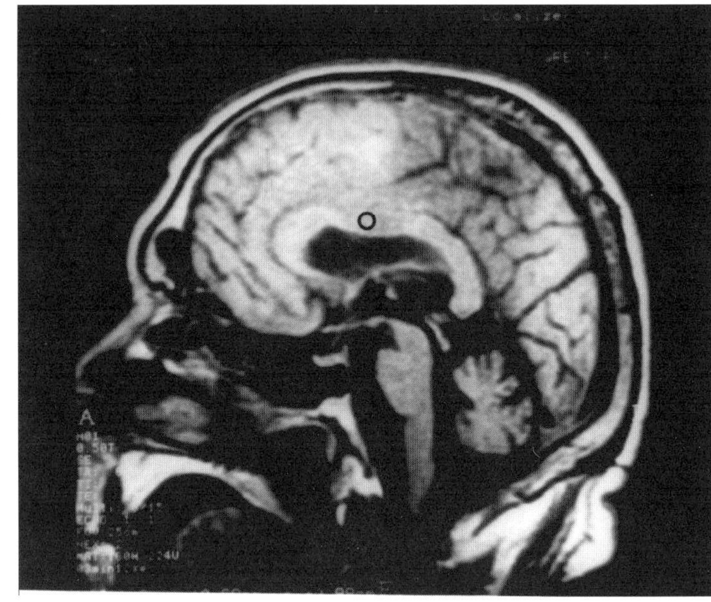

Figure 98a.

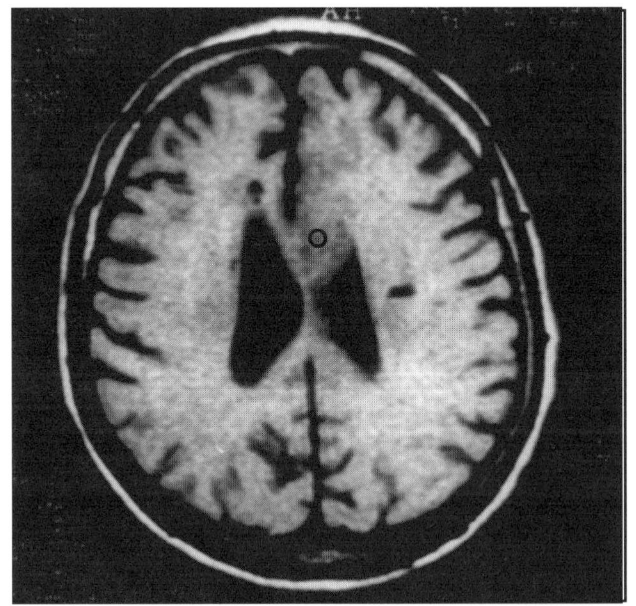

Figure 98b.

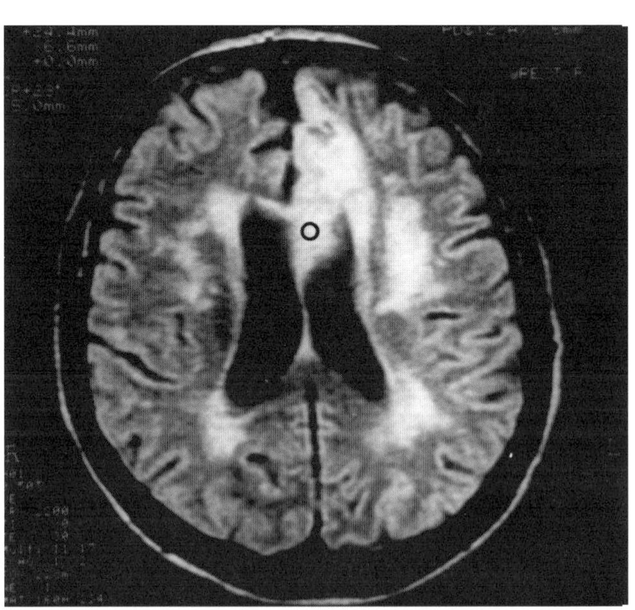

Figure 98c.

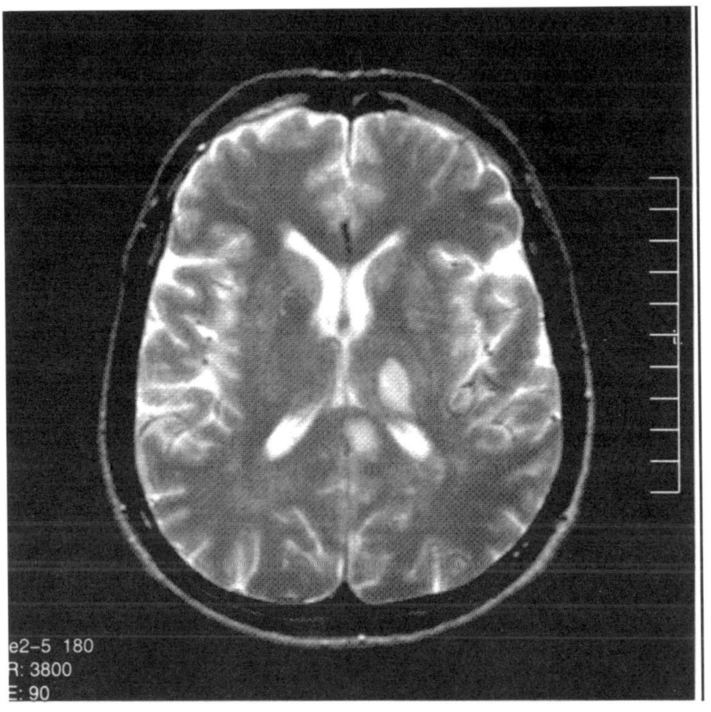

Figure 99a.

Figure 99 a-c. **Acute infarction.** 52-year-old man. T2W image reveals high-signal lesions in the corpus callosum, and left thalamus (a). ADC map reveals a low ADC value of the infarcted area in the corpus callosum: 0.53 X 10^{-3} mm^2/sec, indicating restriction of molecular motion of water (cytotoxic edema). A normal value from the frontal white matter is shown: 0.82 X10^{-3} mm^2/sec (b).

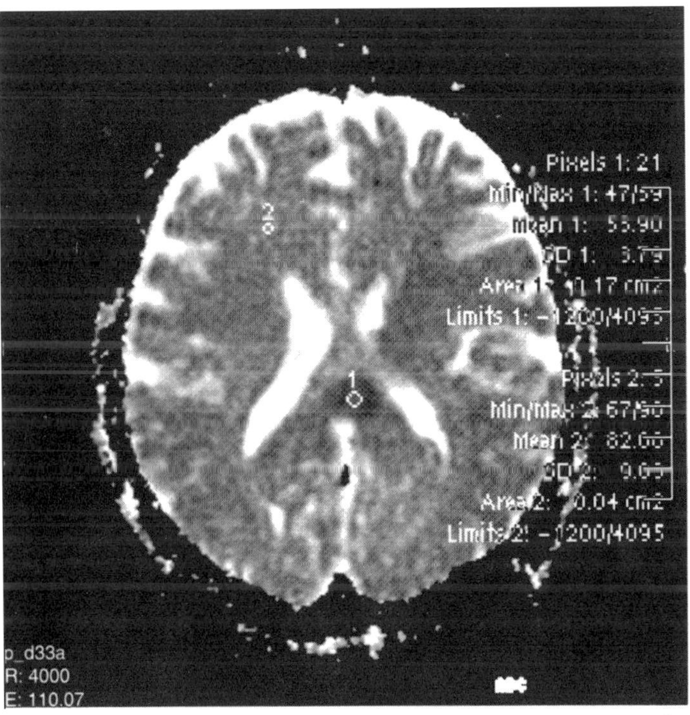

Figure 99b.

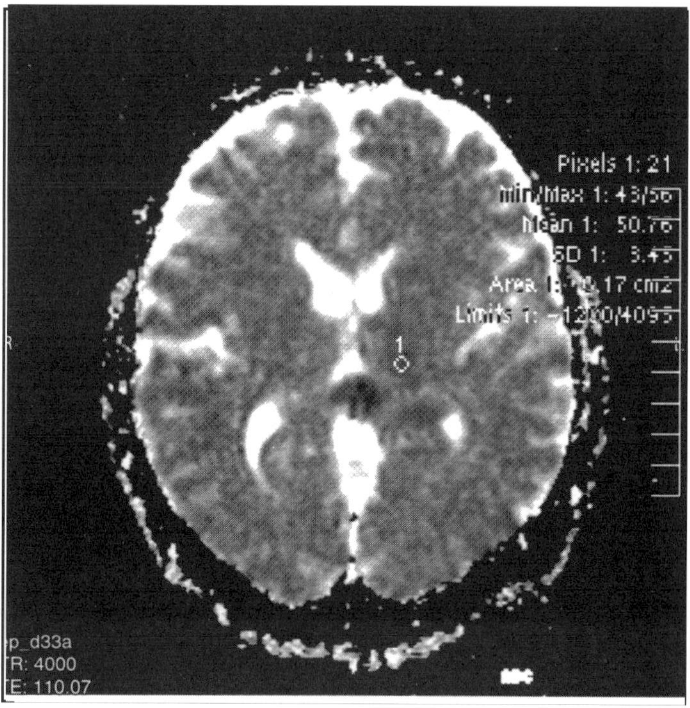

Figure 99c.

ADC value of the thalamic acute infarction is: 0.50 X10^{-3} mm^2/sec (c).

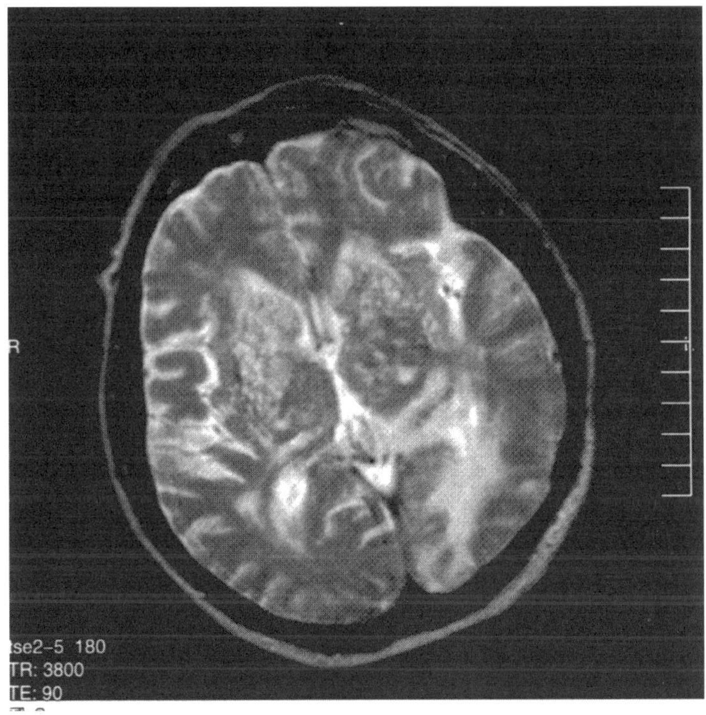

Figure 100a.

Figure 100 a-d. **Acute infarction, leukoariasis, and enlarged Virchow-Robin spaces.** 69-year-old man. T2W image reveals a high signal left occipital lesion. Note extensive dilatation of Virchow-Robin spaces in the periventricular regions (a).

$b=1000P$ sec/mm^2 (true diffusion) image reveals infarcted regions in the left half of the corpus callosum, left occipital lobe, and left internal capsule, manifested by high signal of cytotoxic edema *(P is phase gradient)* (b).

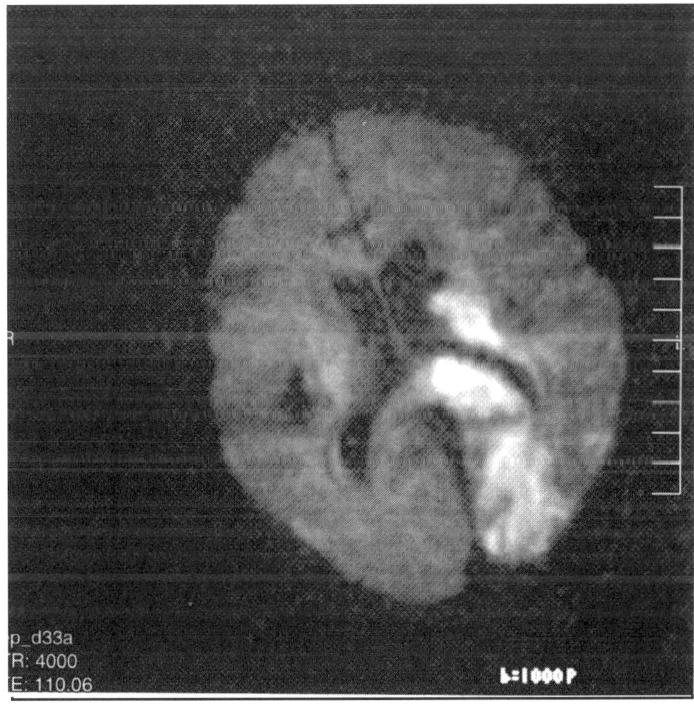

Figure 100b.

ADC map reveals low values in the infarcted regions: 0.42, and 0.47 X10^{-3} mm^2/sec. ADC value from a frontal region with leukoariasis is high: 1.52 X10^{-3} mm^2/sec (c).

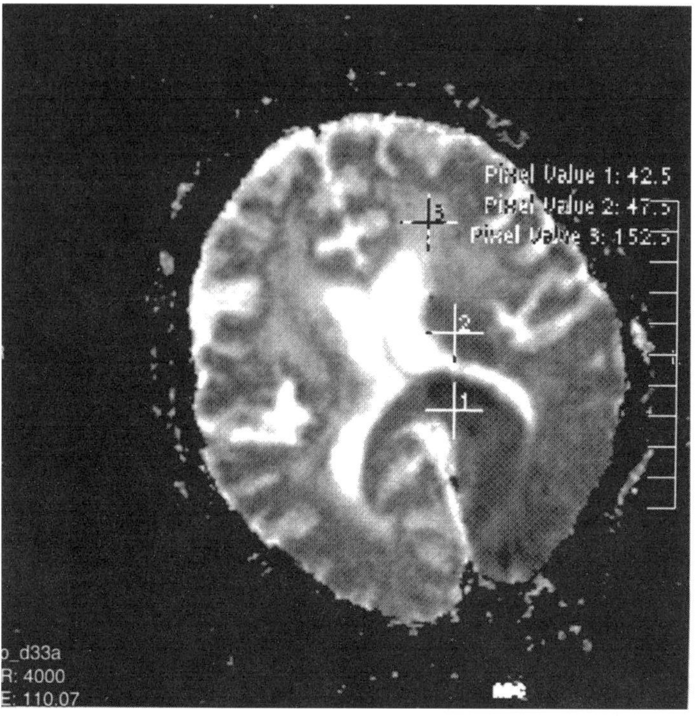

Figure 100c.

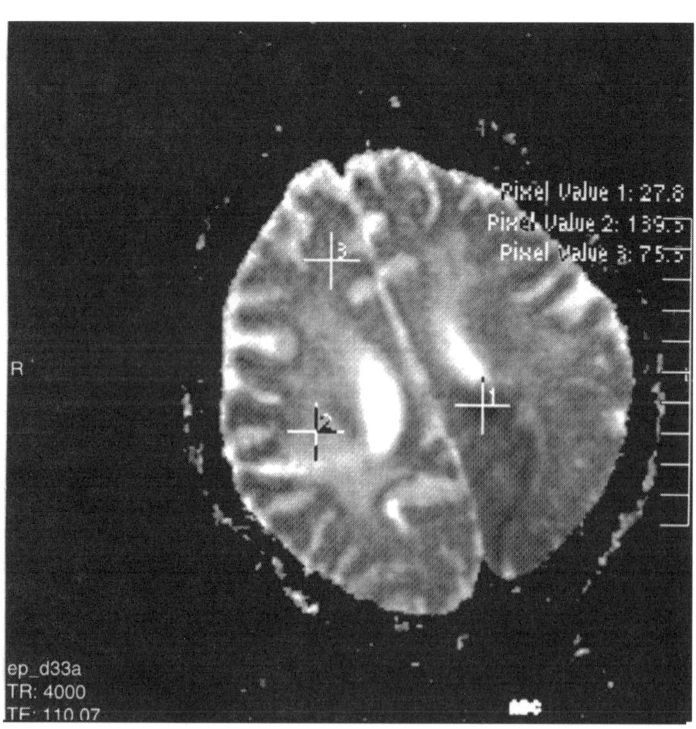

Figure 100d.

ADC value of the infarcted region in the corpus callosum is: 0.27 X10^{-3} mm^2/sec. That of periventricular enlarged Virchow-Robin spaces is: 1.39 X10^{-3} mm^2/sec. A normal parenchymal value is shown from the right frontal white matter: 0.75 X10^{-3} mm^2/sec (d). Note that changes related with leukoariasis, and enlarged Virchow-Robin spaces are not visible in the b=1000S sec/mm^2 (true diffusion) image (b).

Figure 101 a,b. **Acute infarction (corpus callosum).** 6-year-old girl. b=1000P sec/mm^2 (true diffusion) image reveals presence of infarction as a high signal area. High signal reflects restriction of water molecules in the infarcted area due to cytotoxic edema (a). ADC value measurement of the infarcted area by rectangular ROI evaluation reveals 0.47 X10^{-3} mm^2/sec. Normal parenchymal ADC value is shown at the right frontal region: 0.79 X10^{-3} mm^2/sec (b). In infarcts ADC values generally range from 0.14 to 0.50 (**0.32±0.09**) X10^{-3} mm^2/sec. Mean ADC value for cerebral parenchyma usually is: (**0.84±0.11**) X10^{-3} mm^2/sec between the ranges 0.60 to 1.05 X10^{-3} mm^2/sec.

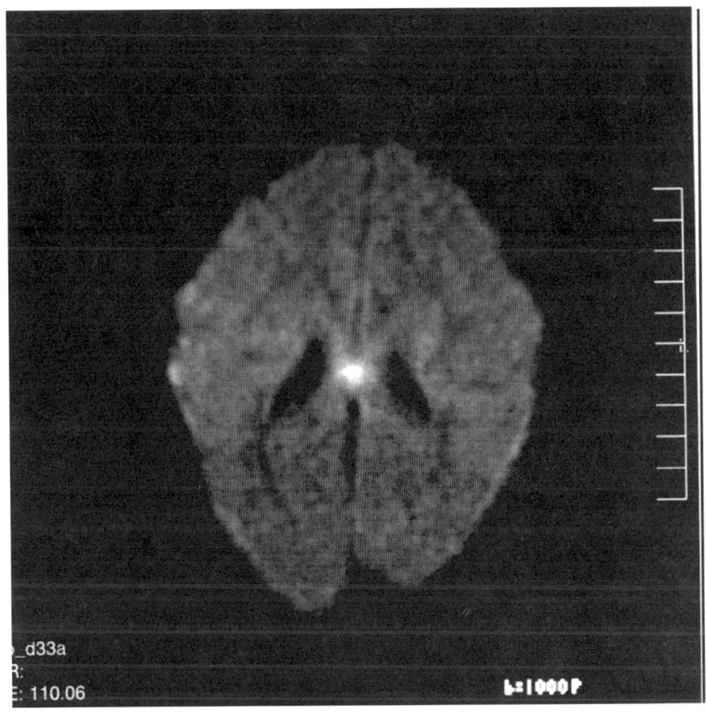

Figure 101a.

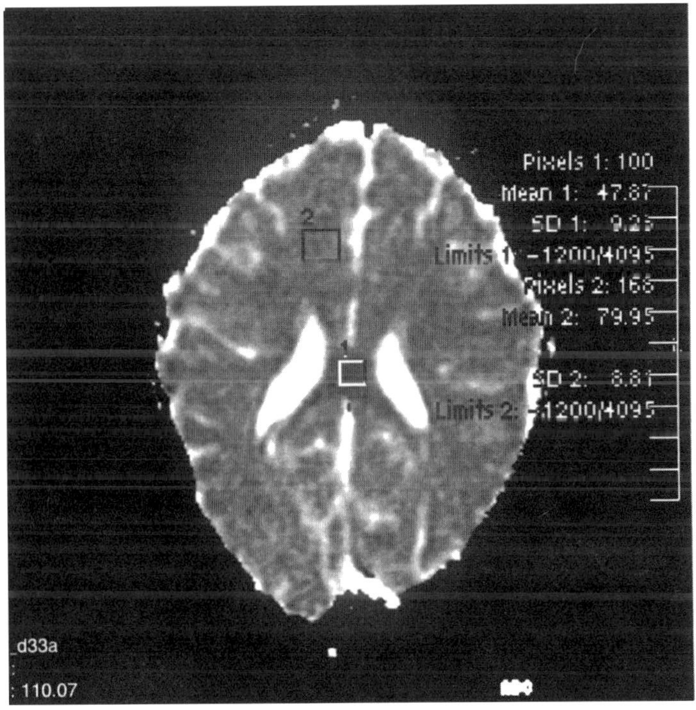

Figure 101b.

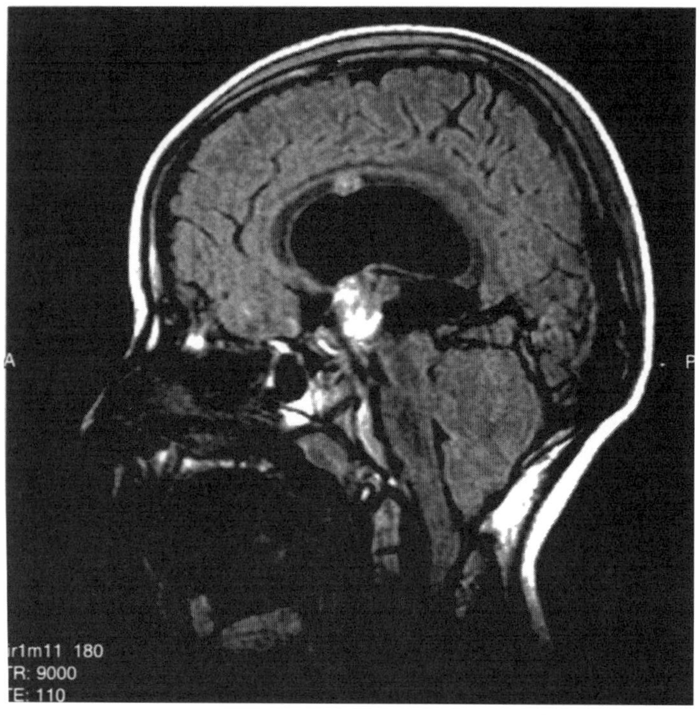

Figure 102a.

Figure 102 a-h. **Chiari II malformation. Endoscopic ventriculostomy.** 8-year-old girl. FLAIR image shows a high-signal change in the corpus callosum due to the endoscopic intervention (a).

PSIF (anisotropic diffusion) images (b-d) show the high signal changes in the corpus callosum. Postintervention defect in the floor of the 3rd ventricle is also seen (b).

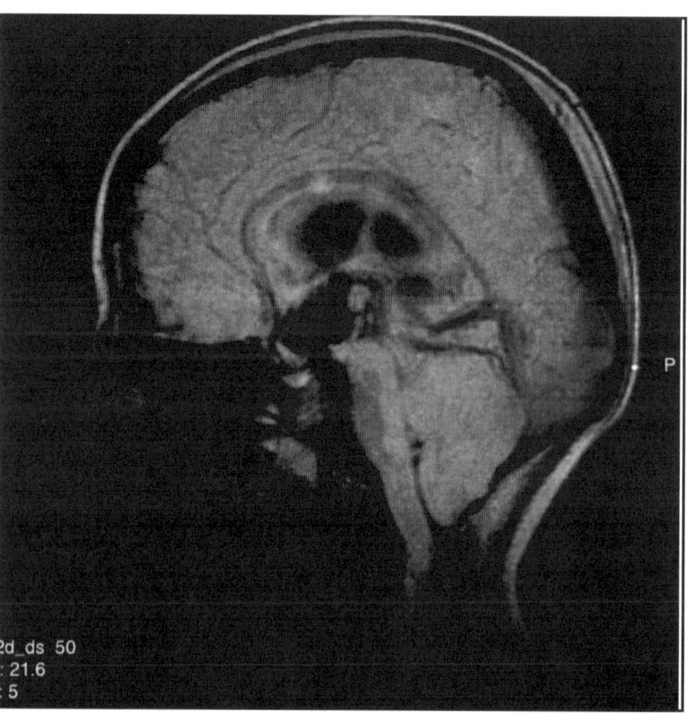

Figure 102b.

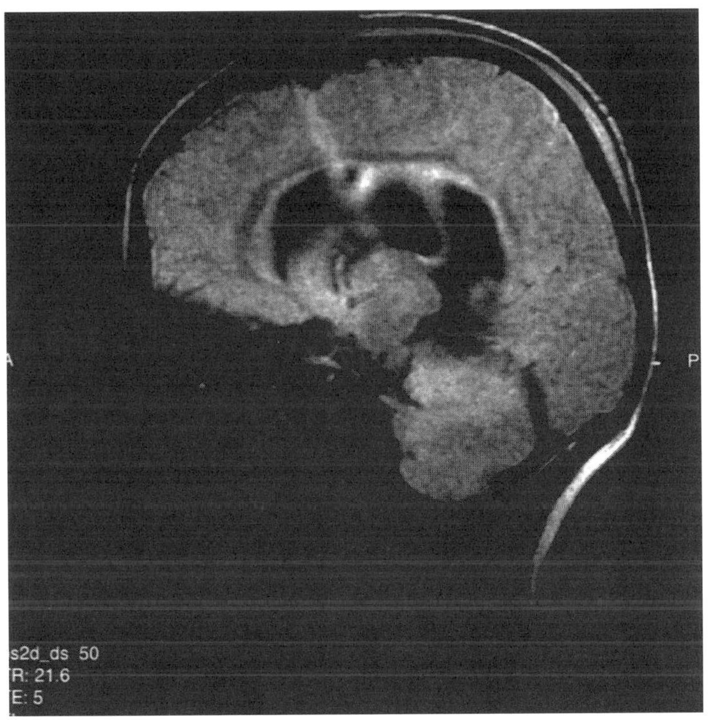

Figure 102c.

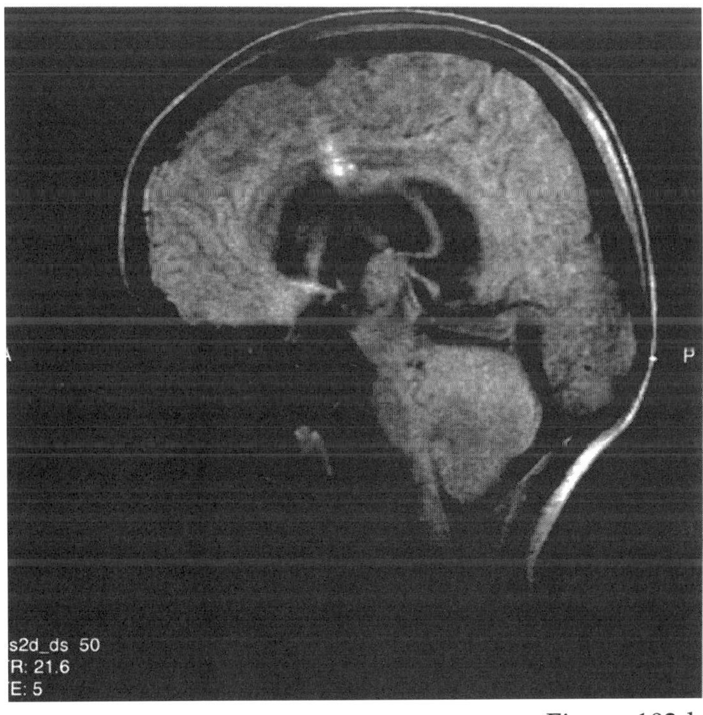

Figure 102d.

b=50T image (T2-weighted) reveals a high signal focus in the corpus callosum (e).

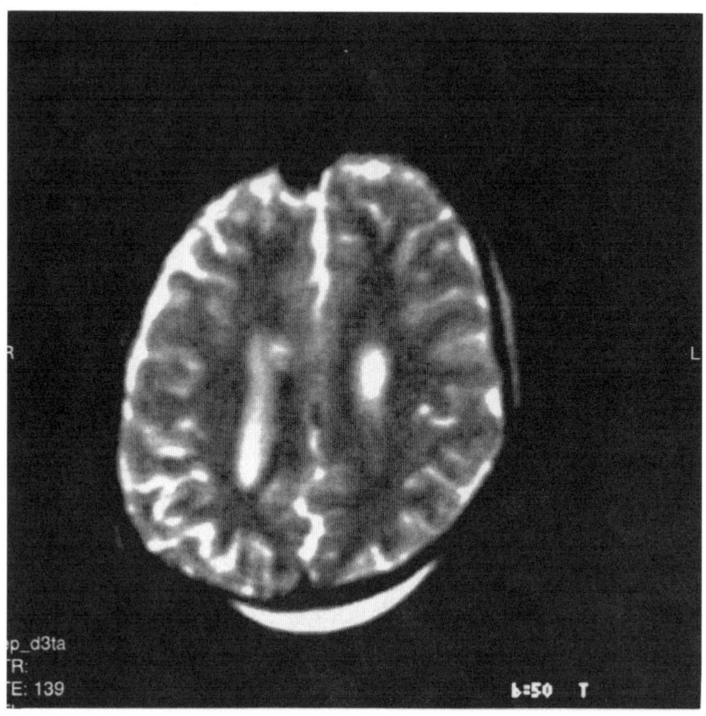

Figure 102e.

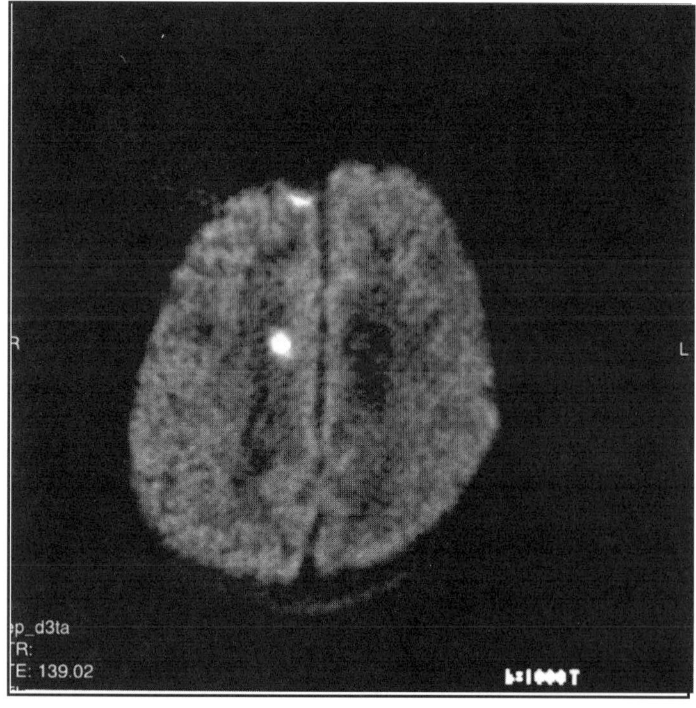

Figure 102f.

b=1000T sec / mm² (true diffusion) image identifies the lesion as an ischemic area, as it has high signal representing cytotoxic edema (f).

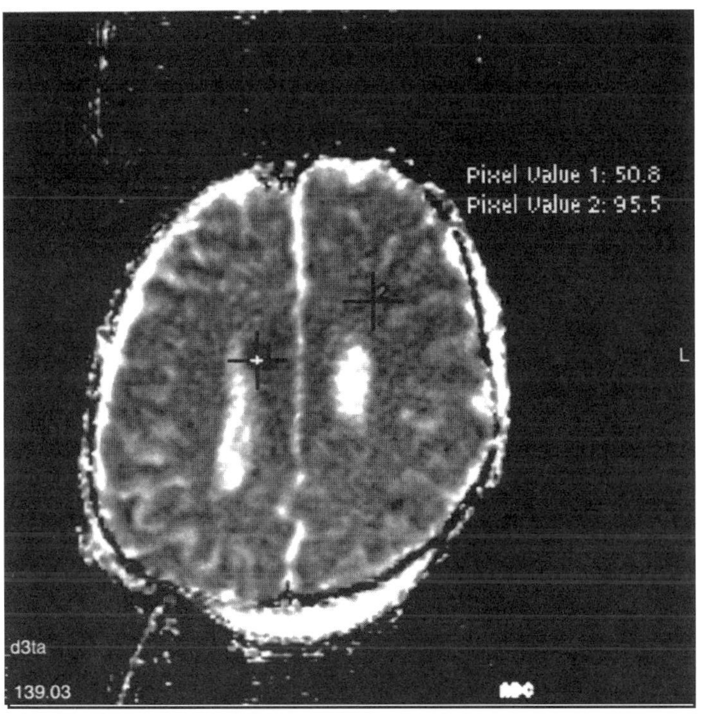

Figure 102g.

The lesion has a low ADC value: 0.50 $\times 10^{-3}$ mm^2/sec, consistent with ischemia. Normal ADC value is shown from the contralateral parenchyma: 0.95 $\times 10^{-3}$ mm^2/sec (g).

CISS (constructive interference of steady state) image, which is a gradient-echo sequence, demonstrates the postintervention defect in the floor of the 3rd ventricle. A gray line of jet flow (arrow) is seen from the ostium revealing effectivity of the endoscopic intervention (h).

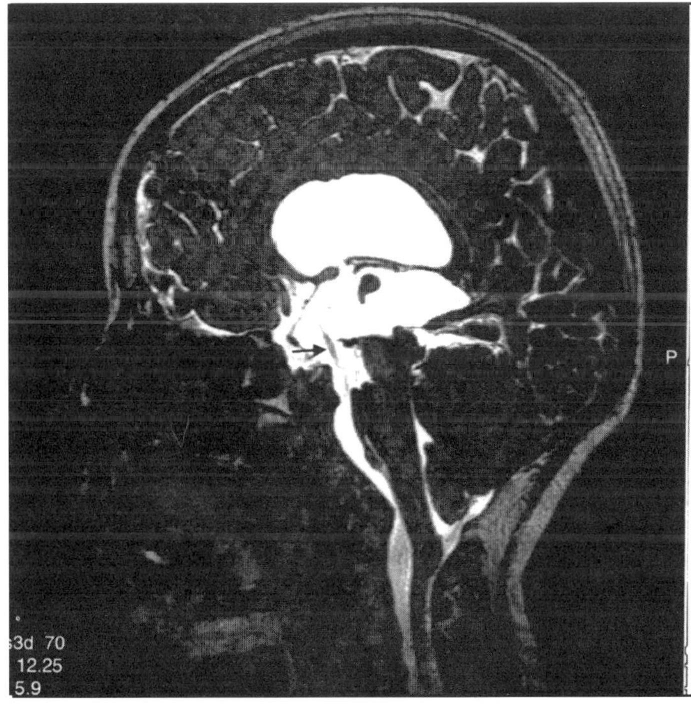

Figure 102h.

Figure 103 a-c. **FLAIR imaging of the corpus callosum in hydrocephalus.** Sagittal FLAIR image is shown from a normal individual with a normal corpus callosum. Its inner layer is seen as a thin hyperintense line (arrows). The normal thickness of this line is approximately between 1.5 to 2.5 mm (a).

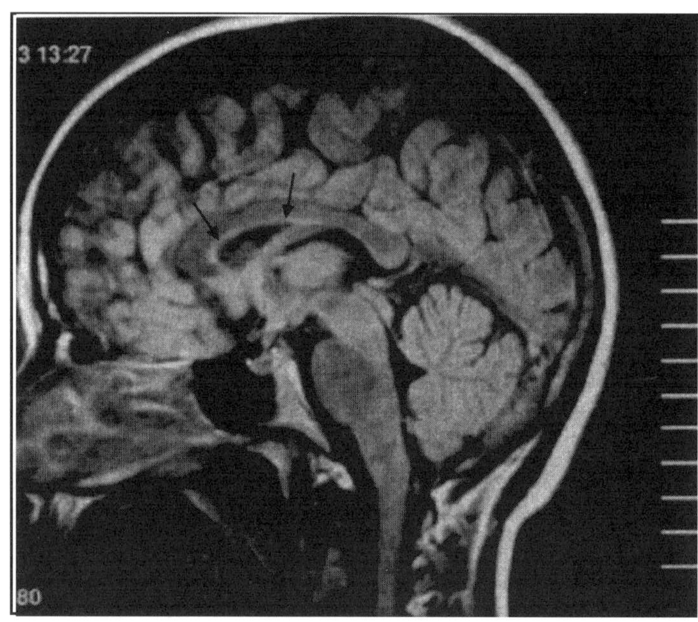

Figure 103a.

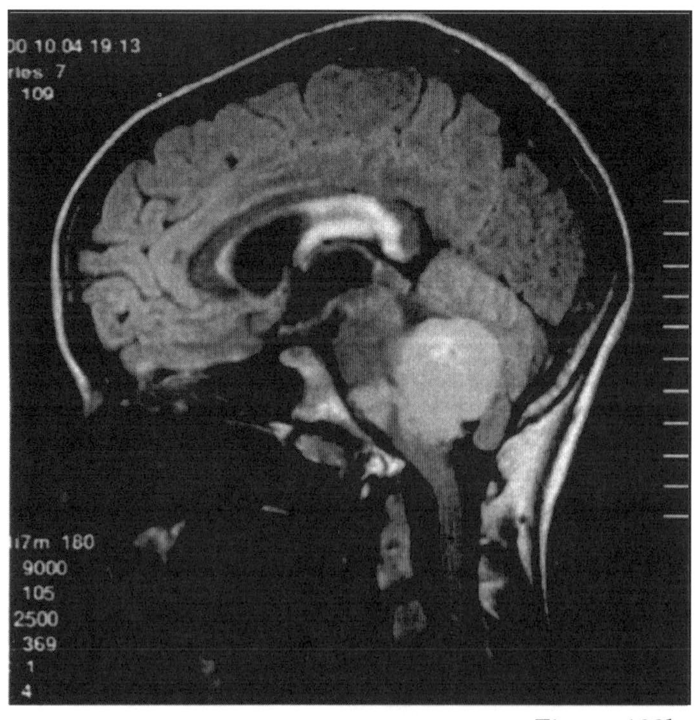

In a patient (23-year-old woman) with ependymoma of the fourth ventricle, the inner layer of the corpus callosum as well as the fornix reveals apparent thickening (8 mm), and prominent high signal. These are consistent with transependymal resorption of CSF. This is a recent finding recognized by increasing utilization of the FLAIR sequence (b).

Figure 103b.

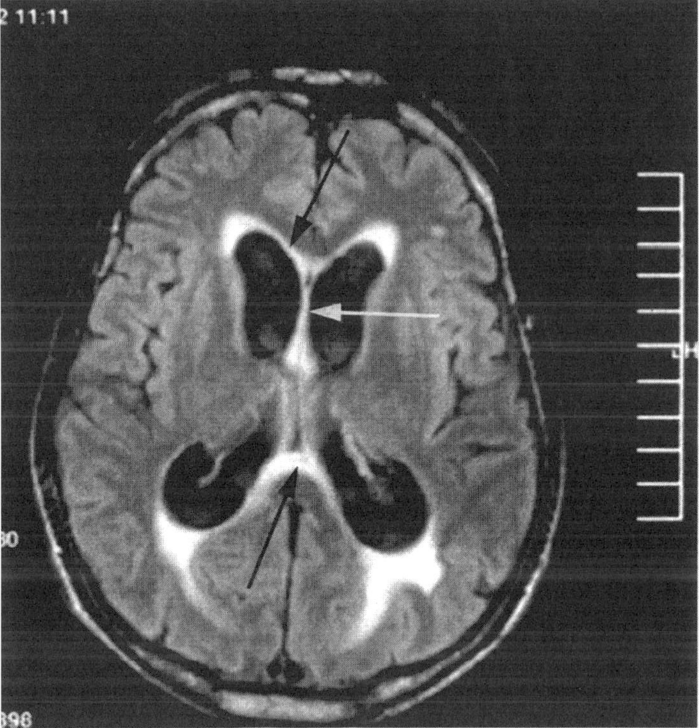

Figure 103c.

Transverse FLAIR image reveals transependymal resorption from the inner callosal layer (black arrows), and from the septum pellucidum (white arrow), in addition to the usually known regions, frontal horns, periatrial regions, occipital and temporal horns (c). (case courtesy of Dr. S. Dzelzite, Riga, Latvia).

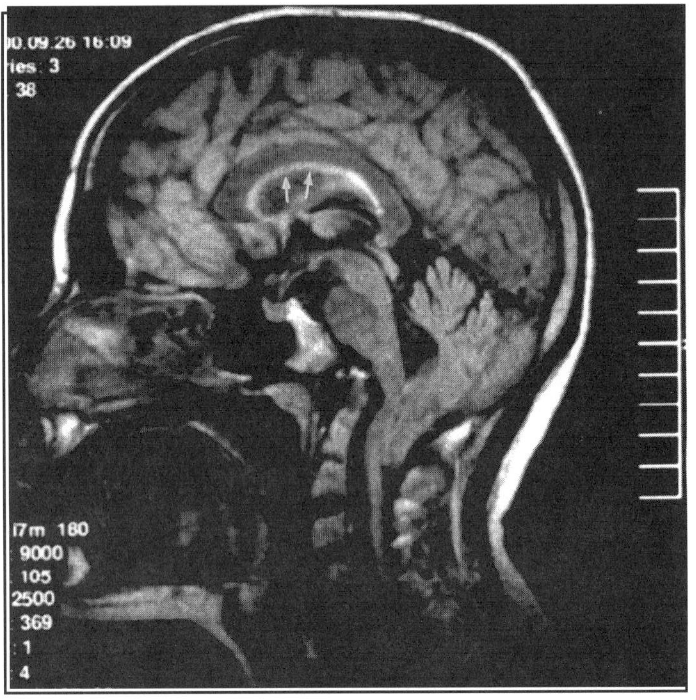

Figure 104a.

Figure 104 a,b. **FLAIR imaging in Chiari I malformation with mild hydrocephalus.** 28-year-old woman. FLAIR image reveals mild hydrocephalus apparently secondary to basilar invajination. Note the bright inner layer of the corpus callosum is thicker than normal (arrows) *(see previous cases)* (a).

Dilatation of the central canal of the spinal cord is associated with the condition. Basilar invagination and compression of the odontoid process upon the medulla oblongata is demonstrated to better advantage (b).

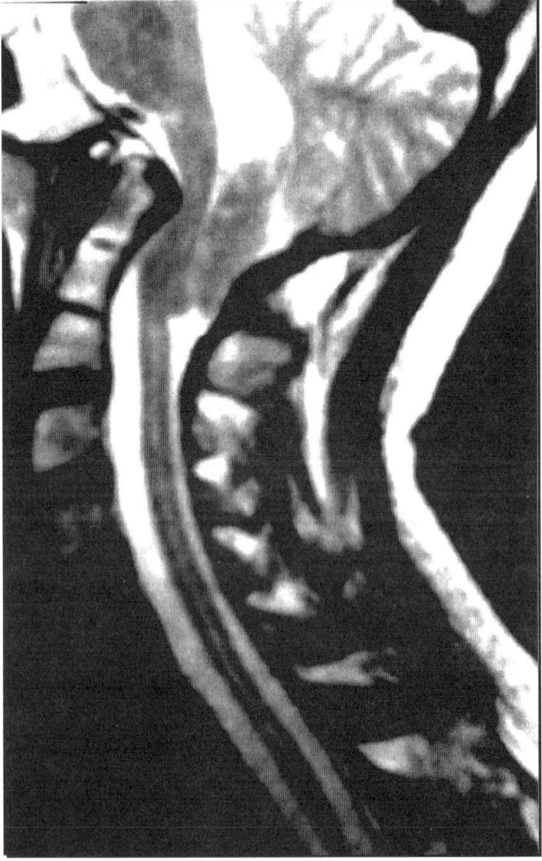

Figure 104b.

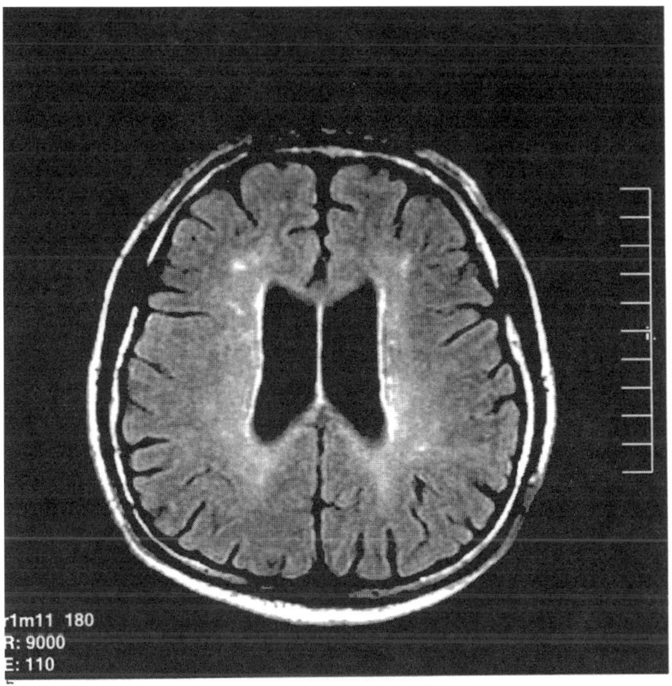

Figure 105 a-d. **Longstanding arrested hydrocephalus.** 27-year-old man. FLAIR image reveals diffuse high signal changes in the periventricular white matter, and corpus callosum (a).

Figure 105a.

ADC map reveals high values: 1.22, 1.14, and 1.23 X10^{-3} mm^2/sec in the periventricular regions (b).

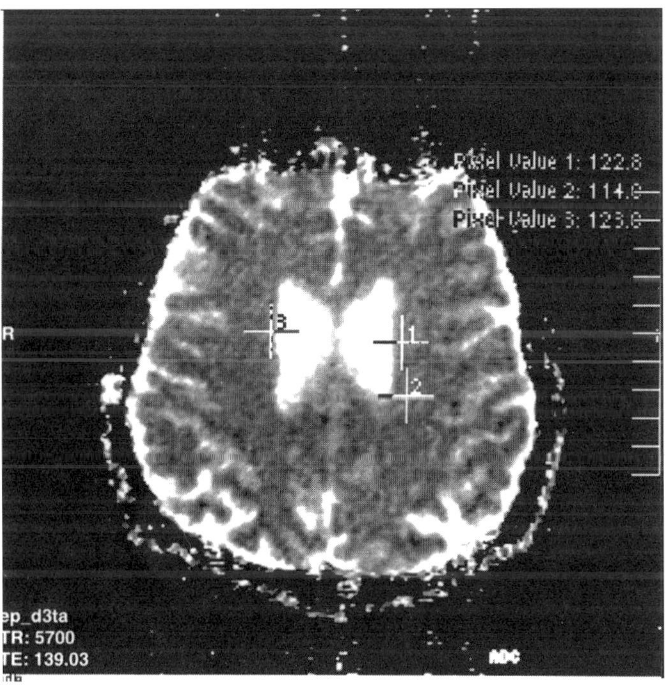

Figure 105b.

High signal in the inner callosal layer is demonstrated by FLAIR image (arrow) (c). Note the changes are less prominent than hydrocephalus due to ependymoma *(see previous cases)*. ADC map reveals a high ADC value in the inner callosal layer: 1.19 X10^{-3} mm^2/sec, and in the right frontal region: 1.17 X10^{-3} mm^2/sec. Normal value from the corpus callosum is shown: 0.79 X10^{-3} mm^2/sec. Also, normal value from CSF is shown: 3.77 X10^{-3} mm^2/sec (d).

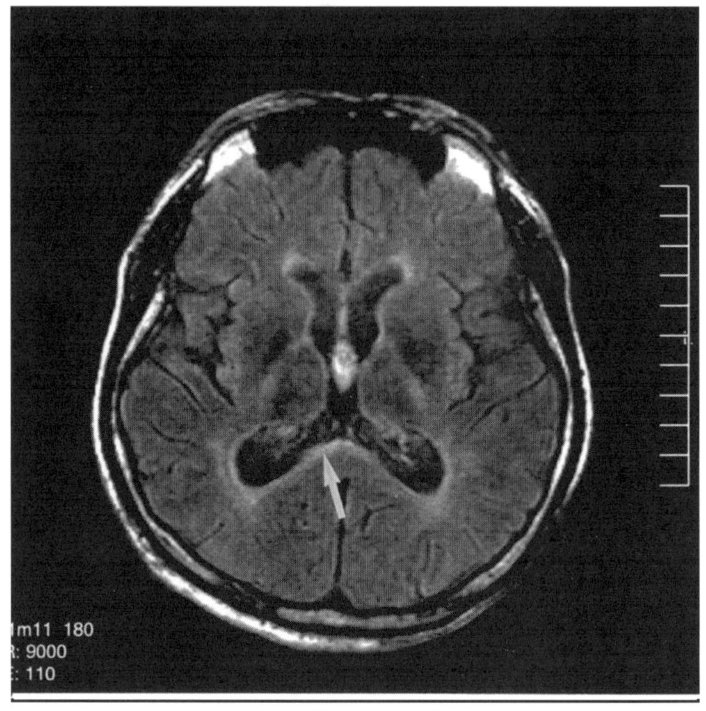

Figure 105c.

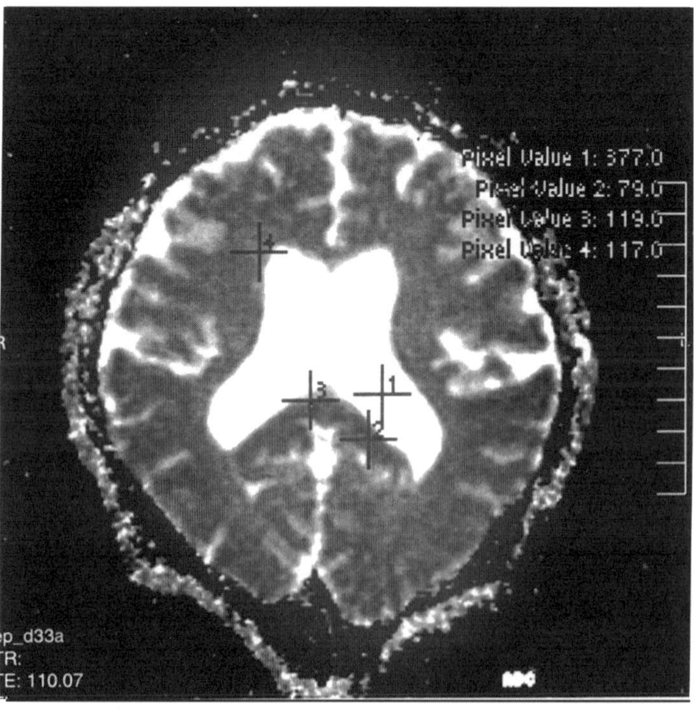

Figure 105d.

LESIONS INDIRECTLY INVOLVING THE CORPUS CALLOSUM

Figure 106 a, b. **Hematoma in the septum pellucidum.** 29-year-old man. *a) SE T1W and b) SE PDW MR images.* The septum pellucidum is filled with a subacute hemorrhagic product (extracellular methemoglobin), which gives bright signal on both imaging sequences (h), and which occurred due to the rupture of an anterior communicating artery aneurysm. The hematoma (h) outlines and slightly displaces the genu of the corpus callosum (g) (a).

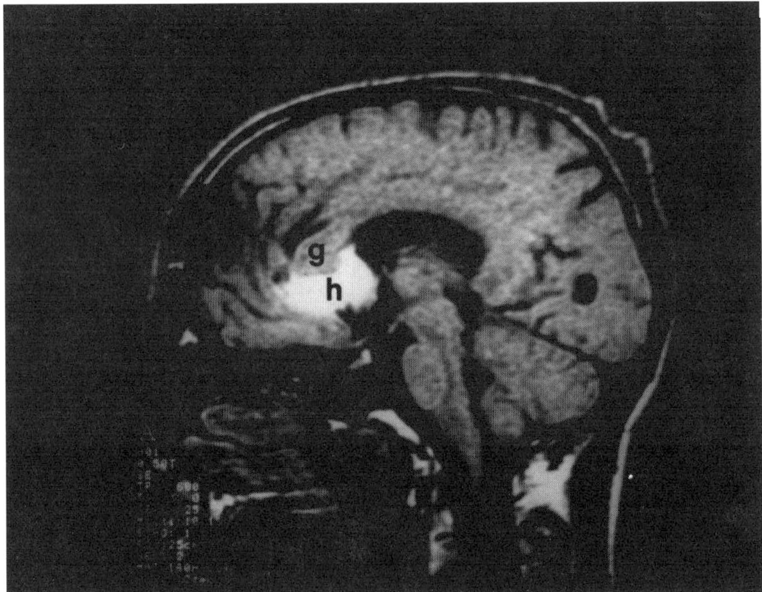

Figure 106a.

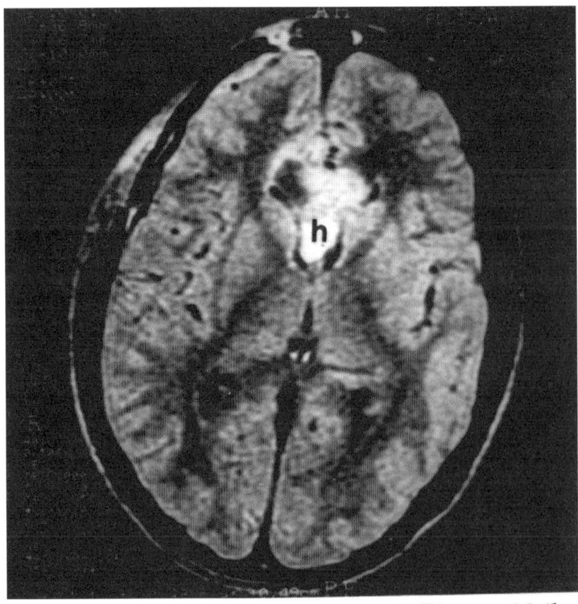

Figure 106b.

Figure 107 a, b. **Glioblastoma multiforme.** 6-year-old boy. *a, b) SE T1W MR images after administration of contrast medium.* There is a large tumor (T) crossing from the right hemisphere to the left. The corpus callosum is pushed backwards (arrows) (a), and not directly involved.

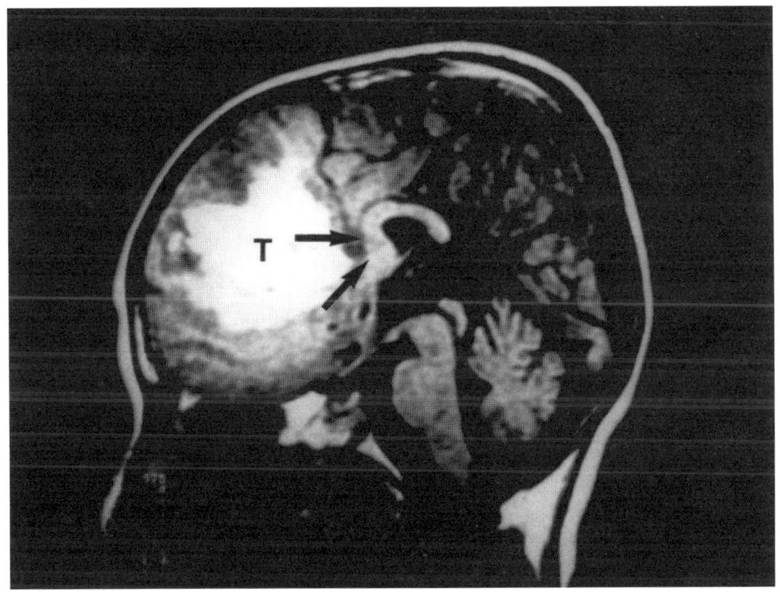

Figure 107a.

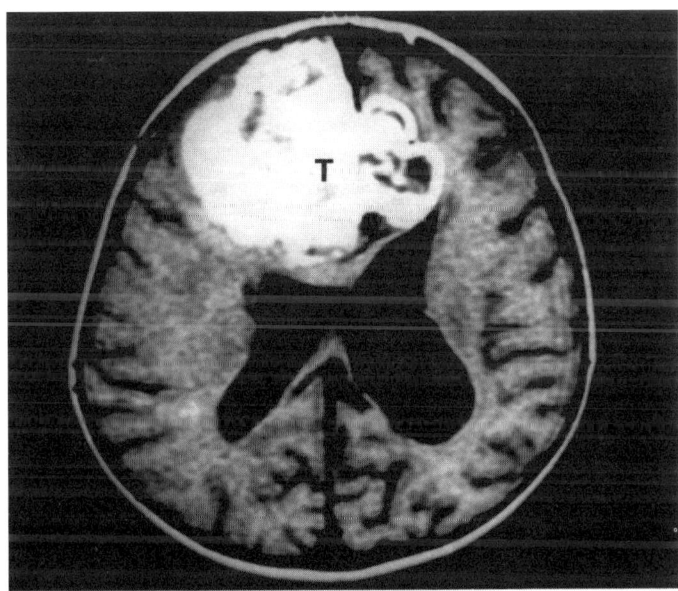

Figure 107b.

Lesions indirectly involving the corpus callosum

Figure 108 a, b. **Giant craniopharyngioma.** 8-year-old boy. *a, b) SE T1W MR images after administration of contrast medium.* A giant craniopharyngioma pushes the corpus callosum upwards (arrows) (a). The lesion is a huge one (large star) with lobulated extensions to the frontal region (small open stars), and to the nasopharynx (asterisk) (a, b). (from reference 3)

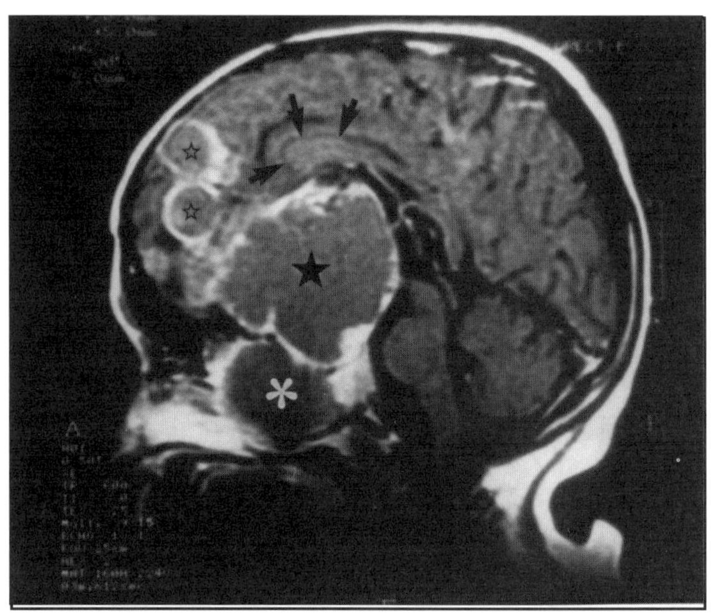

References

1. *Byrne MN, Sessions DG. Nasopharyngeal craniopharyngioma: case report and literature review. Ann Otol Rhinol Laryngol 1990;99:633*
2. *Fitz CR, Mortzman G, Harwood-Nash DC, et al. Computed tomography in cranio-pharyngiomas. Radiology 1978;127:887*
3. *Sener RN. Giant craniopharyngioma extending to the anterior cranial fossa and nasopharynx. AJR 1994;162:441*

Figure 108a.

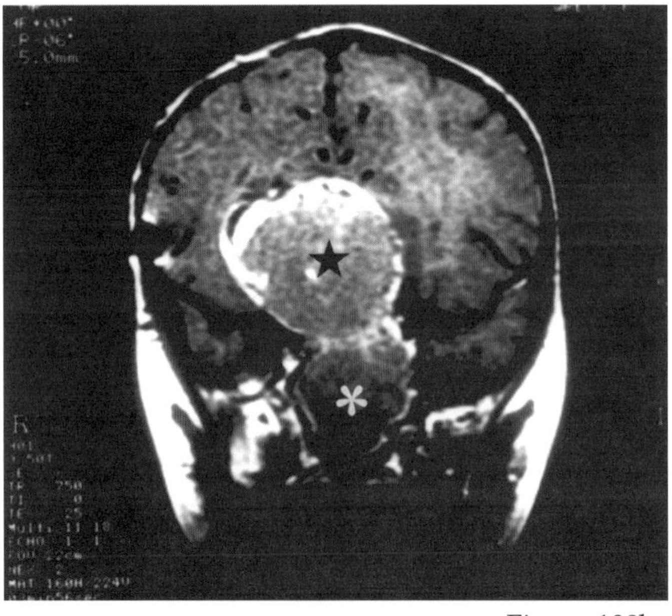

Figure 108b.

Figure 109 a, b. **Cyst of the septum pellucidum.** 9-year-old boy. *a) SE T1W and b) IR T1W MR images.* There is a septum pellucidum cyst, 17mm in diameter (circle) (b), which shows a compression effect upon the inferior surface (effacement) of the body of the corpus callosum. The patient had intermittent headaches, which was attributed to this lesion. A cystic structure between the lateral ventricles, whose walls exhibit lateral bowing and are 10mm apart or greater, is currently considered as a septum pellucidum cyst. Symptomatic septum pellucidum cysts are rare. (from reference 6)

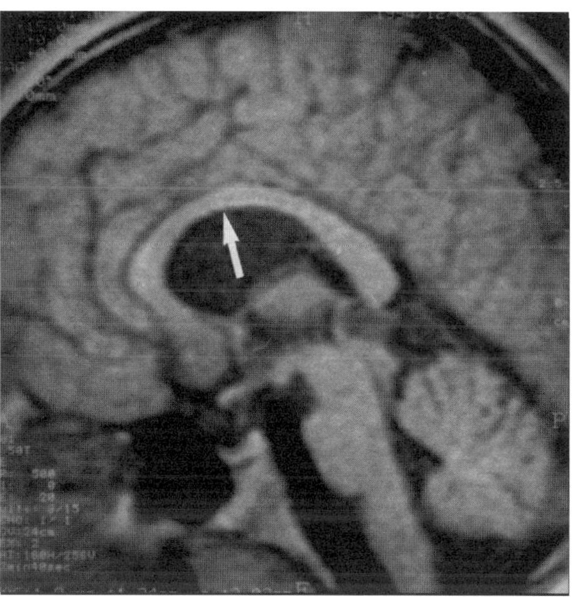

Figure 109a.

References
1. Sarwar M. The septum pellucidum: normal and abnormal. AJNR 1989;10:989
2. Aoki N. Cyst of the septum pellucidum presenting as hemiparesis. Childs Nerv Syst 1986;2:326
3. Lohner Z, Szucs A, Begovics C. Fatal septum pellucidum cyst. Orv Hetil (Hungary) 1989,130.1609
4. Temirov ES, Baliazin VA. Noncommunicating cysts of the septum pellucidum. Zh Vopr Neirokhir (Russia) 1987;4:29
5. Garza-Merkado R. Giant cyst of the septum pellucidum: case report. J Neurosurg 1981;55:646
6. Sener RN. Cysts of the septum pellucidum. Comput Med Imag Graph 1995;19:357

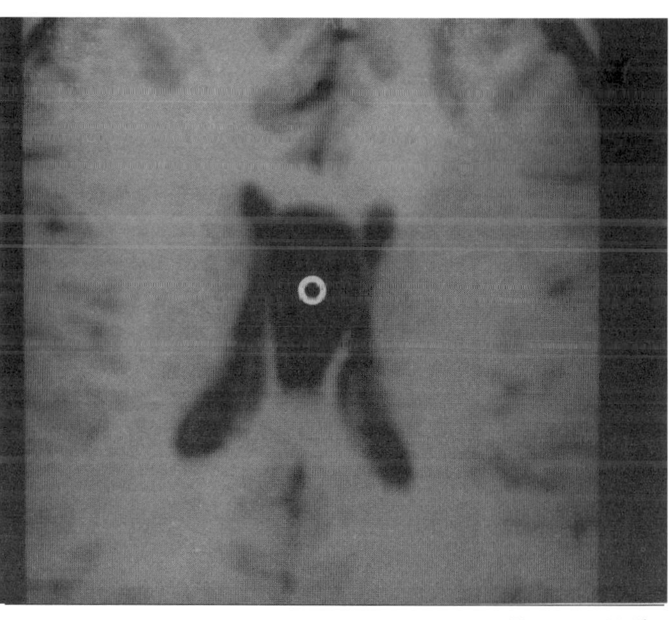

Figure 109b.

Lesions indirectly involving the corpus callosum

Figure 110 a, b. **Small, intraventricular neuroepithelial cyst.** 47-year-old man. *a) SE T1W MR image and b) SE T1W MR image after administration of contrast medium.* There is a small (15mm in diameter) cyst (arrows) (b), which creates a compression at the region of the isthmus of the corpus callosum (arrow) (a). There is no intracystic enhancement, and only the surrounding choroid plexus enhances, which is a normal feature. The lesion was not associated with a parasitic condition, and a 1.5 year follow-up did not reveal any change in size and signal pattern. Such a benign intraventricular cystic structure has been considered as a neuroepithelial (neurogial) cyst.

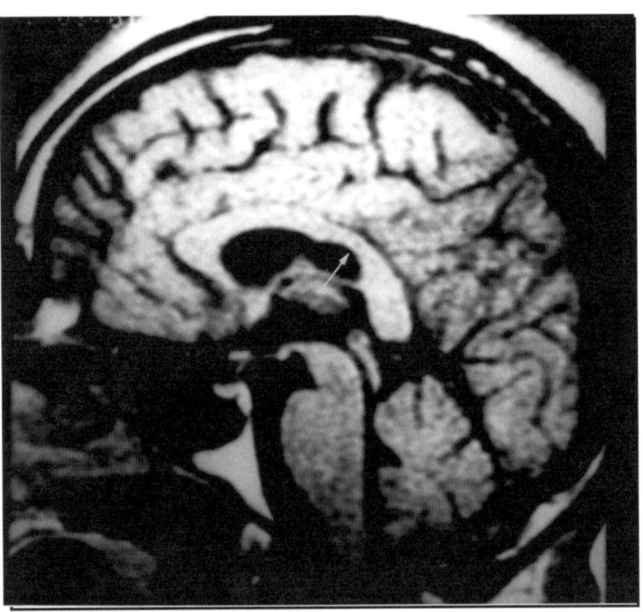

Figure 110a.

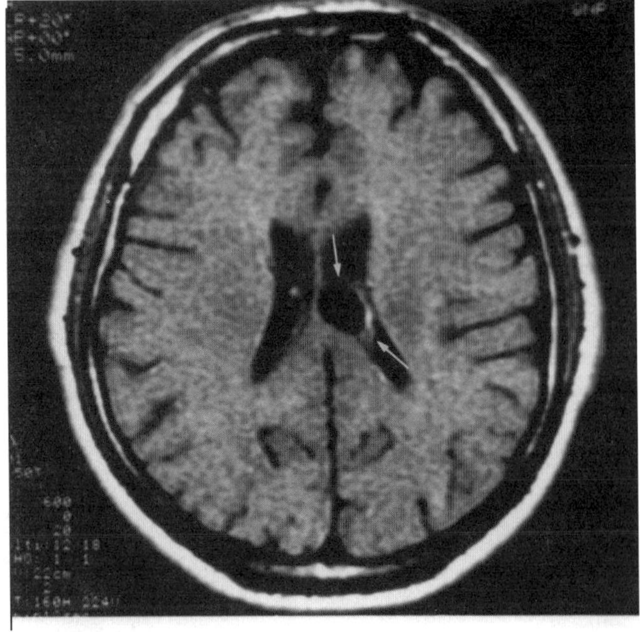

Figure 110b.

Reference

1. *Osborn AG. Diagnostic neuroradiology. St. Louis, Mosby 1994;646*

Figure 111 a, b. **Cyst of the velum interpositum.** 53-year-old woman. a, b) SE T1W MR images after administration of contrast medium. A cyst located in the cistern of the velum interpositum is seen (asterisk) (a, b), which slightly indents the splenium (a). A pineal cyst is excluded, especially by the aid of sagittal images. Note that there is neither intracystic enhancement nor hydrocephalus.

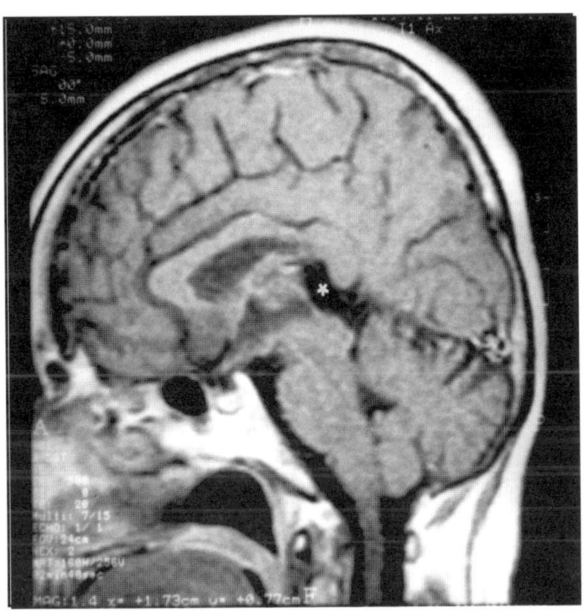

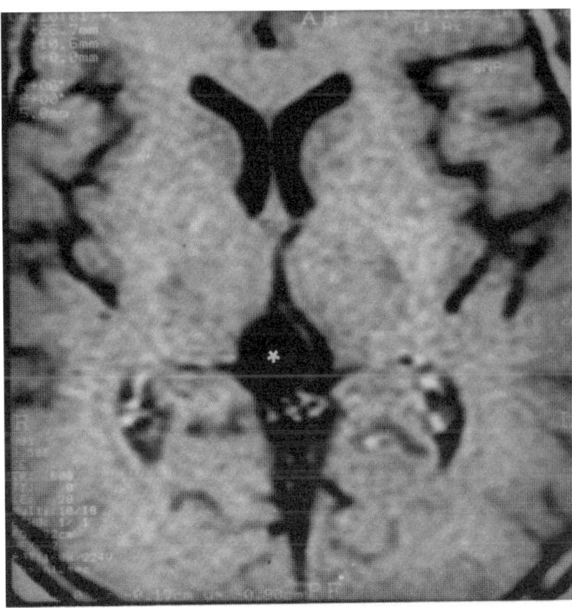

Figure 111a.

Figure 111b.

Figure 112 a, b. **Chiari II malformation.** 2-year-old boy. *a) SE T1W and b) IR T1W MR images.* Typical changes of Chiari II malformation are demonstrated including tectal beaking, a small posterior fossa, dysplastic tentorium and falx. There is hydrocephalus due to aqueduct stenosis, which causes upward displacement and thinning of the corpus callosum (arrows). Note that the caudal parts of the corpus callosum are very thin in this patient.

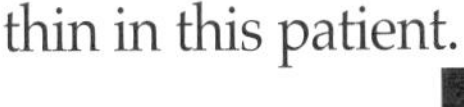

Figure 112a.

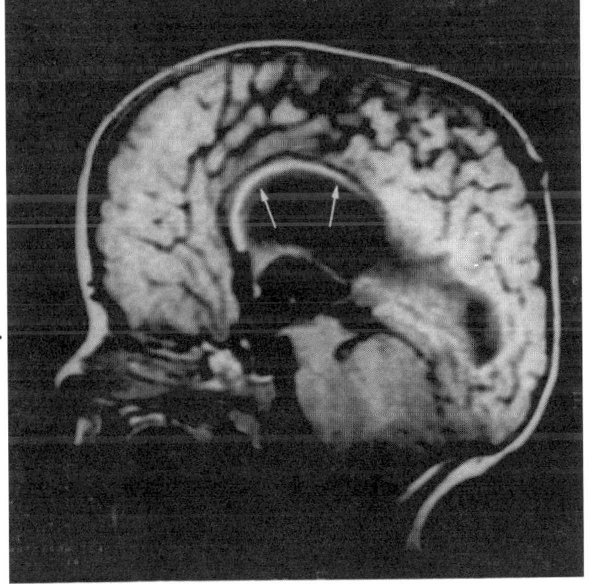

Figure 112b.

Reference
1. *Barkovich AJ. Pediatric neuroimaging. New York, Raven 1995;238*

Figure 113 a-c. **Chiari II malformation (Intrauterine MRI).** Two fetuses in the second trimester. Images with the HASTE (half-fourier single-shot turbo spin eko) sequence reveal a small posterior fossa, and prominantly dilated lateral ventricles (a,b). Note stretching of the very thin corpus callosum (a). A defect in the spine (meningocele) is shown

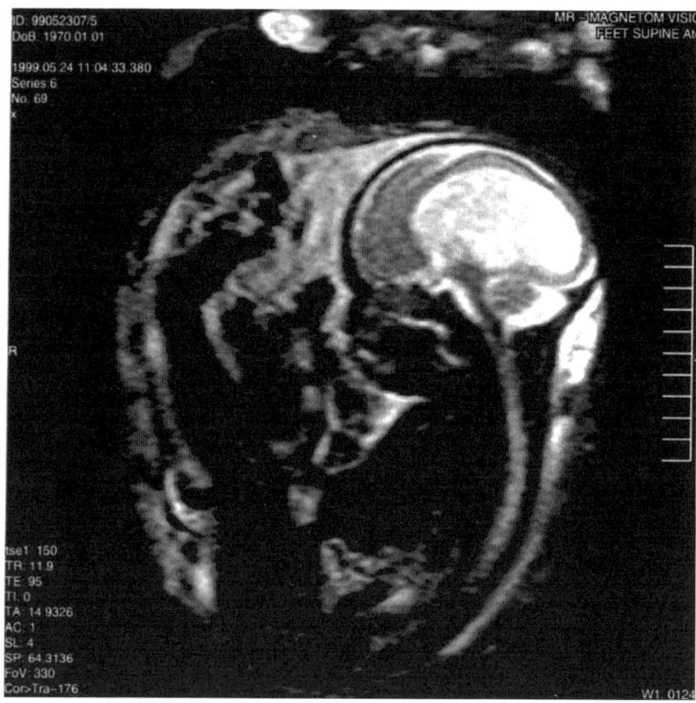

Figure 113a.

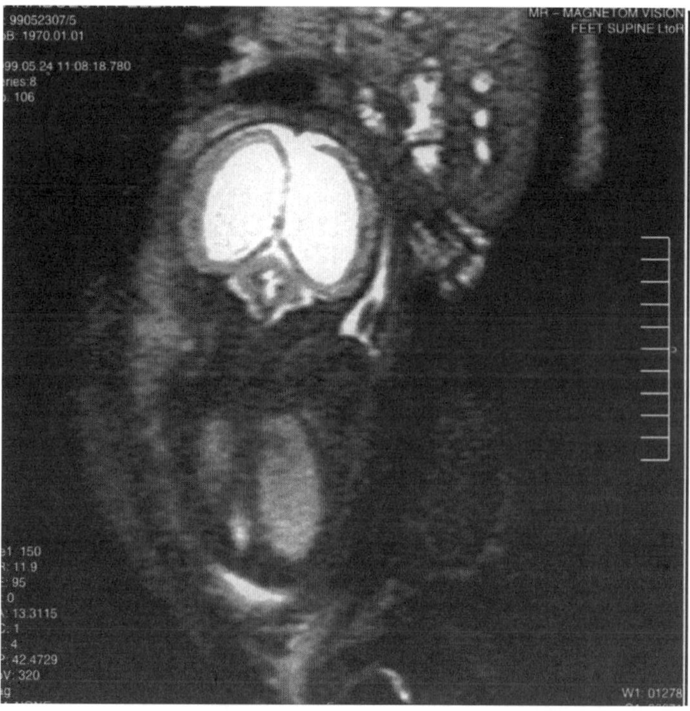

Figure 113b.

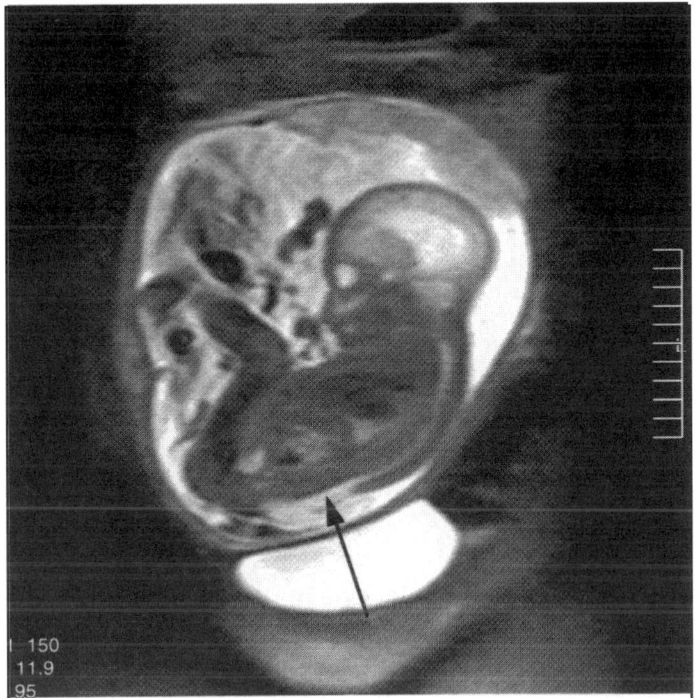

Figure 113c.

in another fetus, again with a small posterior fossa, consistent with Chiari II malformation (c).

References
1. *Levine D, Barnes PD, Sher S, et al. Fetal fast MR imaging: reproducibility, technical quality, and conspicuity of anatomy. Radiology 1998;206:549*
2. *Vimercati A, Greco P, Vera L, et al. The diagnostic role of 'in utero' magnetic resonance imaging. J Perinat Med 1999;27:303*
3. *Liu DPC, Burrowes DM, Qureshi MN. Cyclopia: craniofacial appearance on MR and three-dimensional CT. AJNR 1997;18:543*

Fig.114 a-c. **Chiari II malformation.** 2-year-old girl. T2W image reveals severe hydrocephalus, and stretching of the corpus callosum (a). *Note that absence of the posterior parts of the corpus callosum (dysgenesis) is not uncommon in patients with Chiari II malformation.* T2W and T1W images reveal a cleft in the vermis of the cerebellum (b,c).

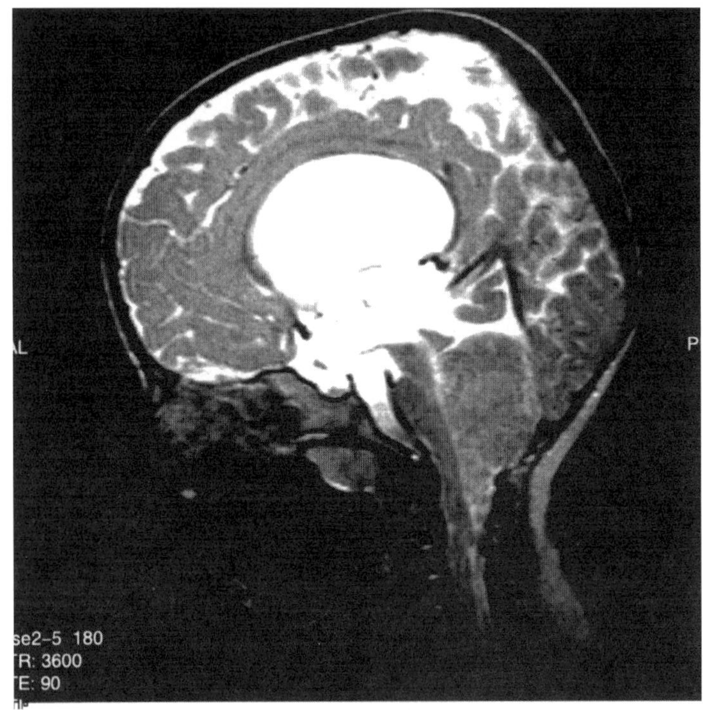

Figure 114a.

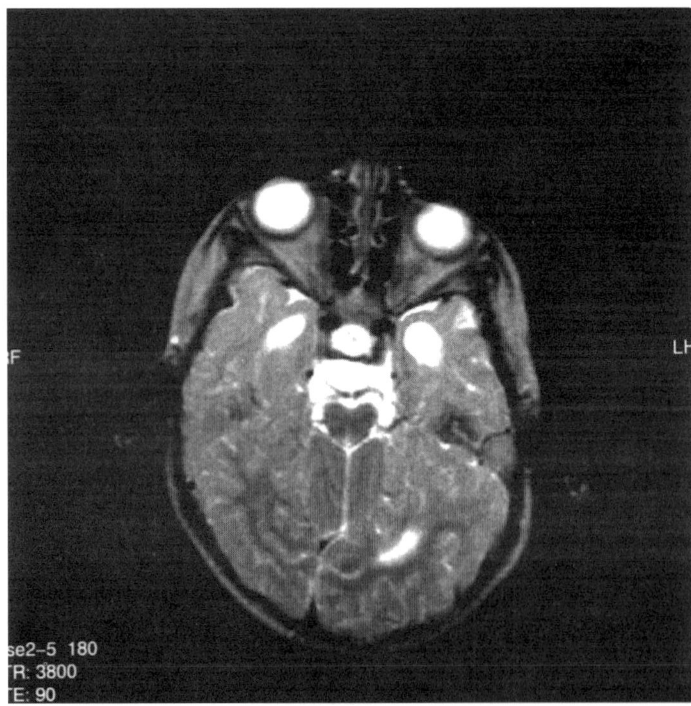

Figure 114b.

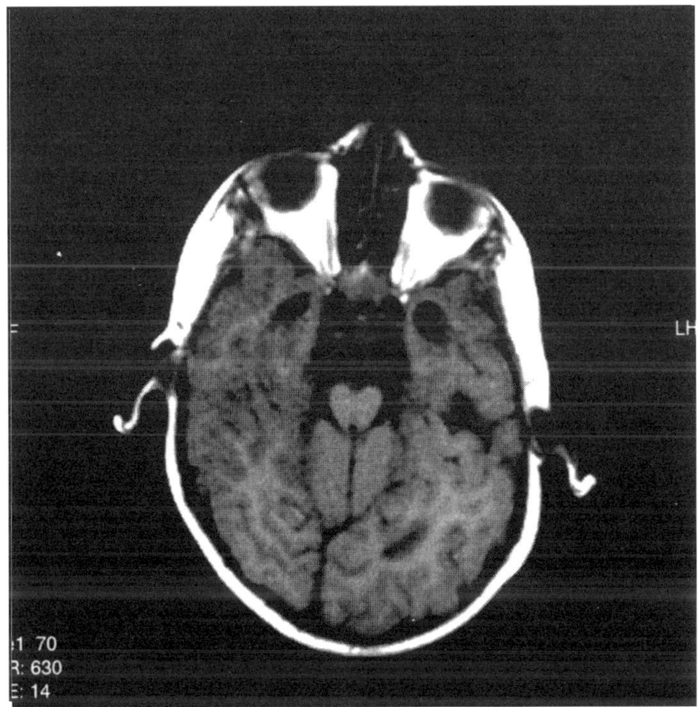

Figure 114c.

Fig.115 a,b. **Chiari II malformation.** 3-year-old girl. T1W image reveals a relatively small appearing corpus callosum without evidence of hydrocephalus (a). T1W image reveals a cleft in the vermis of the cerebellum (b) *(see the previous patient).*

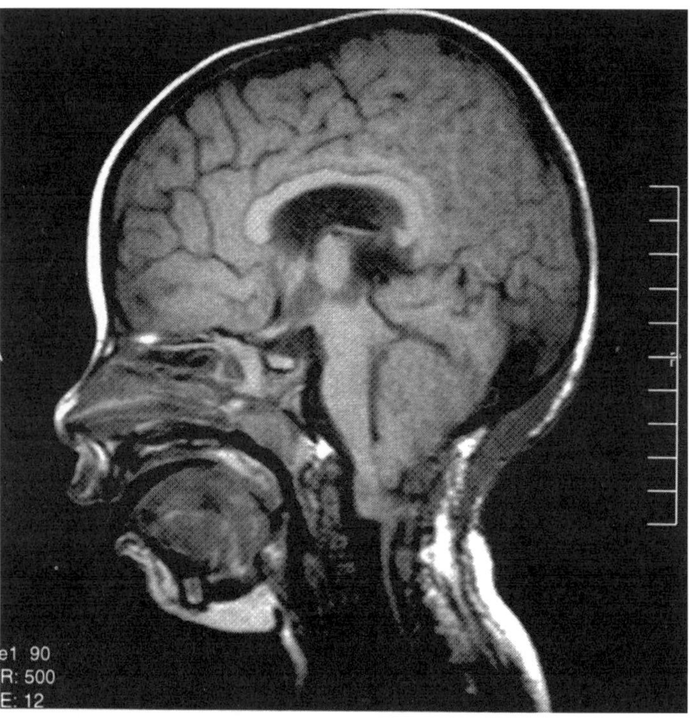

Figure 115a.

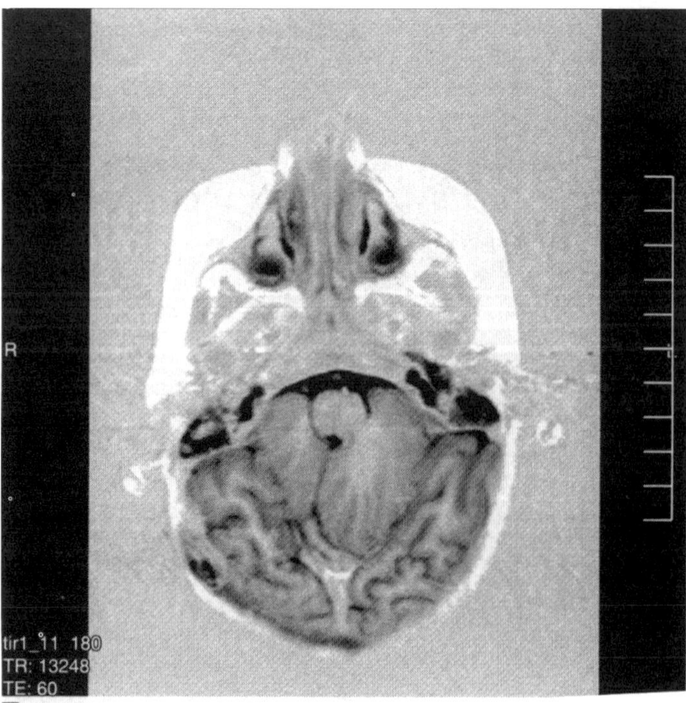

Figure 115b.

Figure 116 a, b. **Dandy-Walker variant.** 2.5-year-old patient. *a) SE T1W and b) IR T1W MR images.* The fourth ventricle is enlarged (a). The vermis show dysplastic folia (a, b). There is a chronic hemorrhagic collection in the posterior fossa and posterior to the occipital lobe as a complication of shunt tube placement (circles) (a). There is hydrocephalus with resultant displacement and thinning of the corpus callosum (arrow) (a).

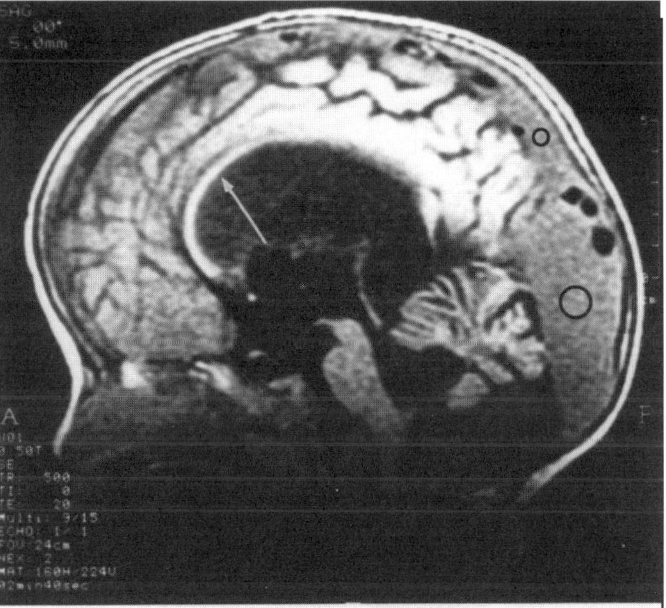

Figure 116a.

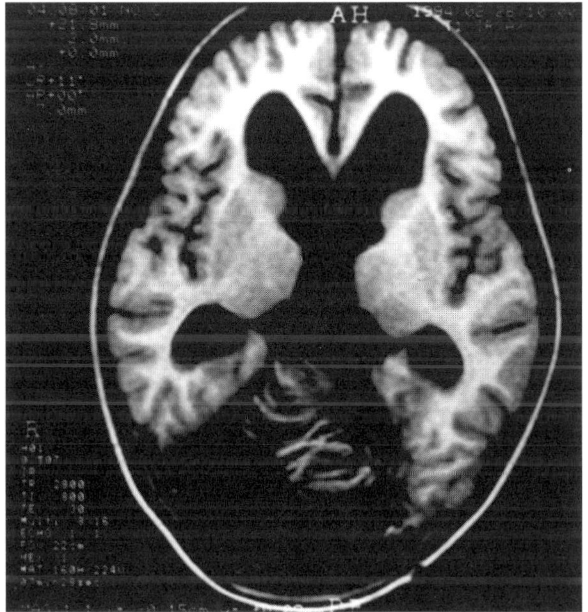

Figure 116b.

Reference
*1.	Barkovich AJ. Pediatric Neuroimaging. New York, Raven 1995;249*

Figure 117 a, b. **Isolated fourth ventricle.** 2-year-old boy. *a) SE T1W and b) SE T2W MR images.* The fourth ventricle shows apparent dilatation (circles) (a, b) due to obstruction of the exit foramina (Magendi and Luschkas), and aqueductal stenosis, and has become isolated. The corpus callosum is displaced and thinned due to hydrocephalus (arrows) (a). Note the appearance of the aqueduct and its similarity to the next patient with isolated aqueductal stenosis (see Fig. 118).

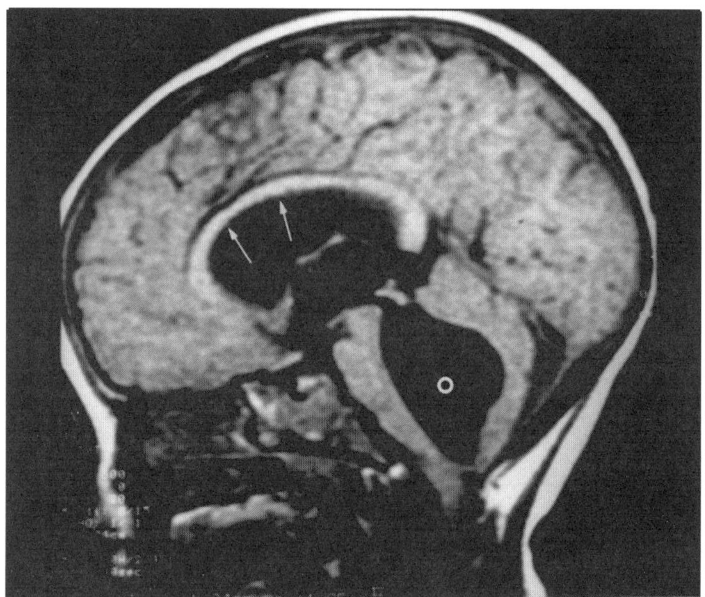

Figure 117a.

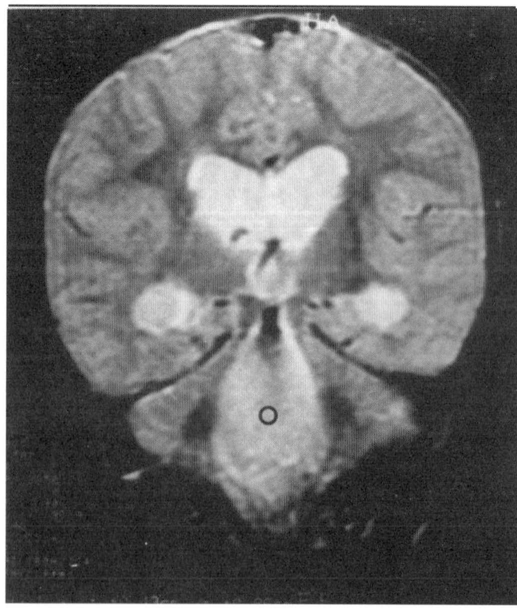

Reference
1. Barkovich AJ. Pediatric neuroimaging. New York, Raven 1995;456

Figure 117b.

Figure 118 a, b. **Aqueduct stenosis.** 1.5-year-old boy. *a, b) SE T1W MR images.* There is triventricular hydrocephalus due to an isolated aqueductal stenosis with resultant displacement and thinning of the corpus callosum (arrows) (a). Note the shape of the aqueduct, which suggest a certain type of stenosing lesion (possibly a web, not identifiable in these images) (see Fig. 117).

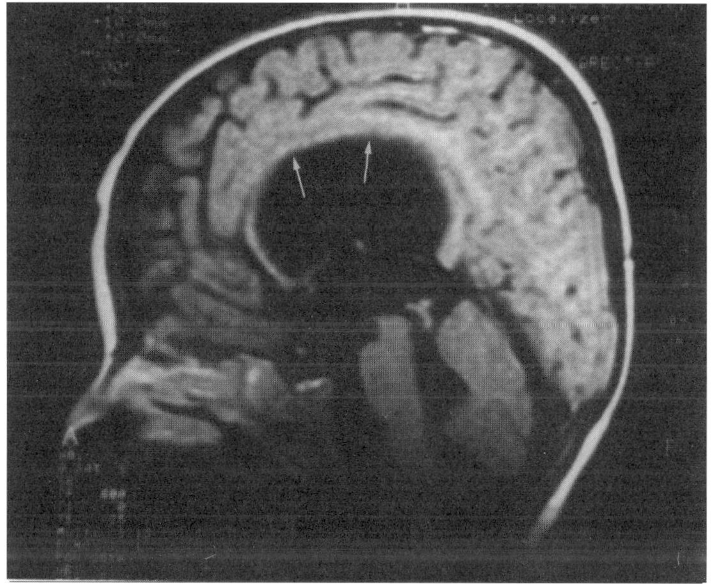

Figure 118a.

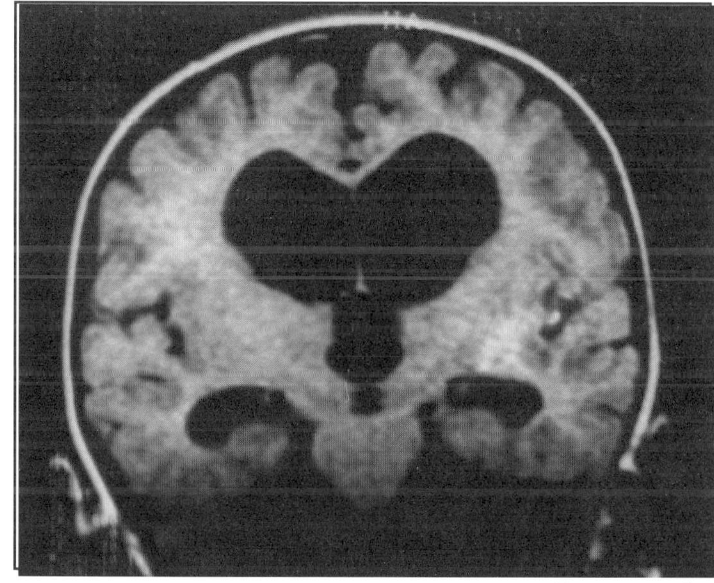

Figure 118b.

Reference
1. *Barkovich AJ. Pediatric neuroimaging. New York, Raven 1995;453*

Lesions indirectly involving the corpus callosum

Figure 119 a-c. **Aqueduct stenosis and temporal hypoplasia.** 13-year-old boy. The aqueduct appears to be stenosed at its lower end. The corpus callosum is diffusely thin, and pushed upwards, secondary to longstanding hydrocephalus on the T1W image (a).

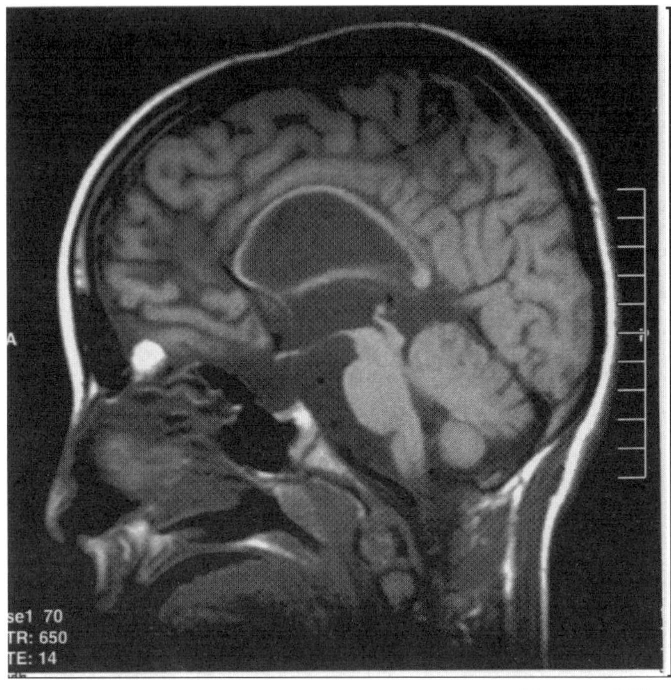

Figure 119a.

The condition is associated with bilateral hypoplasia of the temporal lobes as demonstrated by the T1W image (b), and by the ADC map from a echo-planar diffusion imaging study (c). This condition should be differentiated from bilateral arachnoid cysts. Lack of an impression of external compression effect is in favor of temporal hypoplasia.

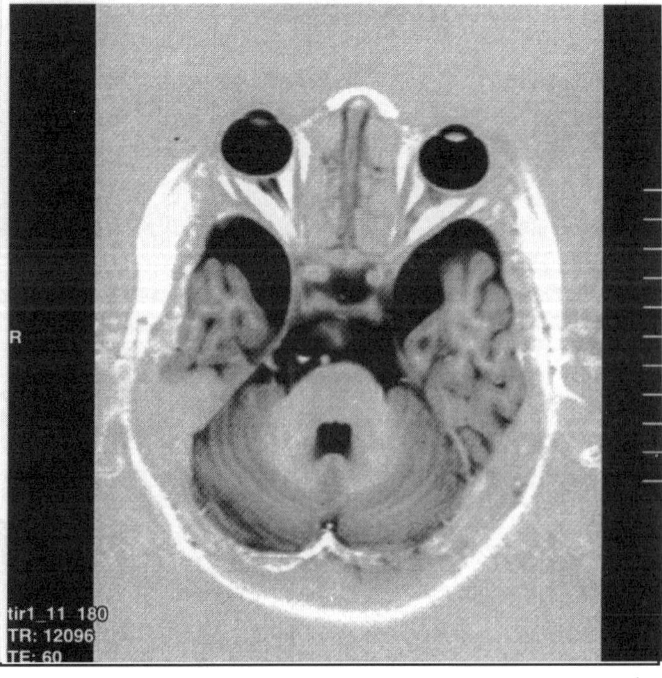

Figure 119b.

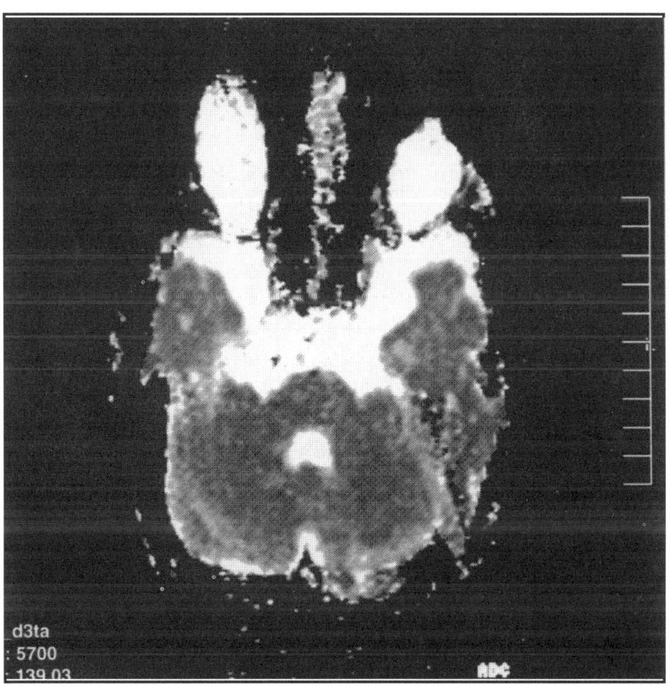

Figure 119c.

Figure 120 a,b. **Aqueduct stenosis.** 3-year-old boy. T2W image reveals stretching and thinning of the corpus callosum due to aqueduct stenosis (a). MR angiography demonstrates upward displacement of the pericallosal and callosomarginal arteries (b).

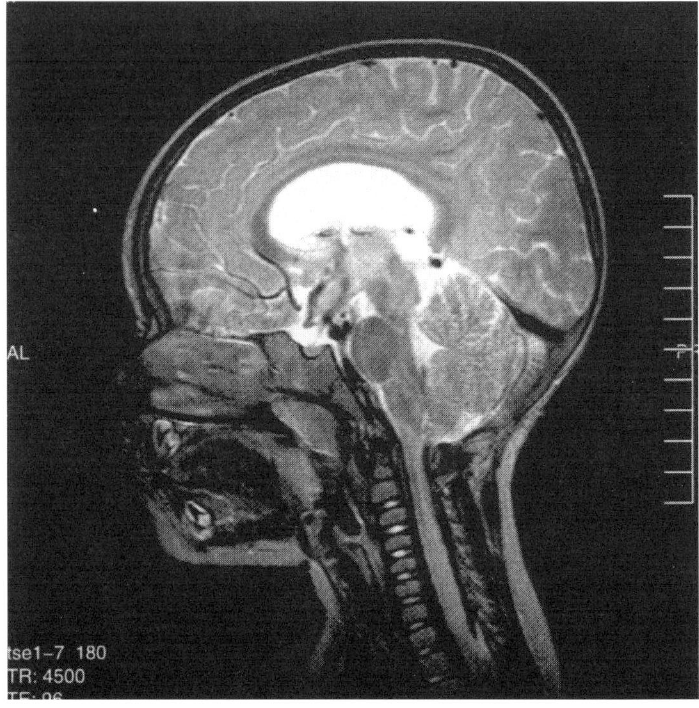

Figure 120a.

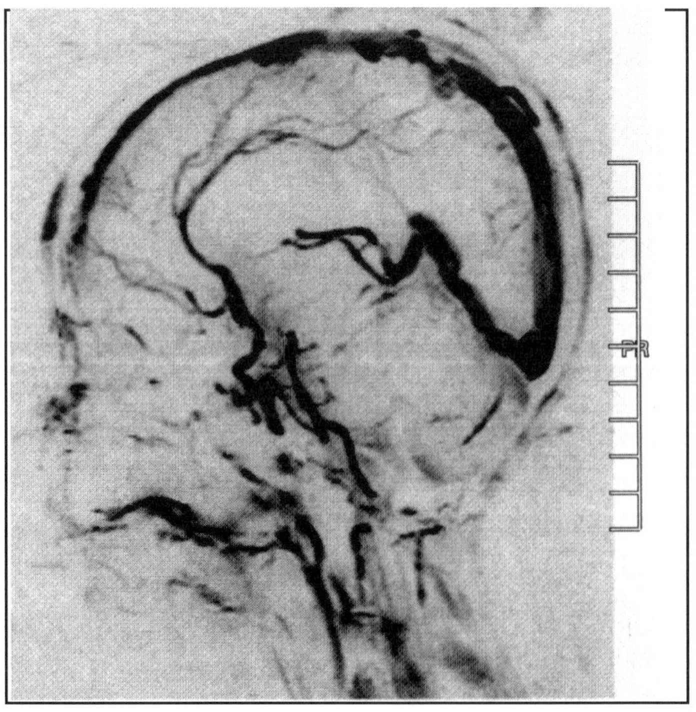

Figure 120b.

Figure 121 a-g. **Pineal cyst compressing the tectum.** 14-year-old girl T1-weighted image reveals a cystic lesion at the pineal region. Hydrocephalus is evident due to tectal compression causing upward displacement and stretching of the corpus callosum (a).

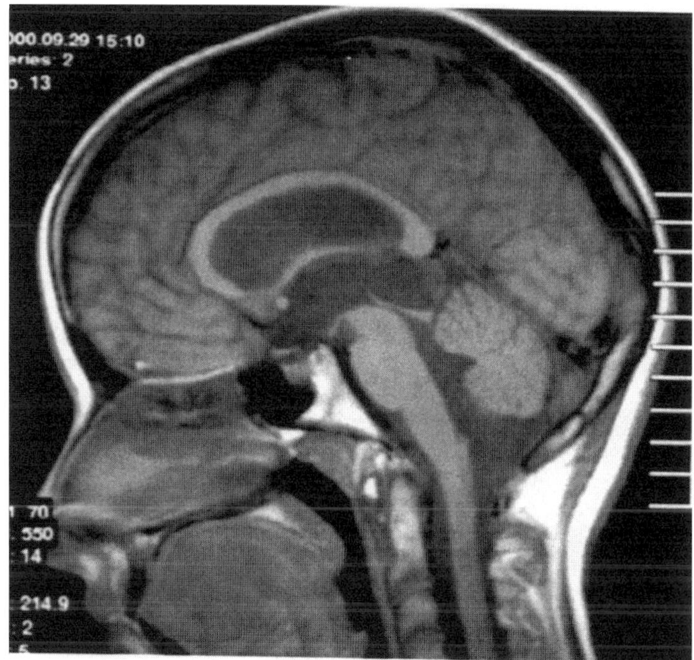

Figure 121a.

Post-contrast T1-weighted image reveals partial enhancement of the pineal tissue (b).

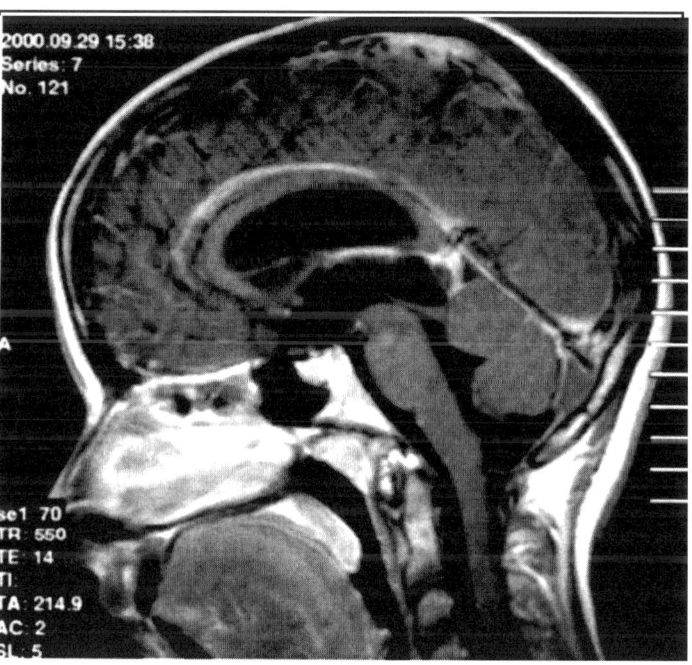

Figure 121b.

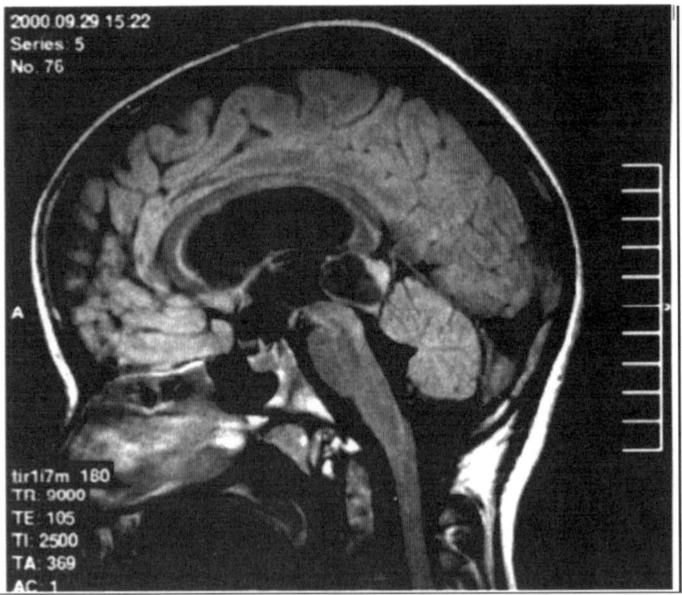

Figure 121c.

FLAIR image demonstrates the pineal tissue to better advantage. The inner layer of the corpus callosum is relatively thick and has high signal, representing transependymal resorption of CSF from its inner surface (c).

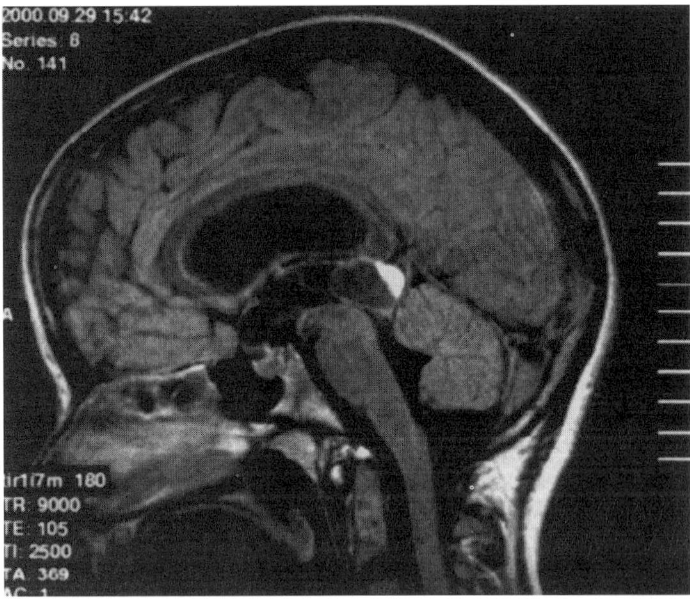

Figure 121d.

Post-contrast FLAIR image reveals apparent enhancement of the pineal tissue to better advantage than the post-contrast T1-weighted image (d).

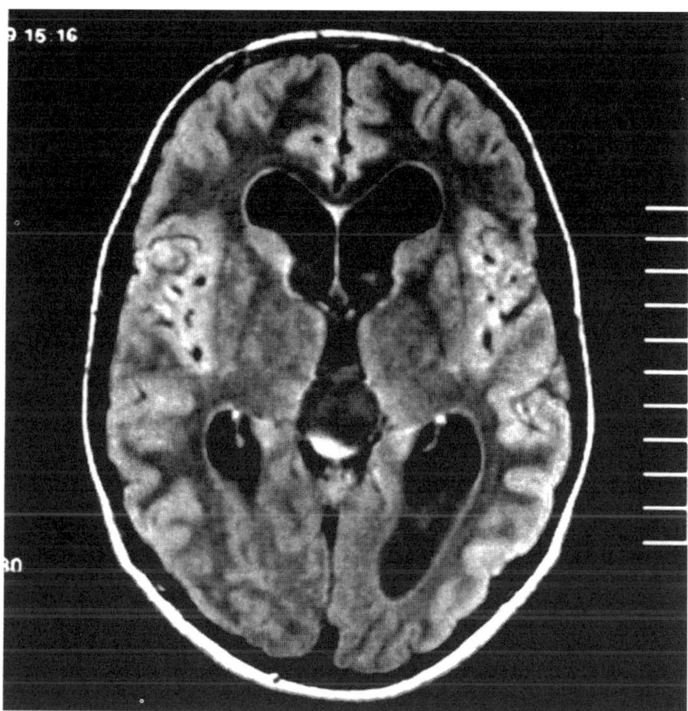

Figure 121e.

FLAIR image in transverse plane shows the cyst, posterior pineal tissue, and hydrocephalus (e).

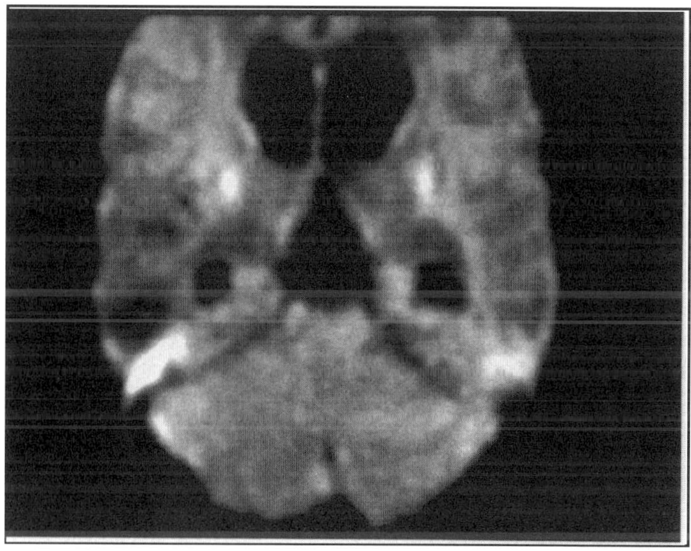

Figure 121f.

Coronal, b=1000 sec/mm^2 (true diffusion) image reveals ventricular dilatation, and the cyst (f).

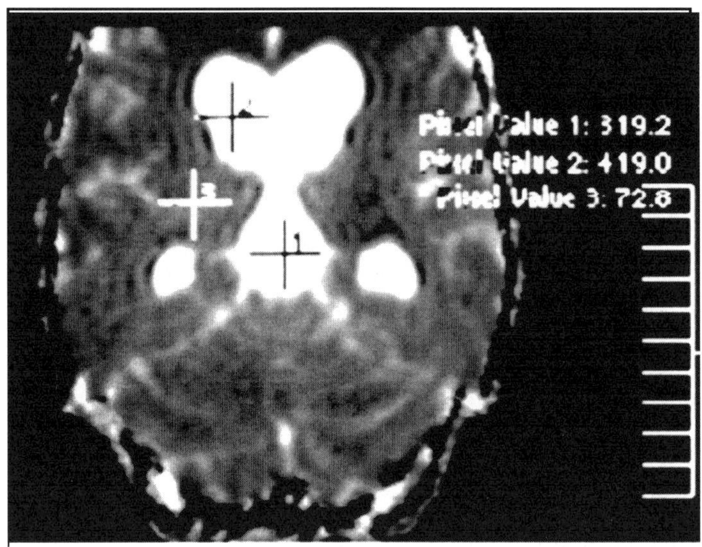

Figure 121g.

ADC map reveals close ADC values of the cyst and CSF: 3.19 X10^{-3} mm^2/sec, and 4.19 X10^{-3} mm^2/sec, respectively (these values are within the normal ranges of CSF). Normal ADC value from the parenchyma is shown: 0.72 X10^{-3} mm^2/sec (g). (case courtesy of Dr. S. Dzelzite, Riga, Latvia).

Figure 122 a-c. **Pineoblastoma.** 12-year-old boy. Post-contrast T1W image reveals the mass with more prominent central enhancement. The corpus callosum is stretched upwards due to hydrocephalus (a).

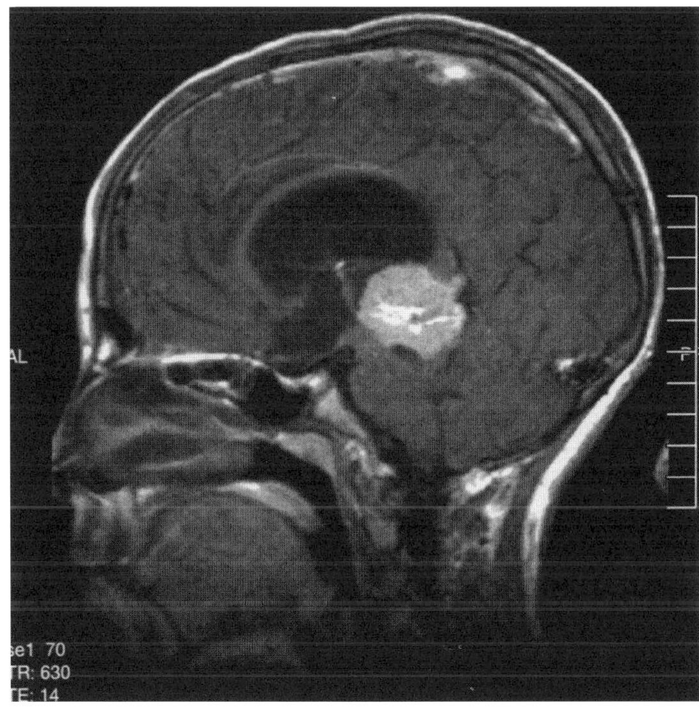

Figure 122a.

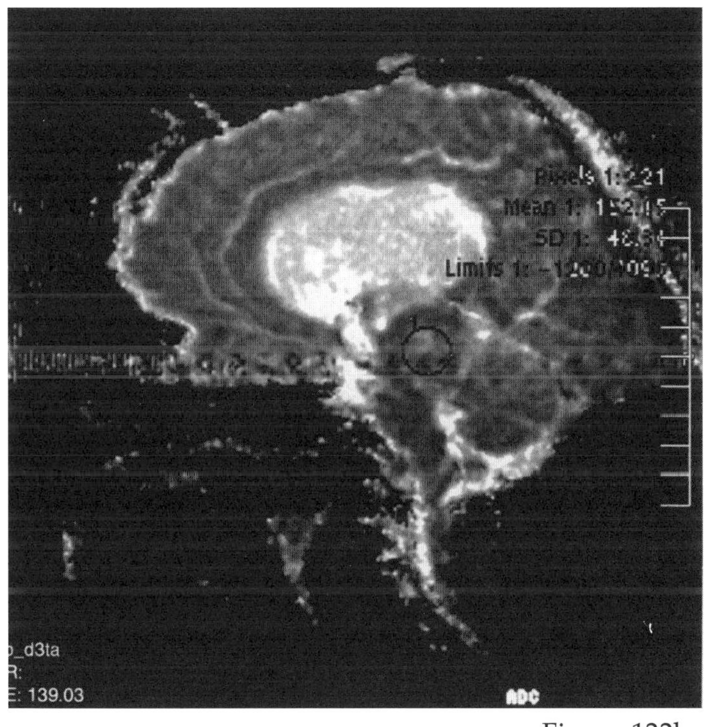

ADC map from diffusion MRI sequence reveals an ADC value of 1.52 X10^{-3} mm^2/sec in the tumor (b).

Figure 122b.

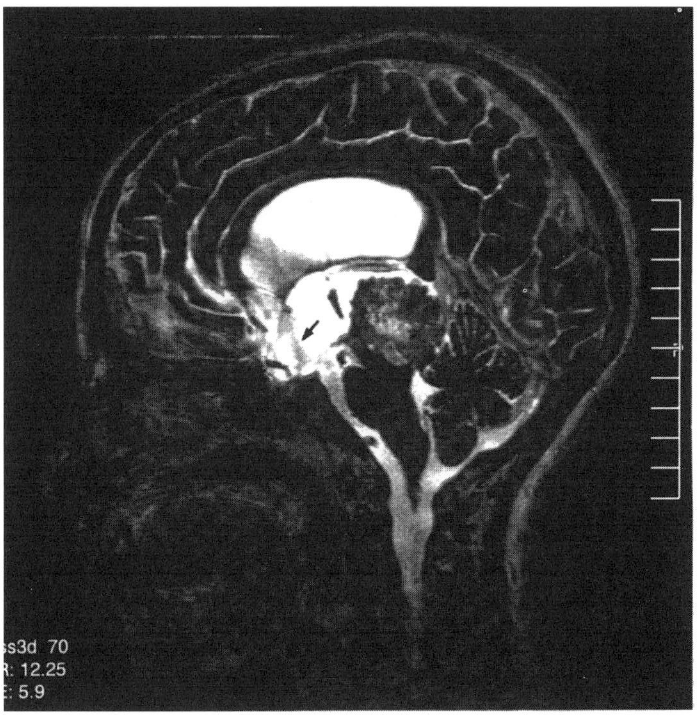

Figure 122c.

CISS (constructive interference of steady state) image following endoscopic intervention, revealing the postintervention ostium in the floor of the 3rd ventricle, and sufficient flow, seen as a gray line (arrow) (c).

Figure 123 a-c. **Pineoblastoma.** 20-year-old man. Post-contrast T1W image reveals the enhancing pineal mass (a).

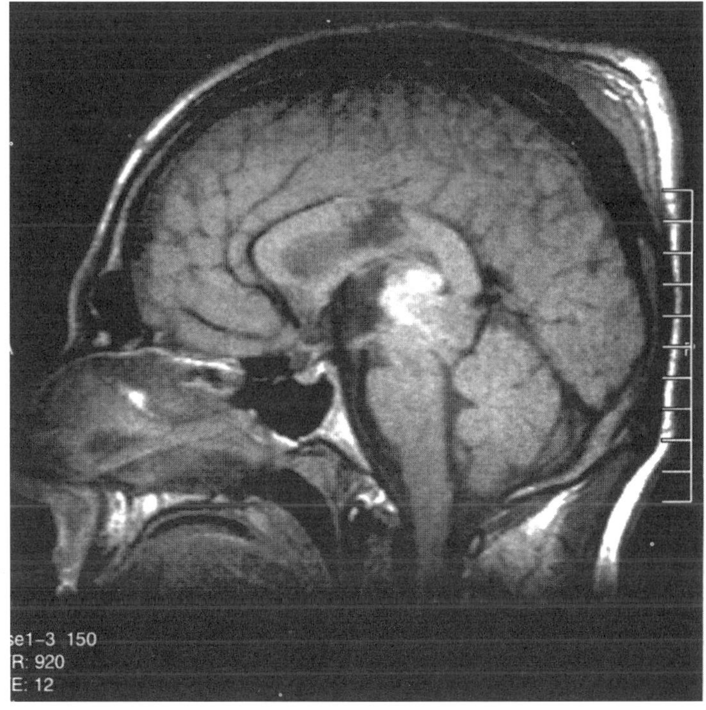

Figure 123a.

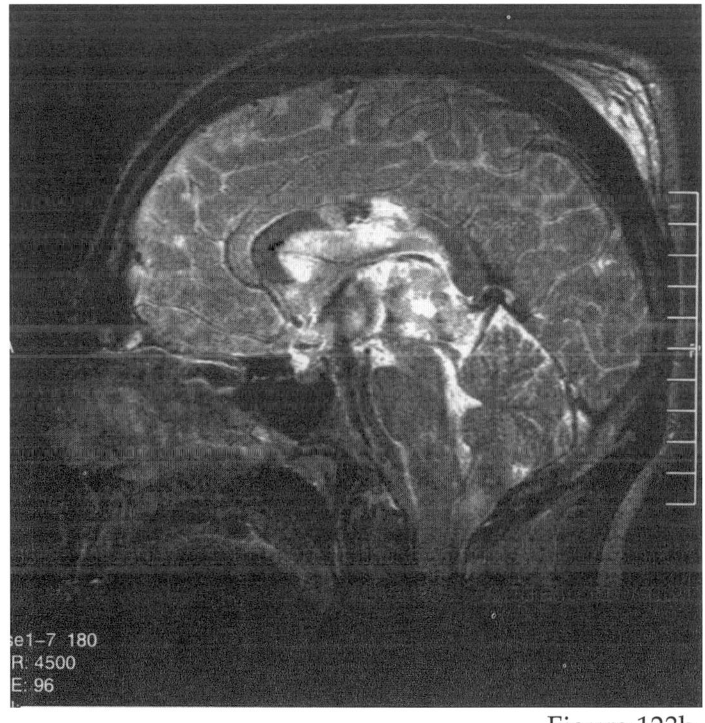

Figure 123b.

T2W image reveals high signal in the tumor (b).

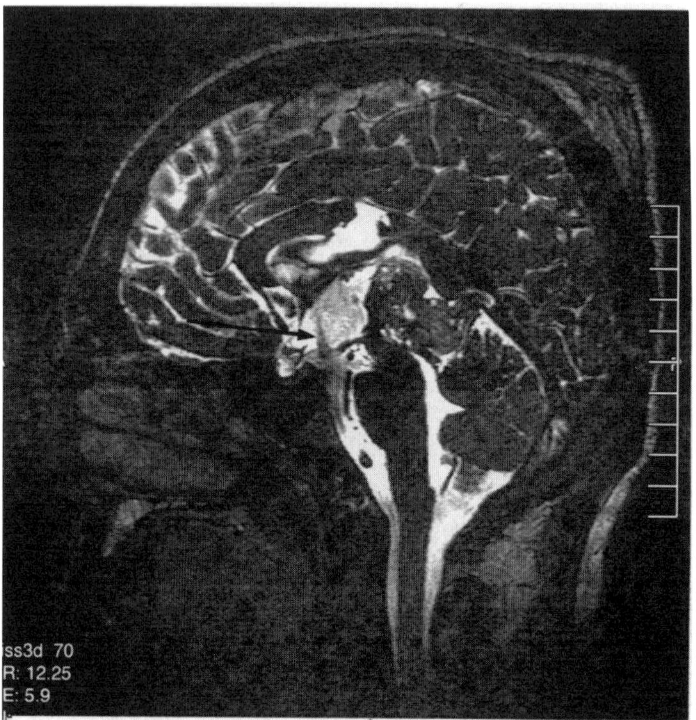

Figure 123c.

CISS (constructive interference of steady state) image following endoscopic intervention, revealing the postintervention ostium in the floor of the 3rd ventricle, and sufficient flow, seen as a gray line (arrow) (c). Note a defect in the corpus callosum due to the intervention (a-c).

Figure 124. **Vein of Galen malformation.** 6-year-old girl. *SE T1W MR image.* The Vein of Galen shows apparent dilatation and compresses the aqueduct (asterisk). The corpus callosum is displaced and thinned due to the resultant hydrocephalus (arrows).

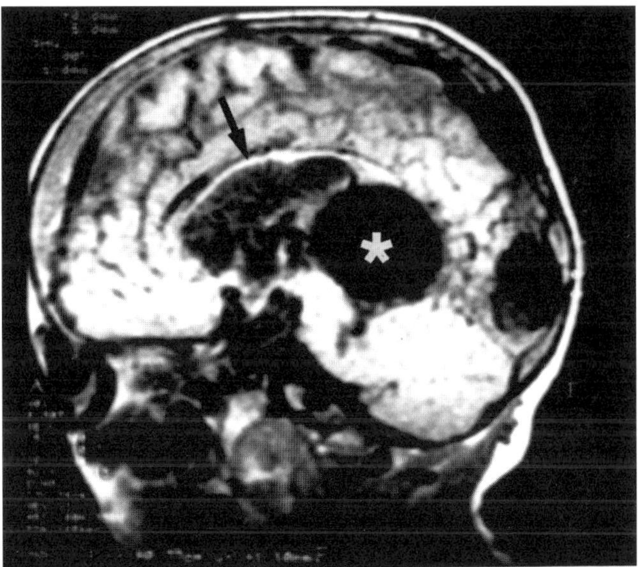

Figure 124.

References

1. *Seidenwurm D, Berenstein A, Hyman A, et al. Vein of Galen malformation: correlation ot clinical presentation, arteriography, and MR imaging. AJNR 1991;12:347-354*
2. *Quisling RG, Mickle JP. Venous pressure measurements in Vein of Galen aneurysms. AJNR 1989;10:411-417*
3. *Sener RN. MR angiography of the Vein of Galen malformation. Clin Imaging 1996;20:243*

Figure 125. **Superior cerebellar arachnoid cyst.** 2-year-old boy. *SE T1W MR image.* There is a large superior cerebellar arachnoid cyst (in the quadrigeminal cistern) compressing the aqueduct and inferiorly displacing the cerebellar vermis (asterisk). The corpus callosum is displaced and thinned due to the resultant hydrocephalus (arrows).

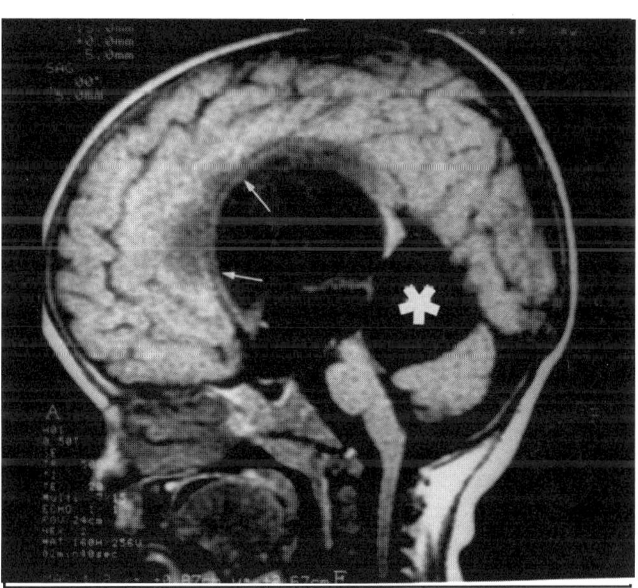

Figure 125.

Reference

1. *Wolpert SM, Barnes PD. MRI in pediatric neuro-radiology. St. Louis, Mosby 1992;117*

Lesions indirectly involving the corpus callosum

Figure 126 a, b. **Suprasellar arachnoid cyst.** 43-year-old man. *a) SE T1W MR images and b) displayed with very narrow window settings.* A large suprasellar arachnoid cyst (c, Fig. b) extends upwards and mimics a third ventricular cyst. The midbrain and aqueduct is pushed backwards (a). The corpus callosum shows displacement and thinning due to the resultant hydrocephalus (arrows) (a).

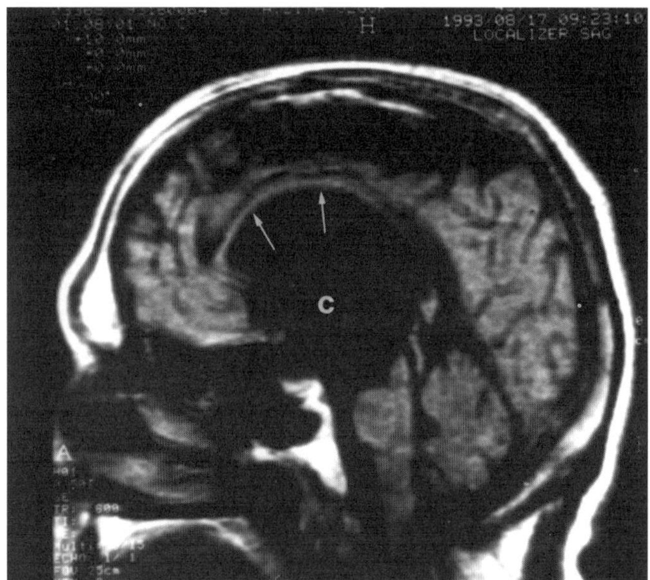

Figure 126a.

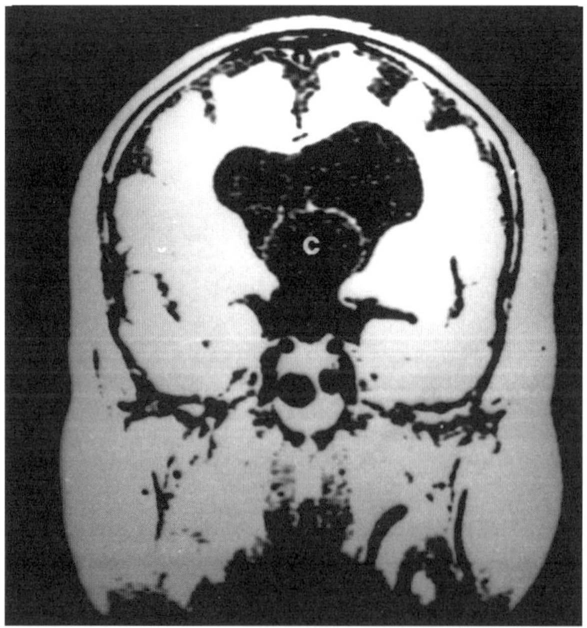

Figure 126b.

Reference
1.   *Barkovich AJ. Pediatric neuroimaging. New York, Raven 1995;448*

Figure 127 a-d. **Choroid plexus carcinoma. Postoperative extravasation of intravenous contrast medium.** 2-year-old girl. Transverse T1W images before (a), and after (b) intravenous administration of contrast medium show the region of operation, and partial excision of the tumor in the choroid plexus of the right lateral ventricle. Extensive extravasation of contrast medium is evident.

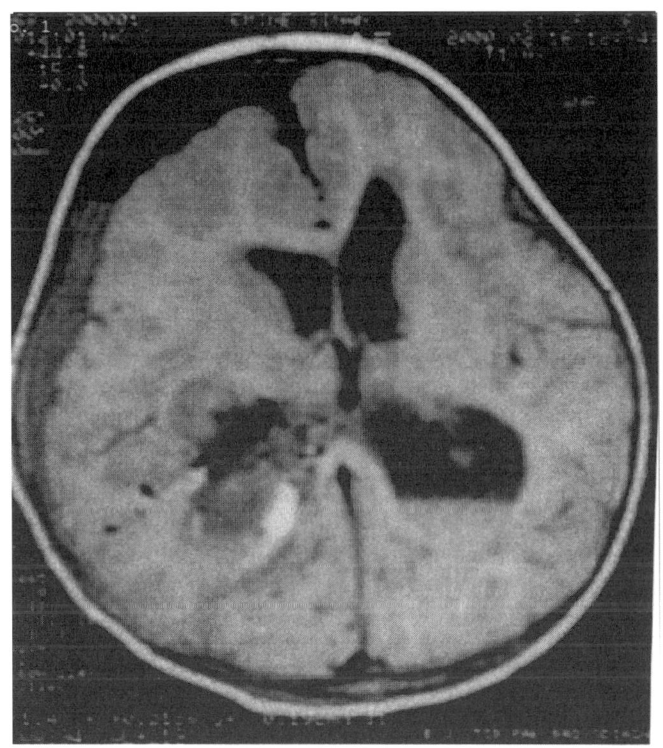

Figure 127a.

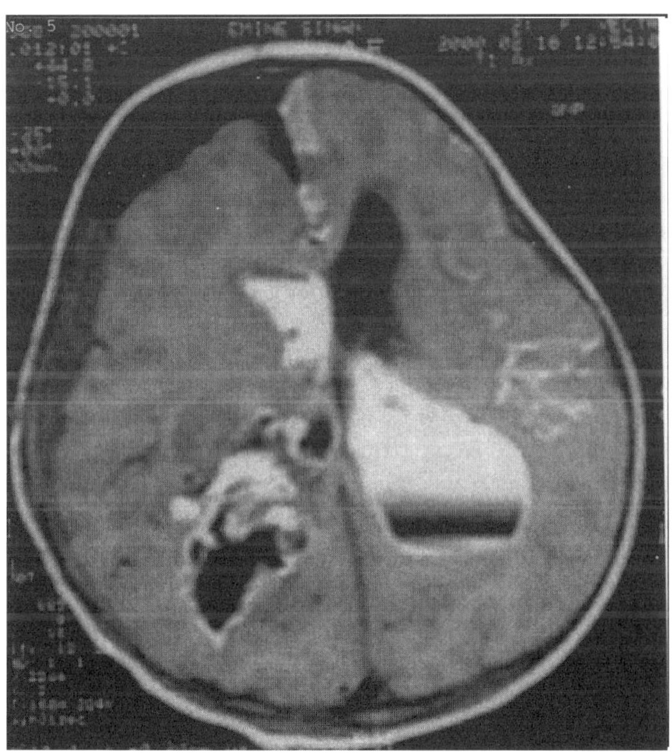

Figure 127b.

Lesions indirectly involving the corpus callosum

Sagittal T1W images before (c), and after (d) intravenous administration of contrast medium reveal extensive extravasation of contast medium to the ventricles, subarachnoid spaces and cisterns. The corpus callosum is pushed upwards due to acute hydrocephalus.

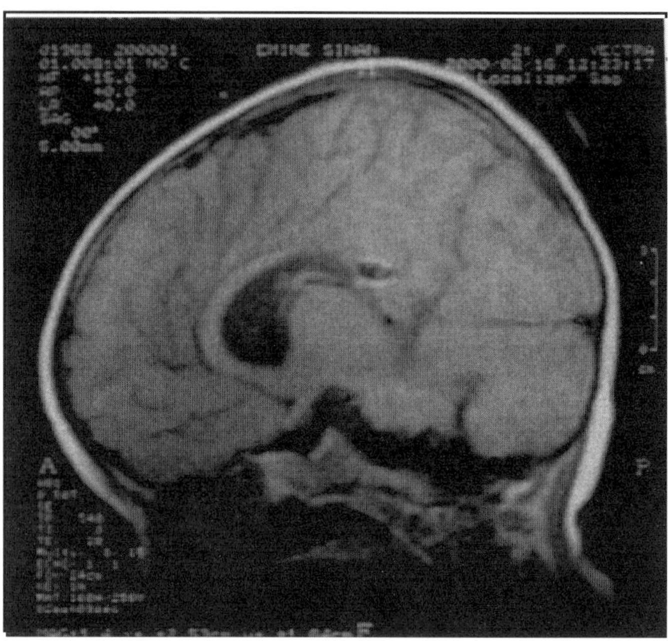

Figure 127c.

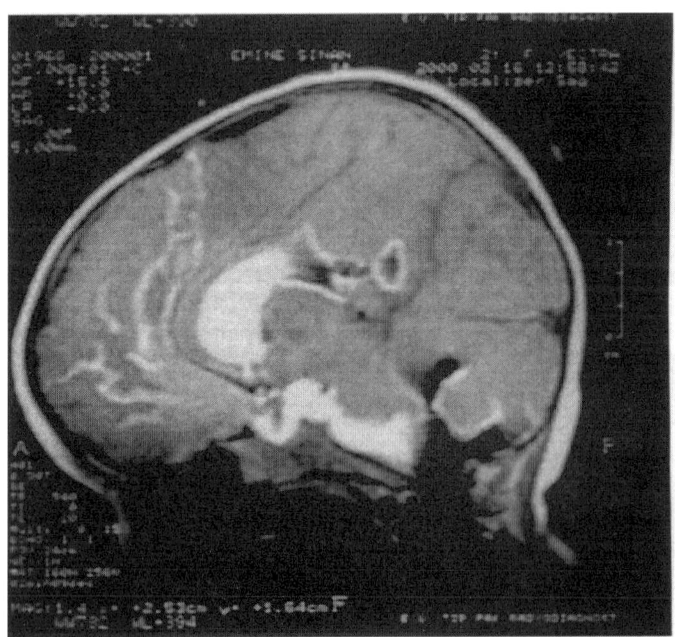

Figure 127d.

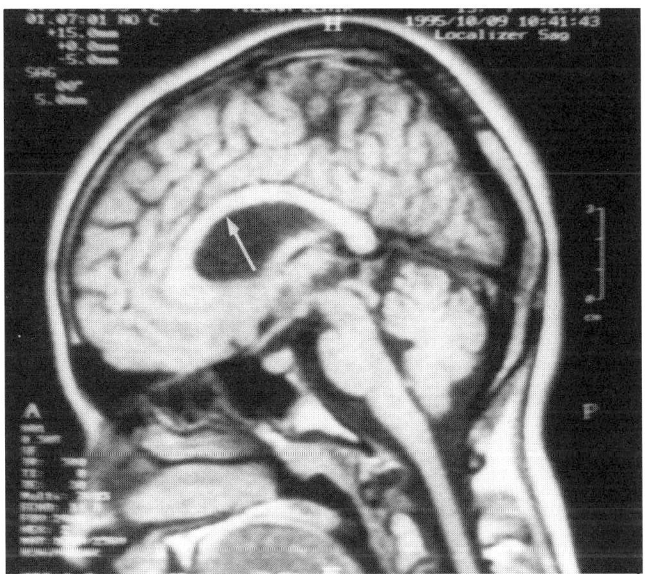

Figure 128a.

Figure 128 a-c. **Unilateral obstruction of the foramen of Monro.** 13-year-old girl. *a) SE T1W MR image, b) SE PDW MR image and c) SE T1W MR image after administration of contrast medium.* There is a compression effect upon the corpus callosum (arrow) (a). The left lateral ventricle is larger than the right, and the septum pellucidum is displaced towards the right (b, c). The condition resulted from unilateral obstruction of the foramen of Monro, probably a congenital stenosis, as contrast-enhanced and other MR images were negative for a tumoral lesion.

Reference

1. Wilberge JE, Vertosick FT, Vries JK. Unilateral hydrocephalus secondary to congenital atresia of the foramen of Monro. J Neurosurg 1983; 59:899

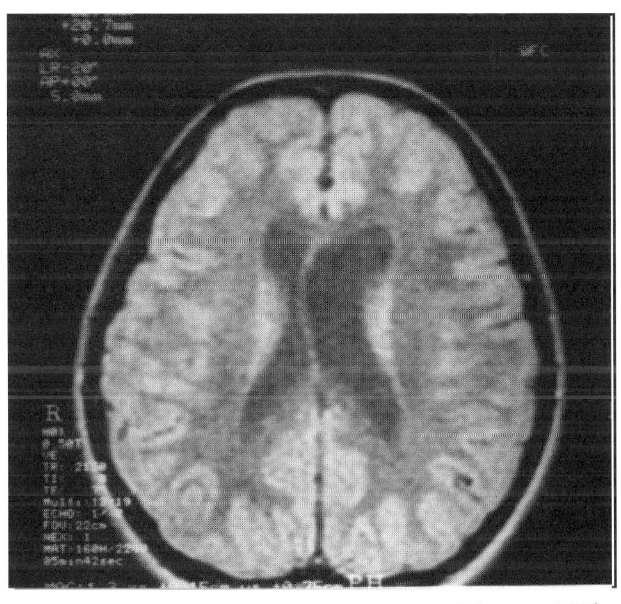

Figure 128b.

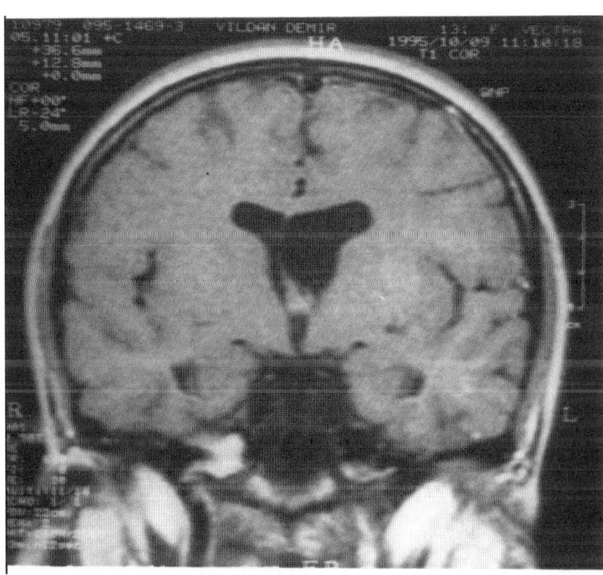

Figure 128c.

Figure 129 a, b. **Cerebral atrophy.** 10-year-old girl. *a) SE T1W and b) SE T2W MR images.* Thinning of the corpus callosum is noted (arrows) (a), secondary to diffuse cerebral atrophy, which is most prominent in the occipital regions (b). History of the patient revealed an abnormality in blood glucose levels during the neonatal period.

Reference
1.   Barkovich AJ. Pediatric neuroimaging. New York, Raven 1995;142

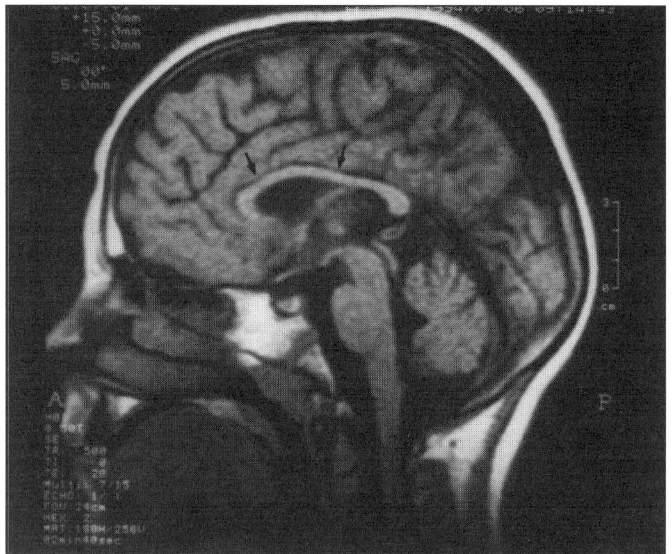

Figure 129a.

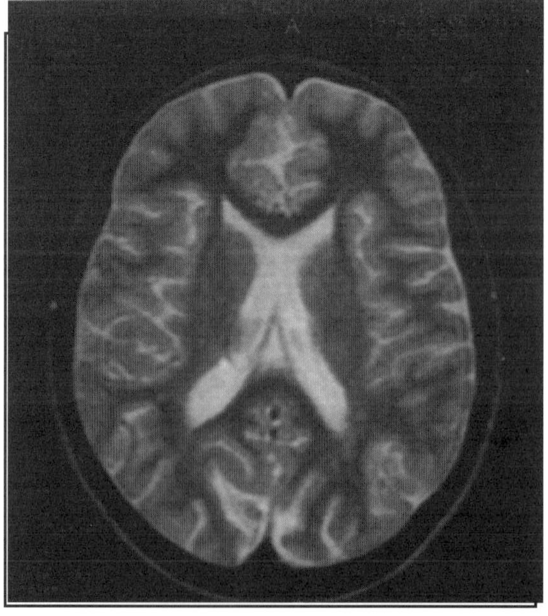

Figure 129b.

Figure 130 a-c. **Alexander's disease (adult form).** 63-year-old man. *a) SE T1W, b, c) SE T2W MR images.* The corpus callosum is atrophic (arrows) (a), and there is diffuse sulcal enlargement. The deep white matter show apparent hyperintense changes, predominantly in the frontal lobes. This condition represents an adult onset of Alexander's disease. The possibility of multiple sclerosis was clinically excluded.

Reference
1.   Osborn AG. Diagnostic neuroradiology. St. Louis, Mosby 1994;730

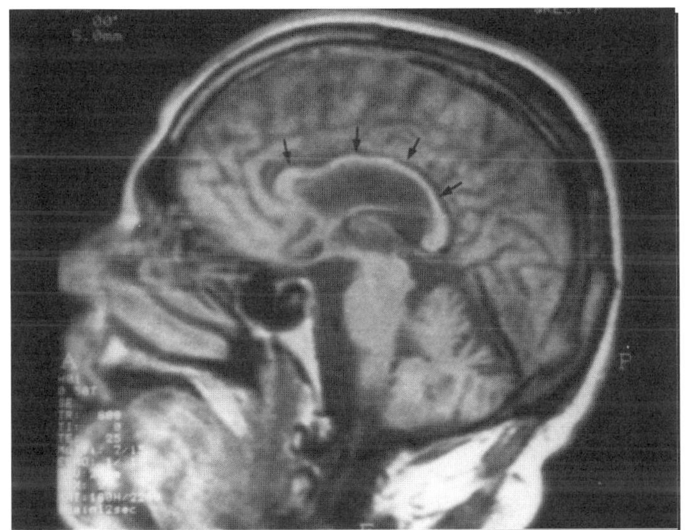

Figure 130a.

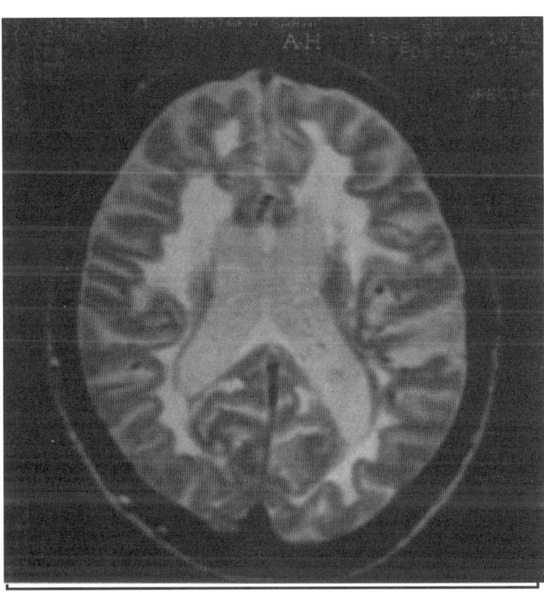

Figure 130b.

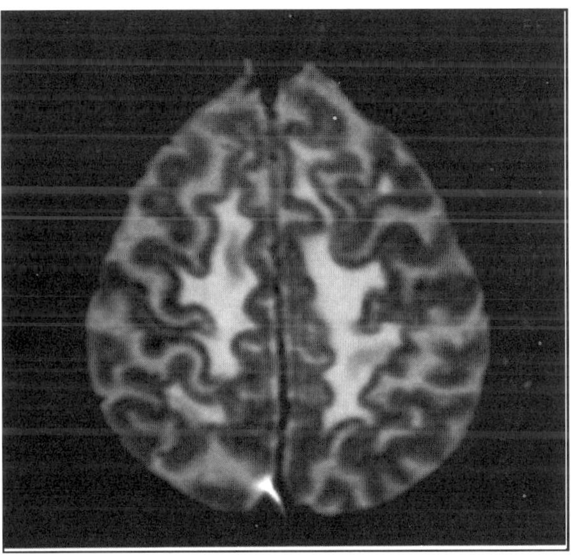

Figure 130c.

Figure 131. **Cerebral atrophy.** 65-year-old woman. *SE T1W MR image.* The corpus callosum has been thinned secondary to cerebral atrophy (arrows). Note that the calvarium is thickened in this patient with Paget's disease.

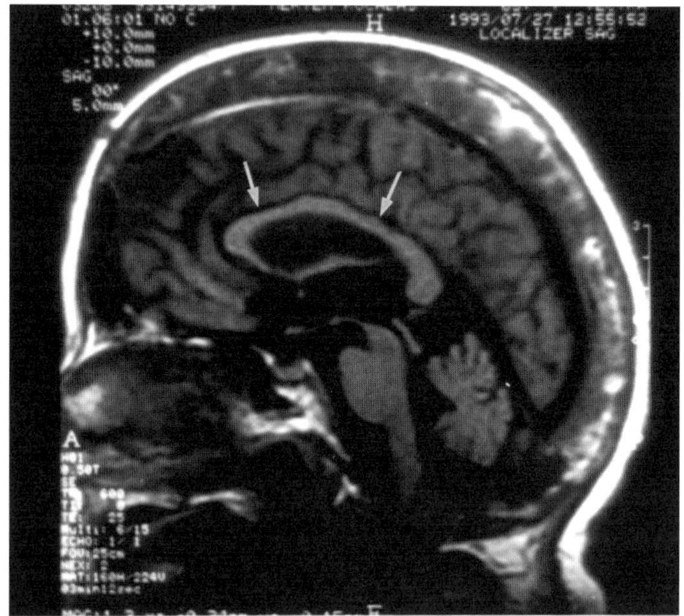

Figure 131.

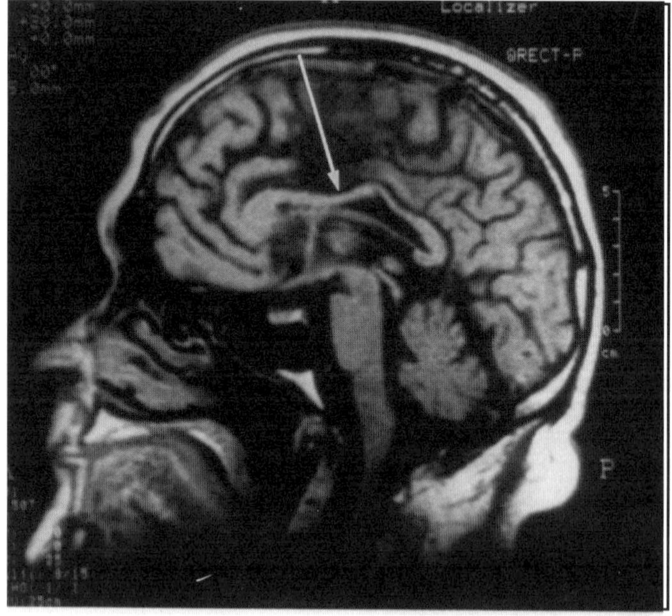

Figure 132.

Figure 132. **Cerebral atrophy.** 72-year-old man. *SE T1W MR image.* There is a very thin corpus callosum (arrow) in this patient with multi-infarct dementia.

Reference
1. Osborn AG. Diagnostic neuroradiology. St. Louis, Mosby 1994;754

GENERAL BIBLIOGRAPHY

1. *HABIB M. THE NEUROLOGICAL BASIS OF DEVELOPMENTAL DYSLEXIA - AN OVERVIEW AND WORKING HYPOTHESIS.* BRAIN 123: 2373-2399, 2000

2. *PIERALLINI A, PANTANO P, FANTOZZI LM, et al. CORRELATION BETWEEN MRI FINDINGS AND LONG-TERM OUTCOME IN PATIENTS WITH SEVERE BRAIN TRAUMA.* NEURORADIOLOGY 42: 860-867, 2000

3. *LUM C, MIKULIS DJ, MCANDREWS M, et al. INVESTIGATING INTERHEMISPHERIC TRANSFER OF INFORMATION IN AGENESIS OF THE CORPUS CALLOSUM USING FUNCTIONAL MRI.* RADIOLOGY 217: 295-296, 2000

4. *THOMPSON PM, MEGA MS, WOODS RP, et al. CORTICAL CHANGE IN ALZHEIMER'S DISEASE DETECTED WITH A DISEASE-SPECIFIC POPULATION-BASED BRAIN ATLAS.* CEREB CORTEX 11: 1-16, 2001

5. *YUCEL M, STUART GW, MARUFF P, et al. HEMISPHERIC AND GENDER-RELATED DIFFERENCES IN THE GROSS MORPHOLOGY OF THE ANTERIOR CINGULATE/PARACINGULATE CORTEX IN NORMAL VOLUNTEERS: AN MRI MORPHOMETRIC STUDY.* CEREB CORTEX 11: 17-25, 2001

6. *FRIESE SA, BITZER M, FREUDENSTEIN D, et al. CLASSIFICATION OF ACQUIRED LESIONS OF THE CORPUS CALLOSUM WITH MRI* NEURORADIOLOGY 42: 795-802, 2000

7. *NANAN R, VON STOCKHAUSEN HB, PETERSEN B, et al. UNUSUAL PATTERN OF LEUKOENCEPHALOPATHY AFTER MORPHINE SULPHATE INTOXICATION.* NEURORADIOLOGY 42: 845-848, 2000

8. *REICHE W, MERKELBACH S, REITH W. NEURORADIOLOGICAL ASPECTS OF MULTIPLE SCLEROSIS.* RADIOLOGE 40: 1045-1056, 2000

9. *YAMAUCHI H, FUKUYAMA H, NAGAHAMA Y, et al. COMPARISON OF THE PATTERN OF ATROPHY OF THE CORPUS CALLOSUM IN FRONTOTEMPORAL DEMENTIA, PROGRESSIVE SUPRANUCLEAR PALSY, AND ALZHEIMER'S DISEASE.* J NEUROL NEUROSUR PS 69: 623-629, 2000

10. *SENER RN. ASSOCIATION OF PERSISTENT FALCINE SINUS WITH DIFFERENT CLINICORADIOLOGIC CONDITIONS: MR IMAGING AND MR ANGIOGRAPHY.* COMPUT MED IMAG GRAP 24: 343-348, 2000

11. *UEMATSU Y, KUBO K, NISHIBAYASHI T, et al. INTERHEMISPHERIC NEUROEPITHELIAL CYST ASSOCIATED WITH AGENESIS OF THE CORPUS CALLOSUM - A CASE REPORT AND REVIEW OF THE LITERATURE.* PEDIATR NEUROSURG 33: 31-36, 2000

12. *HARDAN AY, MINSHEW NJ, KESHAVAN MS. CORPUS CALLOSUM SIZE IN AUTISM.* NEUROLOGY 55: 1033-1036, 2000

13. *TAKAYAMA H, KOBAYASHI M, SUGISHITA M, et al. DIFFUSION-WEIGHTED IMAGING DEMONSTRATES TRANSIENT CYTOTOXIC EDEMA INVOLVING THE CORPUS CALLOSUM IN A PATIENT WITH DIFFUSE BRAIN INJURY.* CLIN NEUROL NEUROSUR 102: 135-139, 2000

General Bibliography

14. *PREIS S, STEINMETZ H, KNORR U, et al. CORPUS CALLOSUM SIZE IN CHILDREN WITH DEVELOPMENTAL LANGUAGE DISORDER.* COGNITIVE BRAIN RES 10: 37-44, 2000

15. *GHARAIBEH WS, ROHLF FJ, SLICE DE, ET AL. A GEOMETRIC MORPHOMETRIC ASSESSMENT OF CHANGE IN MIDLINE BRAIN STRUCTURAL SHAPE FOLLOWING A FIRST EPISODE OF SCHIZOPHRENIA. BIOL PSYCHIAT 48: 398-405, 2000*

16. *HOPKINS WD, RILLING JK. A COMPARATIVE MRI STUDY OF THE RELATIONSHIP BETWEEN NEUROANATOMICAL ASYMMETRY AND INTERHEMISPHERIC CONNECTIVITY IN PRIMATES: IMPLICATION FOR THE EVOLUTION OF FUNCTIONAL ASYMMETRIES.* BEHAV NEUROSCI 114: 739-748, 2000

17. *BLACK SE, MOFFAT SD, YU DC, et al. CALLOSAL ATROPHY CORRELATES WITH TEMPORAL LOBE VOLUME AND MENTAL STATUS IN ALZHEIMER'S DISEASE.* CAN J NEUROL SCI 27: 204-209, 2000

18. *OKUBO S, UEDA M, KAMIYA T, et al. NEUROLOGICAL AND NEURORADIOLOGICAL PROGRESSION IN HEREDITARY SPASTIC PARAPLEGIA WITH A THIN CORPUS CALLOSUM.* ACTA NEUROL SCAND 102: 196-199, 2000

19. *PFEFFERBAUM A, SULLIVAN EV, HEDEHUS M, et al. AGE-RELATED DECLINE IN BRAIN WHITE MATTER ANISOTROPY MEASURED WITH SPATIALLY CORRECTED ECHO-PLANAR DIFFUSION TENSOR IMAGING. MAGNET RESON MED 44: 259-268, 2000*

20. *NAKAMURA M, SAEKI N, IWADATE Y, et al. NEURORADIOLOGICAL CHARACTERISTICS OF PINEOCYTOMA AND PINEOBLASTOMA. NEURORADIOLOGY 42: 509-514, 2000*

21. *REDDY H, LASSONDE M, BEMASCONI N, et al. AN FMRI STUDY OF THE LATERALIZATION OF MOTOR CORTEX ACTIVATION IN ACALLOSAL PATIENTS.* NEUROREPORT 11: 2409-2413, 2000

22. *YAMAUCHI H, FUKUYAMA H, SHIO H. CORPUS CALLOSUM ATROPHY IN PATIENTS WITH LEUKOARAIOSIS MAY INDICATE GLOBAL COGNITIVE IMPAIRMENT. STROKE 31: 1515-1520, 2000*

23. *ALLA P, CARRERE C, DUPONT G, et al. MARCHIAFAVA-BIGNAMI DISEASE: TWO CASES WITH GOOD PROGNOSIS.* PRESSE MED 29: 1170-1172, 2000

24. *HENRY-FEUGEAS MC, AZOUVI P, FONTAINES A, et al. MRI ANALYSIS OF BRAIN ATROPHY AFTER SEVERE CLOSED-HEAD INJURY: RELATION TO CLINICAL STATUS.* BRAIN INJURY 14: 597-604, 2000

25. *MEGURO K, CONSTANS JM, COURTHEOUX P, ET AL. ATROPHY OF THE CORPUS CALLOSUM CORRELATES WITH WHITE MATTER LESIONS IN PATIENTS WITH CEREBRAL ISCHAEMIA.* NEURORADIOLOGY 42: 413-419, 2000

26. *YAMAMOTO T, ASHIKAGA R, ARAKI Y, et al. A CASE OF MARCHIAFAVA-BIGNAMI DISEASE: MRI FINDINGS ON SPIN-ECHO AND FLUID ATTENUATED INVERSION RECOVERY (FLAIR) IMAGES.* EUR J RADIOL 34: 141-143, 2000

27. *FUNNELL MG, CORBALLIS PM, GAZZANIGA MS. INSIGHTS INTO THE FUNCTIONAL SPECIFICITY OF THE HUMAN CORPUS CALLOSUM.* BRAIN 123: 920-926, 2000

28. *ROBICHON F, BOUCHARD P, DEMONET JF, et al. DEVELOPMENTAL DYSLEXIA: RE-EVALUATION OF THE CORPUS CALLOSUM IN MALE ADULTS.* EUR NEUROL 43: 233-237, 2000

29. *BARSI P, KENEZ J, SOLYMOSI D, et al. HIPPOCAMPAL MALROTATION WITH NORMAL CORPUS CALLOSUM: A NEW ENTITY?* NEURORADIOLOGY 42: 339-345, 2000

30. *CERULLO A, MARINI C, CEVOLI S, et al. COLPOCEPHALY IN TWO SIBLINGS: FURTHER EVIDENCE OF A GENETIC TRANSMISSION.* DEV MED CHILD NEUROL 42: 280-282, 2000

31. *YIN R, REDDIHOUGH DS, DITCHFIELD MR, et al. MAGNETIC RESONANCE IMAGING FINDINGS IN CEREBRAL PALSY.* J PAEDIATR CHILD H 36: 139-144, 2000

32. *HECKMANN JG, DRUSCHKY A, KERN PM, et al. GHOST AND MIMICRY TUMORS - PRIMARY CNS LYMPHOMA.* NERVENARZT 71: 305-310, 2000

33. *SUPPRIAN T, BENDSZUS M, HOFMANN E, et al. THE ROLE OF DIFFUSE AXONAL INJURY IN MEDICAL ASSESSMENT OF BRAIN INJURED PATIENTS.* FORTSCHR NEUROL PSYC 68: 121-128, 2000

34. *PARK SA, HAHN JH, KIM JI, et al. MEMORY DEFICITS AFTER BILATERAL ANTERIOR FORNIX INFARCTION.* NEUROLOGY 54: 1379-1382, 2000

35. *CHUA SE, SHARMA T, TAKEI N, et al. A MAGNETIC RESONANCE IMAGING STUDY OF CORPUS CALLOSUM SIZE IN FAMILIAL SCHIZOPHRENIC SUBJECTS, THEIR RELATIVES, AND NORMAL CONTROLS.* SCHIZOPHR RES 41: 397-403, 2000

36. *GE YL, GROSSMAN RI, UDUPA JK, et al. BRAIN ATROPHY IN RELAPSING-REMITTING MULTIPLE SCLEROSIS AND SECONDARY PROGRESSIVE MULTIPLE SCLEROSIS: LONGITUDINAL QUANTITATIVE ANALYSIS.* RADIOLOGY 214: 665-670, 2000

37. *HAUG K, KHAN S, FUCHS S, et al. OFD II, OFD VI, AND JOUBERT SYNDROME MANIFESTATIONS IN 2 SIBS.* AM J MED GENET 91: 135-137, 2000

38. *LEVIN HS, BENAVIDEZ DA, VERGER-MAESTRE K, et al. REDUCTION OF CORPUS CALLOSUM GROWTH AFTER SEVERE TRAUMATIC BRAIN INJURY IN CHILDREN.* NEUROLOGY 54: 647-653, 2000

39. *BONIOLI E, DI STEFANO A, COSTABEL S, et al. PARTIAL AGENESIS OF CORPUS CALLOSUM IN LEOPARD SYNDROME.* INT J DERMATOL 38: 855-856, 1999

40. *KOHLER CG, ANCES BM, COLEMAN AR, et al. MARCHIAFAVA-BIGNAMI DISEASE: LITERATURE REVIEW AND CASE REPORT.* NEUROPSY NEUROPSY BE 13: 67-76, 2000

41. *FRANKLIN MS, KRAEMER GW, SHELTON SE, et al. GENDER DIFFERENCES IN BRAIN VOLUME AND SIZE OF CORPUS CALLOSUM AND AMYGDALA OF RHESUS MONKEY MEASURED FROM MRI IMAGES.* BRAIN RES 852: 263-267, 2000

42. *GUYE M, GASTAUT JL, BARTOLOMEI F. EPILEPSY AND PERISYLVIAN LIPOMA/CORTICAL DYSPLASIA COMPLEX.* EPILEPTIC DISORD 1: 69-73, 1999

43. *DORION AA, CHANTOME M, HASBOUN D, et al. HEMISPHERIC ASYMMETRY AND CORPUS CALLOSUM MORPHOMETRY: A MAGNETIC RESONANCE IMAGING STUDY.* NEUROSCI RES 36: 9-13, 2000

General Bibliography

44. *FABRI M, POLONARA G, QUATTRINI A, et al. ROLE OF THE CORPUS CALLOSUM IN THE SOMATOSENSORY ACTIVATION OF THE IPSILATERAL CEREBRAL CORTEX: AN FMRI STUDY OF CALLOSOTOMIZED PATIENTS. EUR J NEUROSCI 11: 3983-3994, 1999*

45. *NARR KL, THOMPSON PM, SHARMA T, et al. MAPPING MORPHOLOGY OF THE CORPUS CALLOSUM IN SCHIZOPHRENIA. CEREB CORTEX 10: 40-49, 2000*

46. *BARONE R, NIGRO F, TRIULZI F, et al. CLINICAL AND NEURORADIOLOGICAL FOLLOW-UP IN MUCOPOLYSACCHARIDOSIS TYPE III (SANFILIPPO SYNDROME). NEUROPEDIATRICS 30: 270-274, 1999*

47. *LEVINE D, BARNES PD, MADSEN JR, et al. CENTRAL NERVOUS SYSTEM ABNORMALITIES ASSESSED WITH PRENATAL MAGNETIC RESONANCE IMAGING. OBSTET GYNECOL 94: 1011-1019, 1999*

48. *MANES F, PIVEN J, VRANCIC D, et al. AN MRI STUDY OF THE CORPUS CALLOSUM AND CEREBELLUM IN MENTALLY RETARDED AUTISTIC INDIVIDUALS. J NEUROPSYCH CLIN N 11: 470-474, 1999*

49. *KHURANA DS, STRAWSBURG RH, ROBERTSON RL, et al. MRI SIGNAL CHANGES IN THE WHITE MATTER AFTER CORPUS CALLOSOTOMY. PEDIATR NEUROL 21: 691-695, 1999*

50. *MOSTOFSKY SH, WENDLANDT J, CUTTING L, et al. CORPUS CALLOSUM MEASUREMENTS IN GIRLS WITH TOURETTE SYNDROME. NEUROLOGY 53: 1345-1347, 1999*

51. *LEVENTER RJ, PHELAN EM, COLEMAN LT, et al. CLINICAL AND IMAGING FEATURES OF CORTICAL MALFORMATIONS IN CHILDHOOD. NEUROLOGY 53: 715-722, 1999*

52. *ISHII K, IKEJIRI Y, SASAKI M, et al. REGIONAL CEREBRAL GLUCOSE METABOLISM AND BLOOD FLOW IN A PATIENT WITH MARCHIAFAVA-BIGNAMI DISEASE. AM J NEURORADIOL 20: 1249-1251, 1999*

53. *BENAVIDEZ DA, FLETCHER JM, HANNAY HJ, et al. CORPUS CALLOSUM DAMAGE AND INTERHEMISPHERIC TRANSFER OF INFORMATION FOLLOWING CLOSED HEAD INJURY IN CHILDREN. CORTEX 35: 315-336, 1999*

54. *AUER-GRUMBACH M, FAZEKAS F, RADNER H, et al. TROYER SYNDROME: A COMBINATION OF CENTRAL BRAIN ABNORMALITY AND MOTOR NEURON DISEASE? J NEUROL 246: 556-561, 1999*

55. *WINKLER PA, WEIS S, WENGER E, et al. TRANSCALLOSAL APPROACH TO THE THIRD VENTRICLE: NORMATIVE MORPHOMETRIC DATA BASED ON MAGNETIC RESONANCE IMAGING SCANS, WITH SPECIAL REFERENCE TO THE FORNIX AND FORNICEAL INSERTION. NEUROSURGERY 45: 309-317, 1999*

56. *BAKSHI R, SHAIKH ZA, KAMRAN S, et al. MRI FINDINGS IN 32 CONSECUTIVE LIPOMAS USING CONVENTIONAL AND ADVANCED SEQUENCES. J NEUROIMAGING 9: 134-140, 1999*

57. *ROBICHON F, GIRAUD K, BERBON M, et al. SEXUAL DIMORPHISM IN ANTERIOR SPEECH REGION: AN MRI STUDY OF CORTICAL ASYMMETRY AND CALLOSAL SIZE. BRAIN COGNITION 40: 241-246, 1999*

58. *LAZAR LM, MILROD LM, SOLOMON GE, et al. ASYNCHRONOUS PENTOBARBITAL-INDUCED BURST SUPPRESSION WITH CORPUS CALLOSUM HEMORRHAGE. CLIN NEUROPHYSIOL 110: 1036-1040, 1999*

59. *TOMABECHI C, TAKANO K, SUZUKI N, et al. A CASE OF SYMPTOMATIC INTERHEMISPHERIC ARACHNOID CYST IN THE ELDERLY.* NEUROL SURG TOKYO 27: 377-381, 1999

60. *TEKGUL H, DIZDARER G, YALMAN O, et al. ASSOCIATED BRAIN ABNORMALITIES IN PATIENTS WITH CORPUS CALLOSUM ANOMALIES. TURKISH J PEDIATR 41: 173-180, 1999*

61. *GIEDD JN, BLUMENTHAL J, JEFFRIES NO, et al. DEVELOPMENT OF THE HUMAN CORPUS CALLOSUM DURING CHILDHOOD AND ADOLESCENCE: A LONGITUDINAL MRI STUDY.* PROG NEURO-PSYCHOPH 23: 571-588, 1999

62. *GABRIEL S, GROSSMANN A, HOPPNER J, et al. MARCHIAFA-BIGNAMI-SYNDROME. EXTRAPONTINE MYELINOLYSIS IN CHRONIC ALCOHOLISM. NERVENARZT 70: 349-356, 1999*

63. *OKA S, MIYAMOTO O, JANJUA NA, et al. RE-EVALUATION OF SEXUAL DIMORPHISM IN HUMAN CORPUS CALLOSUM.* NEUROREPORT 10: 937-940, 1999

64. *KEENE DL, JIMENEZ C, HSU E. MRI DIAGNOSIS OF GLIOMATOSIS CEREBRI.* PEDIATR NEUROL 20: 148-151, 1999

65. *TAKAO T, KAKU S, TASHIMA T, et al. CEREBRAL B-CELL LYMPHOMA FOLLOWING TREATMENT FOR TOLOSA-HUNT SYNDROME.* CLIN NEUROPATHOL 18: 87-92, 1999

66. *KIVITIE-KALLIO S, AUTTI T, SALONEN O, et al. MRI OF THE BRAIN IN THE COHEN SYNDROME: A RELATIVELY LARGE CORPUS CALLOSUM IN PATIENTS WITH MENTAL RETARDATION AND MICROCEPHALY. NEUROPEDIATRICS 29: 298-301, 1998*

67. *TSUMOTO T, NISHIOKA K, NAKAKITA K, et al. ACQUIRED STUTTERING ASSOCIATED WITH CALLOSAL INFARCTION: A CASE REPORT.* NEUROL SURG TOKYO 27: 79-83, 1999

68. *PELTZ MT, CASCIU L, MANCONI FM, et al. DISTRIBUTION OF WHITE MATTER LESIONS IN MULTIPLE SCLEROSIS AND SYSTEMIC LUPUS ERYTHEMATOSUS - DIFFERENTIATION USING MRI.* RIV NEURORADIOL 11: 17-19, 1998

69. *EDWARDS SGM, GONG QY, LIU C, et al. INFRATENTORIAL ATROPHY ON MAGNETIC RESONANCE IMAGING AND DISABILITY IN MULTIPLE SCLEROSIS.* BRAIN 122: 291-301, 1999

70. *RORICHT S, MEYER BU, IRLBACHER K, et al. IMPAIRMENT OF CALLOSAL AND CORTICOSPINAL SYSTEM FUNCTION IN ADOLESCENTS WITH EARLY-TREATED PHENYLKETONURIA: A TRANSCRANIAL MAGNETIC STIMULATION STUDY.* J NEUROL 246: 21-30, 1999

71. *RUIZ-MARTINEZ J, PEREZ-BALSA AM, RUIBAL M, et al. MARCHIAFAVA-BIGNAMI DISEASE WITH WIDESPREAD EXTRACALLOSAL LESIONS AND FAVOURABLE COURSE. NEURORADIOLOGY 41: 40-43, 1999*

72. *KIM SS, CHANG KH, KIM ST, et al. FOCAL LESION IN THE SPLENIUM OF THE CORPUS CALLOSUM IN EPILEPTIC PATIENTS: ANTIEPILEPTIC DRUG TOXICITY?* AM J NEURORADIOL 20: 125-129, 1999

73. *SUZUKI K, YAMADORI A, ENDO K, et al. DISSOCIATION OF LETTER AND PICTURE NAMING RESULTING FROM CALLOSAL DISCONNECTION. NEUROLOGY 51: 1390-1394, 1998*

General Bibliography

74. *AY H, FURIE KL, YAMADA K, et al. DIFFUSION-WEIGHTED MRI CHARACTERIZES THE ISCHEMIC LESION IN TRANSIENT GLOBAL AMNESIA. NEUROLOGY 51: 901-903, 1998*

75. *ROUSSEAUX M, GODEFROY O, CABARET M. REANALYSIS OF LEARNING DISORDERS IN RUPTURED ANEURYSM OF THE ANTERIOR COMMUNICATING ARTERY. REV NEUROL 154: 508-522, 1998*

76. *FREI KP, PATRONAS NJ, CRUTCHFIELD KE, et al. MUCOLIPIDOSIS TYPE IV - CHARACTERISTIC MRI FINDINGS. NEUROLOGY 51: 565-569, 1998*

77. *BRISSE H, SEBAG G, FALLET C, et al. PRENATAL MRI DIAGNOSIS OF CORPUS CALLOSUM AGENESIS: STUDY OF 20 CASES WITH PATHOLOGIC COMPARISONS. J RADIOL 79: 659-666, 1998*

78. *GONCALVES-FERREIRA AJ, HERCULANO-CARVALHO M, MELANCIA JL, ET AL. CORPUS CALLOSUM: MICROSURGICAL ANATOMY AND MRI. STEREOT FUNCT NEUROS 69: 248-248, 1997*

79. *RAYBAUD C, GIRARD N. MRI ANATOMICAL STUDY OF TELENCEPHALIC COMMISSURAL AGENESIS AND DYSPLASIA (AGENESIA OF THE CORPUS CALLOSUM AND RELATED ANOMALIES). CLINICAL CORRELATIONS AND MORPHOGENETIC INTERPRETATION. NEUROCHIRURGIE 44: 38-60, 1998*

80. *CHRISTIAENS JL, BLOND S. ACQUIRED LESIONS OF THE CORPUS CALLOSUM. NEUROCHIRURGIE 44: 116-124, 1998*

81. *JAN M, KAKOU M, VELUT S. SURGICAL APPROACHES OF THE CORPUS CALLOSUM. NEUROCHIRURGIE 44: 133-137, 1998*

82. *YDINGOZ U, MIDIA M. CENTRAL NERVOUS SYSTEM INVOLVEMENT IN INCONTINENTIA PIGMENTI: CRANIAL MRI OF TWO SIBLINGS. NEURORADIOLOGY 40: 364-366, 1998*

83. *GABRIELLI O, COPPA GV, MANZONI M, et al. MINOR CEREBRAL ALTERATIONS OBSERVED BY MAGNETIC RESONANCE IMAGING IN SYNDROMIC CHILDREN WITH MENTAL RETARDATION. EUR J RADIOL 27: 139-144, 1998*

84. *MEYER BU, RORICHT S, NIEHAUS L. MORPHOLOGY OF ACALLOSAL BRAINS AS ASSESSED BY MRI IN SIX PATIENTS LEADING A NORMAL DAILY LIFE. J NEUROL 245: 106-110, 1998*

85. *BAKSHI R, GLASS J, LOUIS BN, et al. MAGNETIC RESONANCE IMAGING FEATURES OF SOLITARY INFLAMMATORY BRAIN MASSES. J NEUROIMAGING 8: 8-14, 1998*

86. *SUPIOT F, GUILLAUME MP, HERMANUS N, et al. TOXOPLASMA ENCEPHALITIS IN A HIV PATIENT: UNUSUAL INVOLVEMENT OF THE CORPUS CALLOSUM. CLIN NEUROL NEUROSUR 99: 287-290, 1997*

87. *HADECKE J, BUCHFELDER M, TRIEBEL HJ, et al. MULTIPLE INTRACRANIAL LIPOMA: A CASE REPORT. NEUROSURG REV 20: 282-287, 1997*

88. *MASUZAWA H, KUBO T, KANAZAWA I, et al. SHEARING INJURIES OF PARASAGITTAL WHITE MATTER, CORPUS CALLOSUM AND BASAL GANGLIA: POSSIBLE RADIOLOGICAL EVIDENCES OF HEMIPLEGIA IN DIFFUSE AXONAL INJURY. NEUROL SURG TOKYO 25: 689-694, 1997*

89. *MATARO M, GARCIASANCHEZ C, JUNQUE C, et al. MAGNETIC RESONANCE IMAGING MEASUREMENT OF THE CAUDATE NUCLEUS IN ADOLESCENTS WITH ATTENTION-DEFICIT HYPERACTIVITY DISORDER AND ITS RELATIONSHIP WITH NEUROPSYCHOLOGICAL AND BEHAVIORAL MEASURES.* ARCH NEUROL-CHICAGO 54: 963-968, 1997

90. *TEICHER MH, ITO Y, GLOD CA, et al. PRELIMINARY EVIDENCE FOR ABNORMAL CORTICAL DEVELOPMENT IN PHYSICALLY AND SEXUALLY ABUSED CHILDREN USING EEG COHERENCE AND MRI.* ANN NY ACAD SCI 821: 160-175, 1997

91. *BERGUI M, BRADAC GB, LEOMBRUNI S, et al. MRI AND CT IN AN AUTOSOMAL-DOMINANT, ADULT-ONSET LEUKODYSTROPHY.* NEURORADIOLOGY 39: 423-426, 1997

92. *YASUDA Y, WATANABE T, TANAKA H, et al. AMNESIA FOLLOWING INFARCTION IN THE RIGHT RETROSPLENIAL REGION.* CLIN NEUROL NEUROSUR 99: 102-105, 1997

93. *CIONI G, DIPACO MC, BERTUCCELLI B, et al. MRI FINDINGS AND SENSORIMOTOR DEVELOPMENT IN INFANTS WITH BILATERAL SPASTIC CEREBRAL PALSY.* BRAIN DEV-JPN 19: 245-253, 1997

94. *ASHIKAGA R, ARAKI Y, ISHIDA O. MRI OF HEAD INJURY USING FLAIR.* NEURORADIOLOGY 39: 239-242, 1997

95. *UTSUNOMIYA H, OGASAWARA T, HAYASHI T, et al. DYSGENESIS OF THE CORPUS CALLOSUM AND ASSOCIATED TELENCEPHALIC ANOMALIES: MRI.* NEURORADIOLOGY 39: 302-310, 1997

96. *SISODIYA SM, FREE SL. DISPROPORTION OF CEREBRAL SURFACE AREAS AND VOLUMES IN CEREBRAL DYSGENESIS - MRI-BASED EVIDENCE FOR CONNECTIONAL ABNORMALITIES.* BRAIN 120: 271-281, 1997

97. *MERCURI E, JONGMANS M, HENDERSON S, et al. EVALUATION OF THE CORPUS CALLOSUM IN CLUMSY CHILDREN BORN PREMATURELY: A FUNCTIONAL AND MORPHOLOGICAL STUDY.* NEUROPEDIATRICS 27: 317-322, 1996

98. *SCHAEFER GB, BODENSTEINER JB, BUEHLER BA, et al. THE NEUROIMAGING FINDINGS IN SOTOS SYNDROME.* AM J MED GENET 68: 462-465, 1997

99. *DEMAEREL P, VANDEGAER P, WILMS G, et al. INTERHEMISPHERIC LIPOMA WITH VARIABLE CALLOSAL DYSGENESIS: RELATIONSHIP BETWEEN EMBRYOLOGY, MORPHOLOGY, AND SYMPTOMATOLOGY.* EUR RADIOL 6: 904-909, 1996

100. *ANLAR B, SAATCI I, KOSE G, et al. MRI FINDINGS IN SUBACUTE SCLEROSING PANENCEPHALITIS.* NEUROLOGY 47: 1278-1283, 1996

101. *ATKINSON DS, ABOUKHALIL B, CHARLES PD, et al. MIDSAGITTAL CORPUS CALLOSUM AREA, INTELLIGENCE, AND LANGUAGE DOMINANCE IN EPILEPSY.* J NEUROIMAGING 6: 235-239, 1996

102. *RAJAPAKSE JC, GIEDD JN, RUMSEY JM, et al. REGIONAL MRI MEASUREMENTS OF THE CORPUS CALLOSUM: A METHODOLOGICAL AND DEVELOPMENTAL STUDY.* BRAIN DEV-JPN 18: 379-388, 1996

103. *JANOWSKY JS, KAYE JA, CARPER RA. ATROPHY OF THE CORPUS CALLOSUM IN ALZHEIMER'S DISEASE VERSUS HEALTHY AGING.* J AM GERIATR SOC 44: 798-803, 1996

General Bibliography

104. *LEONARD G, ZATORRE RJ, LEBLANC R, ET AL. LANGUAGE LATERALIZATION AND CALLOSAL AGENESIS.* NEUROCASE 2: 175-181, 1996

105. *AUTTI T, RAININKO R, VANHANEN SL, et al. MRI OF NEURONAL CEROID LIPOFUSCINOSIS .1. CRANIAL MRI OF 30 PATIENTS WITH JUVENILE NEURONAL CEROID LIPOFUSCINOSIS.* NEURORADIOLOGY 38: 476-482, 1996

106. *SHINOMIYA N, NAGAYAMA T, FUJIOKA Y, et al. MRI IN THE MILD TYPE OF MUCOPOLYSACCHARIDOSIS II (HUNTER'S SYNDROME). NEURORADIOLOGY 38: 483-485, 1996*

107. *NISHIO S, MORIOKA T, TAKESHITA I, et al. GLIAL TUMOURETTES (GLIAL MICROTUMOURS): THEIR CLINICAL AND HISTOPATHOLOGICAL MANIFESTATIONS.* ACTA NEUROCHIR 138: 818-823, 1996

108. *PFEFFERBAUM A, LIM KO, DESMOND JE, et al. THINNING OF THE CORPUS CALLOSUM IN OLDER ALCOHOLIC MEN: A MAGNETIC RESONANCE IMAGING STUDY.* ALCOHOL CLIN EXP RES 20: 752-757, 1996

109. *AGUIAR MD, CAVALCANTI M, BARBOSA H, et al. AICARDI SYNDROME AND CHOROID PLEXUS PAPILLOMA: A RARE ASSOCIATION. CASE REPORT ARQ NEURO-PSIQUIAT 54: 313-317, 1996*

110. *SERVAN J, VERSTICHEL P, ELGHOZI D, et al. HEMISPHERIC DISCONNECTION SYNDROME FOLLOWING A PARTIAL CALLOSAL INFARCT: NEUROPSYCHOLOGICAL AND MRI STUDY.* REV NEUROL 152: 165-173, 1996

111. *KAMAKI M, KAWAMURA M, MORIYA H, et al. CALLOSAL BLEEDING IN A CASE OF MARCHIAFAVA-BIGNAMI DISEASE.* J NEUROL SCI 136: 86-89, 1996

112. *HOMMER D, MOMENAN R, RAWLINGS R, et al. DECREASED CORPUS CALLOSUM SIZE AMONG ALCOHOLIC WOMEN.* ARCH NEUROL-CHICAGO 53: 359-363, 1996

113. *BLANCHET B, ROLAND J, BRAUN M, et al. ANATOMY AND MRI ANATOMY OF THE CEREBRAL INTER-HEMISPHERIC COMMISSURES. J NEURORADIOLOGY 22: 237-251, 1995*

114. *GIEDD JN, RUMSEY JM, CASTELLANOS FX, et al. A QUANTITATIVE MRI STUDY OF THE CORPUS CALLOSUM IN CHILDREN AND ADOLESCENTS. DEV BRAIN RES 91: 274-280, 1996*

115. *VERMERSCH P, ROCHE J, HAMON M, et al. WHITE MATTER MAGNETIC RESONANCE IMAGING HYPERINTENSITY IN ALZHEIMER'S DISEASE: CORRELATIONS WITH CORPUS CALLOSUM ATROPHY.* J NEUROL 243: 231-234, 1996

116. *WILLNOW S, KIESS W, BUTENANDT O, et al. ENDOCRINE DISORDERS IN SEPTO-OPTIC DYSPLASIA (DE MORSIER SYNDROME) - EVALUATION AND FOLLOW UP OF 18 PATIENTS.* EUR J PEDIATR 155: 179-184, 1996

117. *FERRARIO VF, SFORZA C, SERRAO G, et al. SHAPE OF THE HUMAN CORPUS CALLOSUM IN CHILDHOOD - ELLIPTIC FOURIER ANALYSIS ON MIDSAGITTAL MAGNETIC RESONANCE SCANS.* INVEST RADIOL 31: 1-5, 1996

118. *SATOH H, UOZUMI T, KIYA K, et al. MRI OF PINEAL REGION TUMOURS: RELATIONSHIP BETWEEN TUMOURS AND ADJACENT STRUCTURES. NEURORADIOLOGY 37: 624-630, 1995*

119. RILEY EP, MATTSON SN, SOWELL ER, et al. ABNORMALITIES OF THE CORPUS-CALLOSUM IN CHILDREN PRENATALLY EXPOSED TO ALCOHOL. ALCOHOL CLIN EXP RES 19: 1198-1202, 1995

120. MATSUMOTO K, TOMITA S, HIGASHI H, et al. IMAGE-GUIDED STEREOTAXIC BIOPSY FOR BRAIN-TUMORS - EXPERIENCE OF 71 CASES. NEUROL SURG TOKYO 23: 897-903, 1995

121. NAGUMO T, YAMADORI A. CALLOSAL DISCONNECTION SYNDROME AND KNOWLEDGE OF THE BODY - A CASE OF LEFT HAND ISOLATION FROM THE BODY SCHEMA WITH NAMES. J NEUROL NEUROSUR 59: 548-551, 1995

122. GIEDD JN, KOZUCH P, KAYSEN D, et al. RELIABILITY OF CEREBRAL MEASURES IN REPEATED EXAMINATIONS WITH MAGNETIC RESONANCE IMAGING. PSYCHIAT RES-NEUROIM 61: 113-119, 1995

123. NAKAMURA A, IZUMI K, UMEHARA F, et al. FAMILIAL SPASTIC PARAPLEGIA WITH MENTAL IMPAIRMENT AND THIN CORPUS CALLOSUM. J NEUROL SCI 131: 35-42, 1995

124. COPPOLA R, MYSLOBODSKY M, WEINBERGER DR. MIDLINE ABNORMALITIES AND PSYCHOPATHOLOGY - HOW RELIABLE IS THE MIDSAGITTAL MAGNETIC RESONANCE WINDOW INTO THE BRAIN. PSYCHIAT RES-NEUROIM 61: 33-42, 1995

125. PATEL PJ, KOLAWOLE TM, MALABAREY TM, et al. ADRENOLEUKODYSTROPHY - CT AND MRI FINDINGS. PEDIATR RADIOL 25: 256-258, 1995

126. VANZANDIJCKE M, CASSELMAN J. INVOLVEMENT OF CORPUS CALLOSUM IN AMYOTROPHIC LATERAL SCLEROSIS SHOWN BY MRI NEURORADIOLOGY 37: 287-288, 1995

127. STROTTMANN JM, GINSBERG LE, STANTON C. LANGERHANS CELL HISTIOCYTOSIS INVOLVING THE CORPUS-CALLOSUM AND CEREBELLUM - GADOLINIUM-ENHANCED MRI. NEURORADIOLOGY 37: 289-292, 1995

128. WANG ZP, OSAWA M, FUKUYAMA Y. MORPHOMETRIC STUDY OF THE CORPUS CALLOSUM IN FUKUYAMA TYPE CONGENITAL MUSCULAR-DYSTROPHY BY MAGNETIC-RESONANCE-IMAGING. BRAIN DEV-JPN 17: 104-110, 1995

129. CASTELLANOS FX, GIEDD JN, ECKBURG P, et al. QUANTITATIVE MORPHOLOGY OF THE CAUDATE-NUCLEUS IN ATTENTION-DEFICIT HYPERACTIVITY DISORDER. AM J PSYCHIAT 151: 1791-1796, 1994

130. IAI M, TANABE Y, GOTO M, et al. A COMPARATIVE MAGNETIC RESONANCE IMAGING STUDY OF THE CORPUS-CALLOSUM IN NEUROLOGICALLY NORMAL CHILDREN AND CHILDREN WITH SPASTIC DIPLEGIA. ACTA PAEDIATR 83: 1086-1090, 1994

131. CHATEIL JF, GIRAULT JM, PEDESPAN JM, et al. AGYRIA-PACHYGYRIA IN CHILDREN - IMAGING FINDINGS. ARCH PEDIATRIE 1: 551-560, 1994

132. NALD MR, SCHAEFER GB, OLNEY AH, et al YPOPLASIA OF THE CEREBELLAR VERMIS AND CORPUS-CALLOSUM IN THROMBOCYTOPENIA WITH ABSENT RADIUS SYNDROME ON MRI STUDIES. M J MED GENET 50: 46-50, 1994

133. PALMERI S, BATTISTI C, FEDERICO A, ET AL. HYPOPLASIA OF THE CORPUS CALLOSUM IN NIEMANN-PICK TYPE-C DISEASE. NEURORADIOLOGY 36: 20-22, 1994

General Bibliography

134. *BODENSTEINER J, SCHAEFER GB, BREEDING L, et al. HYPOPLASIA OF THE CORPUS CALLOSUM - A STUDY OF 445 CONSECUTIVE MRI SCANS. J CHILD NEUROL 9: 47-49, 1994*

135. *CURATOLO P, CILIO MR, DELGIUDICE E, et al. FAMILIAL WHITE-MATTER HYPOPLASIA, AGENESIS OF THE CORPUS CALLOSUM, MENTAL-RETARDATION AND GROWTH DEFICIENCY - A NEW DISTINCTIVE SYNDROME.* NEUROPEDIATRICS 24: 77-82, 1993

136. *CASTROGAGO M, RODRIGUEZNUNEZ A, EIRIS J, et al. FAMILIAL AGENESIS OF THE CORPUS CALLOSUM - A NEW FORM.* ARCH FR PEDIATR 50: 327-330, 1993

137. *XIONG L, RAUCH RA, HAGINO N, et al. AN ANIMAL MODEL OF CORPUS CALLOSUM IMPINGEMENT AS SEEN IN PATIENTS WITH NORMAL PRESSURE HYDROCEPHALUS.* INVEST RADIOL 28: 46-50, 1993

138. *POZZILLI C, FIESCHI C, PERANI D, et al. RELATIONSHIP BETWEEN CORPUS CALLOSUM ATROPHY AND CEREBRAL METABOLIC ASYMMETRIES IN MULTIPLE SCLEROSIS.* J NEUROL SCI 112: 51-57, 1992

139. *KURODA Y, KAWASAKI T, HARAOKA S, ET AL. AUTOPSY REPORT OF PRIMARY CNS B-CELL LYMPHOMA INDISTINGUISHABLE FROM MULTIPLE SCLEROSIS - DIAGNOSIS WITH THE IMMUNOGLOBULIN GENE REARRANGEMENTS ANALYSIS.* J NEUROL SCI 111: 173-179, 1992

140. *MELIN GI, KELLER MS. PERICALLOSAL LIPOMA EXTENDING THROUGH THE CHOROIDAL FISSURE - US/CT/MRI CORRELATION.* NEURORADIOLOGY 34: 402-403, 1992

141. *HAEUSLER G, FRISCH H, GUCHEV Z, et al. HYPOPLASIA OF THE CORPUS CALLOSUM AND GROWTH HORMONE DEFICIENCY IN THE XXXXY SYNDROME.* AM J MED GENET 44: 230-232, 1992

142. *HAMANO K, MATSUBARA T, SHIBATA S, et al. AICARDI SYNDROME ACCOMPANIED BY AUDITORY DISTURBANCE AND MULTIPLE BRAIN TUMORS.* BRAIN DEV-JPN 13: 438-441, 1991

143. *DORAISWAMY PM, FIGIEL GS, HUSAIN MM, et al. AGING OF THE HUMAN CORPUS CALLOSUM - MAGNETIC RESONANCE IMAGING IN NORMAL VOLUNTEERS.* J NEUROPSYCH CLIN N 3: 392-397, 1991

144. *PETER JC, SINCLAIRSMITH C, DEVILLIERS JC. MIDLINE DERMAL SINUSES AND CYSTS AND THEIR RELATIONSHIP TO THE CENTRAL NERVOUS SYSTEM.* EUR J PEDIATR SURG 1: 73-79, 1991

145. *JIOKIKTJIEN C, VALK J, RAMAEKERS G. MALFORMATION OR DAMAGE OF THE CORPUS CALLOSUM - A CLINICAL AND MRI STUDY.* BRAIN DEV-JPN 10: 92-99, 1988

146. *REINARZ S, COFFMAN C, SMOKER WRK, et al. MRI OF THE CORPUS CALLOSUM - NORMAL AND PATHOLOGICAL ANATOMY.* AM J NEURORADIOL 7: 543-543, 1986